Handbook of Nutrition and Pregnancy

Handbook of Nutrition and Pregnancy

Editor: Jena Lin

AMERICAN
MEDICAL PUBLISHERS
www.americanmedicalpublishers.com

AMERICAN
MEDICAL PUBLISHERS
www.americanmedicalpublishers.com

Cataloging-in-Publication Data

Handbook of nutrition and pregnancy / edited by Jena Lin.
p. cm.
Includes bibliographical references and index.
ISBN 978-1-63927-685-1
1. Pregnancy--Nutritional aspects. 2. Prenatal care. 3. Pregnancy.
4. Nutrition--Requirements. I. Lin, Jena.
RG559 .H36 2023
618.24--dc23

American Medical Publishers,
41 Flatbush Avenue,
1st Floor, New York,
NY 11217, USA

ISBN 978-1-63927-685-1 (Hardback)

Contents

Preface

The main aim of this book is to educate learners and enhance their research focus by presenting diverse topics covering this vast field. This is an advanced book which compiles significant studies by distinguished experts in the area of analysis. This book addresses successive solutions to the challenges arising in the area of application, along with it; the book provides scope for future developments.

The requirement of nutrients naturally rises at the time of pregnancy as compared to any other stage of women's life. Additional nutrients are essential throughout the time of gestation for the growth of maternal tissues which support the development of fetus. The constituents which are required for the fast development and growth of fetus rely on the supply from maternal diet. The nutrients required for a pregnant woman consist of zinc, thiamin, protein, vitamin B6, α-linolenic acid, niacin, iodine, folate, riboflavin and iron. The food consisting of these nutrients are beans, dark green or orange vegetables, nuts, grains and meat. Additional energy is needed for tissue deposition, moving a heavier body and an increase in the metabolic rate. Majority of the nutrients for fetal and maternal tissues are needed in the later stage of pregnancy. This book provides significant information to help develop a good understanding of the role of nutrition during pregnancy. Those with an interest in this field of study would find it helpful.

It was a great honour to edit this book, though there were challenges, as it involved a lot of communication and networking between me and the editorial team. However, the end result was this all-inclusive book covering diverse themes in the field.

Finally, it is important to acknowledge the efforts of the contributors for their excellent chapters, through which a wide variety of issues have been addressed. I would also like to thank my colleagues for their valuable feedback during the making of this book.

Editor

1

Maternal Iodine Status and Associations with Birth Outcomes in Three Major Cities in the United Kingdom

Charles J. P. Snart [1,†], Claire Keeble [2,†], Elizabeth Taylor [1], Janet E. Cade [3], Paul M. Stewart [4], Michael Zimmermann [5], Stephen Reid [6], Diane E. Threapleton [1], Lucilla Poston [7], Jenny E. Myers [8], Nigel A. B. Simpson [9,‡], Darren C. Greenwood [1,2,‡] and Laura J. Hardie [1,*,‡]

1 Department of Clinical and Population Science, Leeds Institute of Cardiovascular and Metabolic Medicine, School of Medicine, University of Leeds, Leeds LS2 9JT, UK; medcjps@leeds.ac.uk (C.J.P.S.); E.Taylor@leeds.ac.uk (E.T.); D.E.Threapleton@leeds.ac.uk (D.E.T.); D.C.Greenwood@leeds.ac.uk (D.C.G.)
2 Leeds Institute for Data Analytics, University of Leeds, Leeds LS2 9JT, UK; C.M.Owen@leeds.ac.uk
3 Nutritional Epidemiology Group, School of Food Science & Nutrition, University of Leeds, Leeds LS2 9JT, UK; J.E.Cade@leeds.ac.uk
4 Faculty of Medicine and Health, University of Leeds, Leeds LS2 9JT, UK; P.M.Stewart@leeds.ac.uk
5 Laboratory for Human Nutrition, Institute of Food, Nutrition and Health, Swiss Federal Institute of Technology (ETH), 8092 Zürich, Switzerland; michael.zimmermann@hest.ethz.ch
6 Earth Surface Science Institute, School of Earth and Environment, University of Leeds, Leeds LS2 9JT, UK; S.Reid@leeds.ac.uk
7 Division of Women's Health, Women's Health Academic Centre, King's College London, London SE1 7EH, UK; lucilla.poston@kcl.ac.uk
8 Maternal and Fetal Health Research Centre, Institute of Human Development, University of Manchester, Manchester M13 0JH, UK; Jenny.Myers@manchester.ac.uk
9 Division of Women's and Children's Health, School of Medicine, University of Leeds, Leeds LS2 9JT, UK; N.A.B.Simpson@leeds.ac.uk
* Correspondence: L.J.Hardie@leeds.ac.uk
† These two authors joint first authors.
‡ These three authors joint senior authors.

Abstract: Severe iodine deficiency in mothers is known to impair foetal development. Pregnant women in the UK may be iodine insufficient, but recent assessments of iodine status are limited. This study assessed maternal urinary iodine concentrations (UIC) and birth outcomes in three UK cities. Spot urines were collected from 541 women in London, Manchester and Leeds from 2004–2008 as part of the Screening for Pregnancy End points (SCOPE) study. UIC at 15 and 20 weeks' gestation was estimated using inductively coupled plasma-mass spectrometry (ICP-MS). Associations were estimated between iodine status (UIC and iodine-to-creatinine ratio) and birth weight, birth weight centile (primary outcome), small for gestational age (SGA) and spontaneous preterm birth. Median UIC was highest in Manchester (139 μg/L, 95% confidence intervals (CI): 126, 158) and London (130 μg/L, 95% CI: 114, 177) and lowest in Leeds (116 μg/L, 95% CI: 99, 135), but the proportion with UIC <50 μg/L was <20% in all three cities. No evidence of an association was observed between UIC and birth weight centile (−0.2% per 50 μg/L increase in UIC, 95% CI: −1.3, 0.8), nor with odds of spontaneous preterm birth (odds ratio = 1.00, 95% CI: 0.84, 1.20). Given the finding of iodine concentrations being insufficient according to World Health Organization (WHO) guidelines amongst pregnant women across all three cities, further studies may be needed to explore implications for maternal thyroid function and longer-term child health outcomes.

Keywords: Iodine; pregnancy; birth weight; Insufficiency; SGA; preterm Birth

1. Introduction

Iodine is essential for the synthesis of the thyroid hormones triiodothyronine (T3) and thyroxine (T4) which regulate growth and metabolism [1]. Maternal iodine requirements are increased throughout pregnancy to support the thyroid hormone demands of the developing foetus [2]. The foetus is initially reliant on maternal thyroid hormones, but as the foetal thyroid begins functioning from 15–17 weeks gestation, it depends on the maternal iodine supply to maintain thyroid hormone production throughout the remainder of pregnancy [2]. Iodine requirements increase throughout gestation, and iodine deficiency during pregnancy is associated with a number of adverse outcomes for the child, including increased mortality, decreased cognitive performance and delayed physical development [1,3]. Severe deficiency during pregnancy can result in cretinism, a condition characterised by severe mental impairment, motor spasticity and deaf-mutism [1,3].

The introduction of iodine into livestock feed and the widespread adoption of iodophors in the dairy industry after the 1930s resulted in the reduction of overt signs of iodine deficiency in the United Kingdom (UK) population by the 1960s [4–6]. To date, the UK has not implemented an iodine fortification programme for commercial bread or salt production unlike countries such as Denmark and Australia [7,8]. Some authors have suggested that the use of iodophors in the dairy and bread industries in the UK has declined and been superseded by non-iodine alternatives, potentially reducing these sources of dietary iodine [1,9]. In addition, wider changes in dietary practice such as reduced milk and fish intake, the increased availability of dairy substitutes and an increase in vegetarianism may also be affecting iodine status in the UK population [9].

Although the UK adult population is considered iodine sufficient [10], recent studies have suggested that women may become deficient during pregnancy [11–16]. Few studies have provided an up-to-date measure of iodine status during pregnancy, nor have they attempted to link insufficiency with birth outcomes [12–15]. Additionally, these studies have been geographically limited, with many being set in single cities or regions in southern England [12–16]. Recent nationally-representative data have suggested that women of child-bearing age in the UK may be iodine insufficient, though this study specifically excluded pregnant and lactating women and did not assess birth outcomes [10].

We therefore aimed to assess iodine status in the three UK sites of the Screening for Pregnancy Endpoints (SCOPE) international birth cohort, and assess associations between maternal iodine status and birth outcomes, including birth weight, birth centile, small for gestational age (SGA) and spontaneous preterm birth.

2. Materials and Methods

2.1. Study Design and Participants

We analysed samples from three English centres from the Screening for Pregnancy Endpoints (SCOPE) birth cohort. The SCOPE study was previously reported in detail elsewhere [17]. In brief, the SCOPE study recruited 5690 nulliparous women with singleton pregnancies before 15 weeks' gestation, between November 2004 and January 2011 in New Zealand, Australia, UK and Ireland. The UK women were recruited in the cities of Leeds, Manchester and London between November 2004 and August 2008. Women were excluded if they presented a high risk of SGA, pre-eclampsia or spontaneous preterm birth [17]. The original SCOPE study protocol has been registered at clinicaltrials.gov NCT02357667.

Participants were interviewed during antenatal clinic visits at 15 ($\pm$ 1) and 20 ($\pm$ 1) weeks' gestation. Participant characteristics were recorded including age, ethnicity, diet, body mass index (BMI), smoking, marital status, employment and socioeconomic status. Participant socioeconomic index was scored using the New Zealand Socio-economic Index 1996. Spot urines were collected for 643 women at the three UK cities; 619 samples were collected at 15 weeks and 585 at 20 weeks, with 547 providing samples at both time points.

2.2. Urinary Iodine Measurement

Urinary iodine concentration (UIC) was measured in all samples taken at 15 and 20 weeks of gestation. Assessment of individual iodine status typically requires a series of 24 hour urine collections, however spot urines are considered an acceptable tool for assessing iodine status on a population basis [3]. It is additionally possible to eliminate some inter-individual variation from spot-urine samples by correcting UIC by urinary creatinine concentration (g/L) [18]. We report iodine status results both as the raw iodine concentration (μg/L) and the iodine-creatinine ratio (I:Cr) (μg/g).

Urinary ^{127}iodine concentration was measured at the University of Leeds using inductively coupled plasma-mass spectrometry (ICP-MS) (Thermo iCAP Q, Hemel Hempstead, UK), accredited by the Centers for Disease Control and Prevention (CDC) Ensuring the Quality of Urinary Iodine Procedures (EQUIP) standardisation programme. Test samples, calibration standards, and quality control samples were diluted 1:10 prior to analysis. Individual samples consisted of 500 μL of participant urine, 4000 μL of diluent (1% tetramethylammonium hydroxide (Sigma Aldrich), 0.01% Triton X-100 (Sigma Aldrich)) and 500 μL high purity H_2O (>18.2 MΩ.cm). Tellurium (10 μg/L) (Sigma Aldrich) was included as an internal standard for the ICP-MS analysis. Sample concentration was determined against a urine matrix matched calibration curve spiked with 0, 5, 10, 40, 70, 100, 400 and 800 μg/L iodide (Sigma Aldrich). The accuracy of the results was further validated through the inclusion of internal quality control urines: A (target iodine value: 59.9 μg/L, range: 47.2–72.5), B (98.1 μg/L, 88.3–107.9) and C (158.9 μg/L, 140.2–177.5). External validation of our results was provided by inclusion of the certified reference material Seronorm Trace Metal Urine Level 1 (target value: 105 μg/L, certified iodine range: 84–126), and through participation in the CDC EQUIP programme. Observed values were 63.3 μg/L (n = 99), 98.6 μg/L (n = 99) and 157.9 μg/L (n = 99) for quality control urines A, B and C respectively. The observed value for certified reference material was 102.7 μg/L (n = 33). Assessment of intra-run precision gave coefficients of variation (CV) of 1.42% at 60 μg/L, 1.67% at 98 μg/L and 2.34% at 159 μg/L. Inter-run precision gave a CV of 2.4% at 60 μg/L, 4.7% at 98 μg/L and 6.0% at 159 μg/L. The method limit of quantification was 1.46 μg/L.

Urinary creatinine concentrations were assessed through a standard microplate assay utilising the Jaffe reaction. Assessment of creatinine intra-assay precision gave a CV of 2% at 10 mg/L, 1% at 70 mg/L and 1.1% at 120 mg/L. Assessment of inter-assay precision gave a CV of 14.5% at 10 mg/L, 9.7% at 70 mg/L and 5.5% at 120 mg/L.

2.3. Outcomes

The primary and a priori outcome for the analysis was birth weight centile. Secondary outcomes were birth weight, SGA, and spontaneous preterm birth. SGA was defined as a birth weight centile <10th on a customised centile chart that accounts for maternal height, weight, parity, ethnicity, neonatal gestation at delivery and sex [19]. This definition was selected due to its standard use in obstetrics and applicability to the UK population, and as it is likely to identify foetal growth restriction. Spontaneous preterm birth was defined as spontaneous preterm labour or preterm premature rupture of the membranes resulting in preterm birth at less than 37 weeks' gestation. These birth outcomes were selected due to the key role of dietary iodine and thyroid hormones in regulating neonatal growth, and the existence of prior studies identifying links between birth weight and preterm birth [20–23].

2.4. Statistical Analysis

Prior to analysis, a set of exclusion parameters were applied. Analysis was limited to participants with urine samples at both time points, using the mean UIC per participant [24]. Exploratory data analysis was then conducted to ensure all values were plausible and all combinations of values were possible. Two participants had duplicate measures at the same time point removed and an additional four participants were excluded due to possessing UIC values more than 3 standard deviations outside of the mean UIC on a log scale. Participant characteristics were described, stratified by location.

Geometric mean and median UIC and I:Cr are presented with 95% confidence intervals (CIs), alongside the proportion of participants with estimated UIC < 50 μg/L. All analyses were completed using Stata version 15.1 (StataCorp. Stata statistical software: Release 15.1. College Station, TX: Stata Corporation, Texas, USA, 2017).

Linear regression was used to quantify associations between UIC and I:Cr for continuous birth outcomes (birth weight and birth weight centile) and logistic regression was used for binary outcomes (SGA and spontaneous preterm birth < 37 weeks). Estimates (with 95% CI) are presented based on the arithmetic mean across the two time points for both UIC and I:Cr for mothers providing both samples (primary analysis) and stratified by time point (secondary analyses). All results are presented as unadjusted and adjusted for known confounders. Directed acyclic graphs were used to inform which variables should be included as covariates, and to prevent over-adjustment [25]. Ethnicity, age, geographic location and socioeconomic index were adjusted for by inclusion in the regression model, except where ethnicity was already accounted for in the birth weight centile and SGA outcomes. Maternal height, weight, parity, neonatal gestation at delivery and sex were also taken into account in the definition of birth weight centile and SGA. The robustness of birthweight and spontaneous preterm birth results to additional adjustment for maternal BMI was assessed.

2.5. Ethics Statement

Ethical approval was gained from local research ethics committees for each SCOPE recruitment site (South East Multi-centre Research Ethics Committee/St Thomas Hospital Research Ethics Committee, 2005082; South East Multi-Centre Research Ethics Committee/Central Manchester Research Ethics Committee, 06/MRE01/98). All participants provided written informed consent.

3. Results

3.1. Participant Characteristics

Table 1 shows participant characteristic summary statistics, including but not limited to maternal age, ethnicity, socioeconomic index, marital status, smoking status, alcohol consumption, height, weight and BMI. The mean maternal age at recruitment was 29 years, 457 (84%) were White Caucasian and 397 (73%) non-smokers (see Table 1). Data were available for 541 participants (151 from London, 260 from Manchester, and 130 from Leeds) after exclusions, with a urine sample available from each participant at both 15 and 20 weeks' gestation. A total of 1082 urine samples were analysed for iodine, with the overall geometric mean of 130 μg/L and a median of 134 μg/L.

3.2. Iodine Status

Geometric mean UIC varied by marital status, geographical location, neonatal gestational age at delivery and gestational time point (Table 2). UIC also varied across time points, with the 20 week concentrations being on average lower than the 15-week concentrations. Participants from Leeds had lower mean UIC (110 μg/L, 95% CI: 99, 121) than participants from Manchester (132 μg/L, 95% CI: 123, 143) or London (145 μg/L, 95% CI: 126, 168). Participants delivering preterm (<37 weeks) generally had similar UIC to those who delivered at term. Consistent with UIC, I:Cr was associated with geographical location and marital status, but not time point or gestational age at delivery. Additionally, I:Cr differed by maternal age category, ethnicity, socioeconomic index and maternal smoking status in the first trimester. Of the three sites, participants at Leeds and Manchester had lower geometric mean I:Cr when compared to London, with Leeds having the lowest. Individuals with UIC (<50 μg/L) constituted 9% (95% CI: 7, 12) across all three sites, with these individuals constituting 9%, 7% and 13% of the Leeds, Manchester and London sites respectively.

Table 1. Participant characteristics by location.

Participant Characteristics	Overall (N = 541)	London (N = 151)	Manchester (N = 260)	Leeds (N = 130)
	n (%)	n (%)	n (%)	n (%)
Mean maternal age (years)				
18–24	121 (22)	12 (8)	62 (24)	47 (36)
25–29	160 (30)	37 (25)	84 (32)	39 (30)
30–34	189 (35)	71 (47)	79 (30)	39 (30)
35+	71 (13)	31 (21)	35 (13)	5 (4)
Maternal ethnicity				
White Caucasian	457 (84)	123 (81)	217 (83)	117 (90)
Other	84 (16)	28 (19)	43 (17)	13 (10)
Maternal socioeconomic index (quartiles)				
Q1 (more deprived)	126 (23)	12 (8)	66 (25)	48 (37)
Q2	133 (25)	31 (21)	68 (26)	34 (26)
Q3	145 (27)	52 (34)	62 (24)	31 (24)
Q4 (less deprived)	137 (25)	56 (37)	64 (25)	17 (13)
Marital status				
Single	84 (16)	14 (9)	38 (15)	32 (25)
Married	258 (48	95 (63	114 (44)	49 (38)
Living as married	199 (37)	42 (28)	108 (42)	49 (38)
Maternal smoking status in 1st trimester				
Non-smoker	397 (73)	128 (85)	186 (72)	83 (64)
Smoker	144 (27)	23 (15)	74 (28)	47 (36)
Maternal alcohol consumption in 1st trimester (units/week)				
0	153 (28)	34 (23)	85 (33)	34 (26)
<2	94 (17)	38 (25)	38 (15)	18 (14)
2–7	160 (30)	41 (27)	79 (30)	40 (31)
>7	134 (25)	38 (25)	58 (22)	38 (29)
Gravidity				
1	385 (71)	105 (70)	184 (71)	96 (74)
2	119 (22)	35 (23)	61 (23)	23 (18)
3+	37 (7)	11 (7)	15 (6)	11 (8)
Maternal height (cm)				
<160	103 (19)	31 (21)	53 (20)	19 (15)
160–169	300 (55)	85 (56)	148 (57)	67 (52)
170+	138 (26)	35 (23)	59 (23)	44 (34)
Maternal weight at 1st visit (kg)				
<60	154 (28)	44 (29)	77 (30)	33 (25)
60–69	190 (35)	60 (40)	89 (34)	41 (32)
70–79	107 (20)	34 (23	48 (18)	25 (19)
80+	90 (17)	13 (9)	46 (18)	31 (24)
Maternal body mass index at 1st visit (kg/m^2)				
<20	38 (7)	12 (8)	13 (5)	13 (10)
20–25	289 (53)	84 (56)	143 (55)	62 (48)
25–30	148 (27)	42 (28	69 (27)	37 (28)
30+	66 (12)	13 (9)	35 (13)	18 (14)
Spontaneous preterm delivery (<37 weeks)				
No	523 (97)	144 (95)	252 (97)	127 (98)
Yes	18 (3)	7 (5)	8 (3)	3 (2)
Neonatal sex				
Male	277 (51)	78 (52)	140 (54)	59 (45)
Female	264 (49)	73 (48)	120 (46)	71 (55)

Numbers represent the number of individuals in each category, with the percentage in brackets.

Table 2. Urinary iodine concentration and iodine-to-creatinine ratio by participant characteristics.

Participant Characteristics	Mean Urinary Iodine Concentration (μg/L)			Mean Iodine-to-Creatinine ratio (μg/g)	
	Geometric mean (95% CI)	**Median (95% CI)**	**Percent < 50μg/L (95% CI)**	**Geometric mean (95% CI)**	**Median (95% CI)**
Overall	130 (122, 138)	134 (124, 145)	9 (7, 12)	193 (182, 205)	186 (175, 201)
Maternal age (years)					
18–24	127 (114, 141)	135 (117, 154)	9 (5, 16)	137 (123, 153)	145 (126, 157)
25–29	116 (104, 129)	122 (100, 135)	9 (5, 14)	190 (171, 211)	186 (162, 222)
30–34	138 (124, 154)	140 (119, 164)	11 (7, 16)	228 (208, 251)	219 (201, 254)
35+	147 (122, 176)	144 (122, 191)	6 (2, 14)	232 (197, 272)	210 (175, 249)
Maternal ethnicity					
White Caucasian	130 (122, 139)	134 (124, 147)	10 (7, 13)	201 (189, 214)	190 (176, 209)
Other	127 (112, 143)	124 (103, 147)	4 (1, 10)	155 (135, 178)	160 (142, 193)
Maternal socioeconomic index (quartiles)					
Q1 (More deprived)	125 (112, 139)	128 (109, 163)	6 (2, 11)	157 (141, 174)	153 (144, 182)
Q2	132 (117, 149)	135 (114, 150)	9 (5, 15)	199 (177, 223)	199 (161, 225)
Q3	133 (118, 151)	135 (113, 162)	10 (6, 16)	209 (186, 235)	202 (172, 224)
Q4 (Less deprived)	129 (114, 146)	132 (119, 149)	11 (6, 17)	209 (186, 236)	200 (177, 228)
Marital status					
Single	112 (98, 128)	114 (99, 135)	13 (7, 22)	140 (123, 159)	150 (127, 175)
Married	128 (117, 141)	130 (119, 146)	10 (7, 15)	216 (199, 234)	211 (186, 230)
Living as married	140 (128, 154)	147 (126, 162)	6 (3, 10)	192 (174, 211)	184 (163, 211)
Maternal smoking status in 1st trimester					
Non-smoker	134 (124, 144)	135 (124, 151)	9 (7, 13)	207 (193, 221)	200 (180, 217)
Smoker	119 (108, 132)	126 (111, 143)	8 (4, 14)	160 (145, 177)	154 (143, 180)
Maternal alcohol consumption in 1st trimester (units/week)					
0	133 (120, 148)	135 (117, 161)	7 (4, 12)	183 (166, 202)	184 (163, 212)
<2	124 (107, 143)	125 (99, 153)	11 (5, 19)	193 (168, 222)	186 (161, 206)
2–7	135 (121, 151)	132 (119, 155)	6 (3, 11)	205 (183, 230)	201 (169, 225)
>7	124 (108, 141)	134 (108, 158)	13 (8, 20)	191 (169, 216)	178 (158, 203)
Gravidity					
1	129 (120, 139)	134 (124, 149)	10 (7, 13)	198 (185, 211)	188 (174, 209)
2	131 (117, 147)	125 (115, 151)	7 (3, 13)	183 (161, 209)	183 (147, 210)
3+	130 (104, 163)	120 (102, 174)	8 (2, 22)	179 (148, 218)	188 (154, 217)

Table 2. *Cont.*

Participant Characteristics	Mean Urinary Iodine Concentration (μg/L)			Mean Iodine-to-Creatinine ratio (μg/g)	
	Geometric mean (95% CI)	Median (95% CI)	Percent < 50μg/L (95% CI)	Geometric mean (95% CI)	Median (95% CI)
Maternal height (cm)					
<160	129 (112, 148)	126 (104, 159)	8 (3, 15)	202 (175, 234)	175 (157, 212)
160–169	134 (123, 145)	134 (123, 152)	10 (7, 14)	196 (182, 212)	197 (176, 212)
170+	122 (110, 137)	131 (115, 152)	9 (5, 15)	180 (161, 202)	170 (152, 206)
Maternal weight at 1st visit (kg)					
<60	131 (116, 146)	126 (112, 152)	9 (5, 15)	207 (185, 231)	201 (175, 234)
60-69	124 (112, 137)	125 (111, 141)	8 (5, 13)	195 (177, 214)	190 (170, 209)
70–79	130 (112, 149)	135 (114, 172)	12 (7, 20)	202 (177, 231)	177 (159, 209)
80+	143 (125, 163)	157 (127, 173)	8 (3, 15)	160 (140, 184)	159 (128, 210)
Maternal body mass index at 1st visit (kg/m^2)					
<20	131 (106, 163)	130 (98, 175)	5 (1, 18)	178 (138, 229)	157 (121, 253)
20–25	127 (116, 138)	127 (117, 146)	10 (7, 14)	207 (192, 224)	200 (181, 221)
25–30	128 (115, 143)	134 (115, 151)	9 (5, 15)	186 (167, 209)	177 (161, 205)
30+	149 (128, 174)	164 (126, 182)	8 (3, 17)	162 (139, 190)	161 (132, 210)
Geographical location					
London	145 (126, 168)	130 (114, 177)	13 (8, 20)	242 (210, 279)	228 (181, 273)
Manchester	132 (123, 143)	139 (126, 158)	7 (4, 10)	183 (171, 196)	183 (165, 202)
Leeds	110 (99, 121)	116 (99, 135)	9 (5, 16)	165 (149, 183)	168 (149, 193)
Spontaneous preterm delivery (<37 weeks)					
No	130 (122, 138)	134 (124, 144)	9 (7, 12)	194 (183, 206)	188 (175, 202)
Yes	132 (89, 196)	147 (75, 254)	11 (1, 35)	171 (129, 226)	155 (140, 246)
Neonatal sex					
Male	128 (118, 139)	134 (119, 147)	10 (7, 14)	199 (184, 215)	186 (174, 210)
Female	132 (121, 143)	134 (122, 151)	8 (5, 12)	187 (172, 204)	184 (163, 206)
Appointment					
15 weeks gestation	134 (125, 143)	135 (127, 152)	12 (10, 15)	176 (165, 188)	172 (159, 189)
20 weeks gestation	101 (94, 109)	107 (95, 115)	23 (19, 27)	188 (177, 200)	183 (170, 200)

3.3. Birth Outcomes

Table 3 shows the associations between mean UIC per participant and continuous birth outcomes. There was little evidence of any association between UIC and birth weight (−14 g per 50 µg/L increase in mean UIC, 95% CI: −35, +6). Results were similar when iodine was corrected for creatinine, with no evidence of any association with birth weight (−8 g per 50 µg/g increase in mean I:Cr, 95% CI: −20, +4). When birth weight was considered further as a customised birth centile, again no evidence of an association was found between mean UIC or mean I:Cr. Birth outcome associations with UIC were largely consistent when iodine levels were assessed at individual time points.

Table 3. Change in continuous birth outcomes associated with a 50 µg/L increment in mean urinary iodine concentration or 50 µg/g increment in iodine-to-creatinine ratio. 95% confidence intervals are included in brackets.

		Change in Outcome per 50 µg/L Increment in Urinary Iodine Concentration		**Change in Outcome per 50 µg/g Increment in Iodine-to-Creatinine Ratio**	
	Appointment	**Unadjusted**	**Adjusted** *	**Unadjusted**	**Adjusted** *
Birth weight (g)	15 weeks	−6 g (21, +10)	−7 g (−23, +8)	0 g (−9, +9)	−4 g (−14, +5)
	20 weeks	−9 g (−27, +9)	−13 g (−31, +5)	−3 g (−14, +7)	−8 g (−19, +4)
	Mean	−10 g (−30, +10)	−14 g (−35, +6)	−2 g (−14, +9)	−8 g (−20, +4)
Birth weight centile **	15 weeks	0.0% (−0.8, +0.8)	−0.2% (−0.9, +0.6)	+0.1% (−0.3, +0.6)	0.0% (−0.5, +0.4)
	20 weeks	+0.1% (−0.8, +1.0)	−0.2% (−1.1, +0.7)	0.0% (−0.5, +0.5)	−0.2% (−0.7, +0.4)
	Mean	0.0% (−0.9, +1.0)	−0.2% (−1.3, +0.8)	+0.1% (−0.5, +0.6)	−0.1% (−0.7, +0.5)

* Adjusted for maternal age, city, ethnicity and socioeconomic index. ** Additionally, gestation at delivery, maternal height and weight, parity and child's sex were taken into account in the definition of birth weight centile.

Table 4 shows associations between mean UIC per participant and binary birth outcomes. No evidence of an association was observed between SGA and mean UIC or mean I:Cr. There was no evidence that spontaneous preterm birth was associated with mean iodine concentration, with a 50 µg/L increase in mean UIC associated with 0% increase in the odds of spontaneous preterm birth (95% CI: −16%, +20%), nor was there any evidence found of an association between mean urinary I:Cr and spontaneous preterm birth (odds ratio: 0.91, 95% CI: 0.78, 1.07).

Table 4. Relative increase in odds of binary birth outcomes (odds ratios) associated with a 50 µg/L increment in mean urinary iodine concentration or 50 µg/g increment in iodine-to-creatinine ratio. 95% confidence intervals are included in brackets.

		Odds Ratio per 50 µg/L Increment in Urinary Iodine Concentration		**Odds Ratio per 50 µg/g Increment in Iodine-to-Creatinine Ratio**	
	Visit	Unadjusted	Adjusted *	Unadjusted	Adjusted *
Small for gestational age **	15 weeks	1.03 (0.96, 1.10)	1.05 (0.97, 1.13)	1.00 (0.95, 1.04)	1.01 (0.97, 1.06)
	20 weeks	1.05 (0.97, 1.13)	1.08 (0.99, 1.16)	1.00 (0.95, 1.05)	1.02 (0.97, 1.07)
	Mean	1.05 (0.97, 1.14)	1.09 (1.00, 1.20)	1.00 (0.94, 1.05)	1.02 (0.96, 1.09)
Spontaneous preterm birth (<37 weeks)	15 weeks	1.03 (0.90, 1.18)	1.02 (0.89, 1.17)	0.96 (0.85, 1.09)	0.96 (0.85, 1.08)
	20 weeks	0.98 (0.82, 1.17)	0.97 (0.81, 1.17)	0.89 (0.75, 1.07)	0.89 (0.76, 1.06)
	Mean	1.02 (0.85, 1.22)	1.00 (0.84, 1.20)	0.91 (0.77, 1.08)	0.91 (0.78, 1.07)

* Adjusted for maternal age, city, ethnicity and socioeconomic index. ** Additionally, gestation at delivery, maternal height and weight, parity and child's sex were taken into account in the definition of small-for-gestational-age.

Estimates for birth weight and spontaneous preterm birth outcomes were not substantially changed on adjustment for maternal BMI (data not shown).

4. Discussion

World Health Organization (WHO) guidelines are commonly applied for assessing iodine deficiency disorders [3]. These guidelines define a median population UIC > 100 μg/L as iodine sufficient for school-age children and non-pregnant adults. In addition the proportion of participants with a UIC < 50 μg/L must not exceed 20% of the population to be considered iodine sufficient. Currently, WHO guidelines define iodine status during pregnancy as either sufficient (median UIC 150–249 μg/L) or insufficient (<150 μg/L). Each of the three cities we have assessed in the SCOPE birth cohort would be classed as iodine insufficient under these pregnancy guidelines. Median UIC varied between each city with London and Manchester cohorts giving the highest median UIC, whilst Leeds gave the lowest. On average, UIC decreased between 15 and 20 weeks of pregnancy, though no such decrease was observed when assessing I:Cr.

Despite the presence of iodine insufficiency in the cohort, there was no evidence of any association between UIC or I:Cr and birth outcomes. Only a small number of studies have assessed potential links between UIC in pregnancy and neonatal outcomes [13,20–23], all of which involved populations that were either sufficient [20,23] or borderline sufficient in iodine [13,21,22]. The majority of studies have found no association between UIC and birth weight [13,20,22]. Two studies found positive associations between UIC and birth weight [21,23], but these associations were inconsistent across trimesters.

Charoenratana et al. [20] found that lower UIC was associated with increased odds of preterm birth in Thai women and studies examining links between thyroid hormone concentrations and birth outcomes suggest that pregnant women with hypothyroidism are at greater risk of preterm birth than euthyroid women [26,27]. Whilst these results appear to contradict ours, it should be noted that our study examined gestational time points in the second trimester of pregnancy, whereas Charoenratana et al. measured UIC across all three trimesters and. In addition, a number of other studies have found no evidence of an association between UIC and preterm birth [13,21,22]. Mild iodine deficiency is known to be linked to maternal hypothyroxinemia, a condition characterized by low free T4 levels despite normal free T3 concentrations [28], which in turn has been related to adverse neurodevelopmental outcomes [29]. Conversely, the association between hyperthyroidism and preterm birth is well documented, with the majority of these cases being associated with increased levels of anti-thyroid autoantibodies [27]. However this study was unable to measure thyroid hormone levels, nor examined a hyperthyroid population. We suggest that further studies are warranted in order to clarify the relationship between iodine status and thyroid hormone concentrations with birth outcomes during pregnancy.

Whilst London and Manchester participants had higher UIC values, they also had smaller proportions of participants in the lowest category of socioeconomic status, with London having the smallest. In contrast, Leeds had the highest proportion. As our study found that lower socioeconomic status was associated with lower UIC, our results may suggest that regions of the UK with a greater proportion of citizens with a lower socioeconomic index may be at greater risk of iodine insufficiency. Additionally, participants in the 25–29 age category generally had lower UIC values than participants in other age categories, whilst active smokers generally had lower mean UIC values than non-smokers. Whilst the proportion of participants in each cohort with UIC values <50 μg/L was adequate under WHO guidelines for the general population (<20% of all participants), our observed proportions still constitute a large number of pregnant women who may be at risk for inadequate iodine intakes, if these samples are representative of the UK population as a whole [3].

This study also found that UIC decreased on average between the two time points. A number of changes occur in foetal physiology during the second trimester of pregnancy, with the most notable being the activation of the foetal thyroid between weeks 16–18 of pregnancy [30]. An increase in free T4 allocation to the foetal cerebral cortex also occurs from the mid-point of the first trimester, peaking in weeks 13–20 of pregnancy [30]. These increases in foetal thyroid hormone demand, along with increased iodine trapping and hormone production by the maternal thyroid to meet these demands, could account for the decrease in UIC seen at week 20, compared with week 15. Changes in renal physiology during pregnancy may also have contributed to the observed decrease in UIC [30,31]. Renal iodine clearance via urine increases by roughly 35–50% throughout pregnancy, a change that results in a shortfall in available serum iodine and a compensatory increase of iodine uptake by the thyroid [31]. Previous studies have suggested that the maternal thyroid responds to low iodine status by upregulating thyroid stimulating hormone (TSH) to stimulate increased iodine capture [31]. The decrease in UIC we observe between weeks 15 and 20 may translate into altered TSH, free T3 or T4, but unfortunately this could not be assessed in the present study. A further possibility is that these observed differences were due to differing urine dilutions of participants at these time points. Notably the difference in UIC observed between time points was not observed when using the I:Cr, a correction aimed at reducing inter-individual variability in UIC [22]. This result suggests that iodine excretion may actually remain relatively constant between 15 and 20 weeks.

Our study was limited by a number of factors. Sample collection was restricted to the second trimester of pregnancy, and used spot rather than 24 h urine samples, which are limited in their applicability for assessing iodine status to the population level, rather than providing information on individual chronic iodine intakes. In addition, recruitment was restricted to a small number of UK cities and as a result, the study may have been limited in its assessment of iodine status in surrounding suburban and rural areas. Our study also has a number of strengths. These include the large number of participants available for each of our three geographical sites compared with many prior UK iodine studies, the collection of demographic details through face-to-face interviews with participants, the use of robust analytical procedures for assessing biomarkers of iodine status, and controlling for a number of potentially confounding variables in the statistical modelling. To the best of our knowledge, this is the first study to compare iodine status between geographically separate UK populations.

5. Conclusions

In conclusion, we have demonstrated that the iodine status of pregnant women in our study cohort is generally insufficient by WHO guidelines, with variations in iodine concentrations occurring across different cities in the UK. This finding broadly supports conclusions made by prior UK studies that pregnant women in the UK are insufficient in dietary iodine [10–16]. However, we have not found evidence that this is adversely associated with the birth outcomes assessed in this study. More detailed follow-up of maternal thyroid function, foetal and childhood growth, plus cognitive development are required to assess the long-term implications of this level of iodine insufficiency.

Author Contributions: Conceptualization, D.C.G. and L.J.H.; Methodology, D.C.G., L.J.H., C.J.P.S., E.T., C.K. and D.E.T.; Validation, C.J.P.S., E.T., D.C.G. and C.K.; Formal Analysis, D.C.G., C.K. and D.E.T.; Investigation, C.J.P.S., E.T. and S.R.; Resources, L.J.H., D.C.G., N.A.B.S., L.P. and J.E.M.; Data Curation, D.C.G., C.K. and D.E.T.; Writing—Original Draft Preparation, C.J.P.S. and C.K.; Writing—Review and Editing, C.J.P.S., C.K., E.T., J.E.T., P.M.S., M.Z., S.R., L.P., J.E.M., N.A.B.S., D.E.T., D.C.G. and L.J.H.; Visualization, D.C.G., C.K. and D.E.T.; Supervision, D.C.G. and L.J.H.; Project Administration, L.J.H. and D.C.G.; Funding Acquisition, L.J.H., D.C.G., J.E.C., P.S. and N.A.B.S.

Acknowledgments: We thank the Iodine in Pregnancy Steering Group for input and advice during study conception, funding acquisition and the wider study timeframe. We thank Amanda McKillion and Sarah Meadows at the Elsie Widdowson Laboratory, University of Cambridge, for additional advice on ICP-MS method development and quality control procedures.

References

1. Zimmermann, M.B.; Jooste, P.L.; Pandav, C.S. Iodine-deficiency disorders. *Lancet* **2008**, *372*, 1251–1262. [CrossRef]
2. Delange, F. Iodine requirements during pregnancy, lactation and the neonatal period and indicators of optimal iodine nutrition. *Public Health Nutr.* **2007**, *10*, 1571–1580. [CrossRef] [PubMed]
3. WHO; UNICEF; ICCIDD. *Assessment of Iodine Deficiency Disorders and Monitoring their Elimination*; WHO: Geneva, Switzerland, 2007.

4. Underwood, E.J. Iodine. In *The Mineral Nutrition of Livestock*; Commonwealth Agriculture Bureau: Slough, UK, 1984; pp. 84–85.
5. Wenlock, R.W. Changing patterns of dietary iodine intake in Britain. In *Dietary Iodine and Other Aetiological Factors in Hyperthyroidism*; MRC Conference Report: Southampton, UK, 1987; pp. 1–6.
6. Philips, D.I.W. Iodine, milk, and the elimination of endemic goitre in Britain: The story of an accidental public health triumph. *J. Epidemiol. Community Health* **1997**, *51*, 391–393. [CrossRef]
7. Rasmussen, L.B.; Ovesen, L.; Christensen, T.; Knuthsen, P.; Larsen, E.H.; Lyhnne, N.; Okholm, B.; Saxholt, E. Iodine content in bread and salt in Denmark after iodization and the influence on iodine intake. *Int. J. Food Sci. Nutr.* **2007**, *58*, 231–239. [CrossRef]
8. Seal, J.A.; Doyle, Z.; Burgess, J.R.; Taylor, R.; Cameron, A.R. Iodine status of Tasmanians following voluntary fortification of bread with iodine. *Med. J. Aust.* **2007**, *186*, 69–71.
9. Pearce, N.E. Iodine nutrition in the UK: What went wrong? *Lancet* **2011**, *377*, 1979–1980. [CrossRef]
10. National Diet and Nutrition Survey. NDNS: Results from Years 7 and 8. Public Health England, 2018. Available online: https://www.gov.uk/government/uploads/system/uploads/attachment_data/file/690475/NDNS_survey_results_from_years_7_and_8_of_the_rolling_programme.pdf (accessed on 21 March 2018).
11. Kibirige, M.S.; Hutchison, S.; Owen, C.J.; Delves, H.T. Prevalence of maternal dietary iodine insufficiency in the north east of England: Implications for the fetus. *Arch. Dis. Child. Fetal. Neonatal Ed.* **2004**, *89*, 436–439. [CrossRef]
12. Rayman, M.; Sleeth, M.; Walter, A.; Taylor, A. Iodine deficiency in UK women of child-bearing age. *Proc. Nutr. Soc.* **2008**, *67*, E399. [CrossRef]
13. Bath, S.C.; Steer, C.D.; Golding, J.; Rayman, M.P. Effect of inadequate iodine status in UK pregnant women on cognitive outcomes in their children: Results from the Avon Longitudinal Study of Parents and Children (ALSPAC). *Lancet* **2013**, *382*, 331–337. [CrossRef]
14. Bath, S.C.; Walter, A.; Taylor, A.; Wright, J.; Rayman, M.P. Iodine deficiency in pregnant women living in the South-East of the UK: The influence of diet and nutritional supplements on iodine status. *Br. J. Nutr.* **2014**, *111*, 162–1631. [CrossRef]
15. Bath, S.C.; Furmidge-Owen, V.; Redman, C.W.G.; Rayman, M.P. Gestational changes in iodine status in a cohort study of pregnant women from the United Kingdom: Season as an effect modifier. *Am. J. Clin. Nutr.* **2015**, *101*, 1180–1187. [CrossRef] [PubMed]
16. Knight, B.A.; Shields, B.M.; He, X.; Pearce, E.N.; Braverman, L.E.; Sturley, R.; Vaidya, B. Iodine deficiency amongst pregnant women in South-West England. *Clin. Endocrinol. (Oxf.)* **2017**, *86*, 451–455. [CrossRef] [PubMed]
17. McCowan, L.M.E.; North, R.A.; Taylor, R. ACTRN12607000551493. Australian New Zealand Clinical Trials Registry 2007. Available online: www.anzctr.org.au/trialSearch.aspx (accessed on 12 February 2019).
18. Knudsen, N.; Christiansen, E.; Brandt-Christensen, M.; Nygaard, B.; Perrild, H. Age- and sex-adjusted iodine/creatinine ratio. A new standard in epidemiological surveys? Evaluation of three different estimates of iodine excretion based on casual urine samples and comparison to 24 h values. *Eur. J. Clin. Nutr.* **2000**, *54*, 361–363. [CrossRef] [PubMed]
19. Gardosi, J. Customised fetal growth standards: Rationale and clinical application. *Semin. Perinatol.* **2004**, *28*, 33–40. [CrossRef] [PubMed]
20. Charoenratana, C.; Leelapat, P.; Traisrisilp, K.; Tongsong, T. Maternal iodine insufficiency and adverse pregnancy outcomes. *Matern Child Nutr.* **2016**, *12*, 680–687. [CrossRef] [PubMed]
21. Álvarez-Pedrerol, M.; Guxens, M.; Mendez, M.; Canet, Y.; Martorell, R.; Espada, M.; Plana, E.; Rebagliato, M.; Sunyer, J. Iodine levels and thyroid hormones in healthy pregnant women and birth weight of their offspring. *Eur. J. Endocrinol.* **2009**, *160*, 423–429. [CrossRef] [PubMed]
22. Leon, G.; Murcia, M.; Rebagliato, M.; Álvarez-Pedrerol, M.; Castilla, A.M.; Basterrechea, M.; Iñiguez, C.; Fernández-Somoano, A.; Blarduni, E.; Foradada, C.M.; et al. Maternal thyroid dysfunction during gestation, preterm delivery, and birth weight. The Infancia y Medio Ambiente Cohort, Spain. *Paediatr Perinat Epidemiol.* **2015**, *29*, 113–122. [CrossRef] [PubMed]
23. Casey, B.M.; Dashe, J.S.; Wells, C.E.; McIntire, D.D.; Byrd, W.; Leveno, K.J.; Cunningham, F.G. Subclinical hypothyroidism and pregnancy outcomes. *Obstet Gynecol.* **2005**, *105*, 239–245. [CrossRef] [PubMed]

24. Hynes, K.L.; Otahal, P.; Hay, I.; Burgess, J.R. Mild iodine deficiency during pregnancy is associated with reduced educational outcomes in the offspring: 9-year follow-up of the Gestational Iodine Cohort. *J. Clin. Endocrinol. Metab.* **2013**, *98*, 1954–1962. [CrossRef]
25. Textor, J.; Hardt, J.; Knüppel, S. DAGitty: A graphical tool for analyzing causal diagrams. *Epidemiology* **2011**, *22*, 745. [CrossRef]
26. Stagnaro-Green, A.; Chen, X.; Bogden, J.D.; Davies, T.F.; Scholl, T.O. The thyroid and pregnancy: A novel risk factor for very preterm delivery. *Thyroid* **2005**, *15*, 351–357. [CrossRef]
27. Sheehan, P.M.; Nankervis, A.; Júnior, E.A.; da Silva Costa, F. Maternal thyroid disease and preterm birth: Systematic review and meta-analysis. *J. Clin. Endocrinol. Metab.* **2015**, *100*, 4325–4331. [CrossRef] [PubMed]
28. Glinoer, D. The importance of iodine nutrition during pregnancy. *Public Health Nutr.* **2007**, *10*, 1542–1546. [CrossRef] [PubMed]
29. Henrichs, J.; Bongers-Schokking, J.J.; Schenk, J.J.; Ghassabian, A.; Schmidt, H.G.; Visser, T.J.; Hooijkaas, H.; de Muinck Keizer-Schrama, S.M.; Hofman, A.; Jaddoe, V.V.; et al. Maternal thyroid function during early pregnancy and cognitive functioning in early childhood: The generation R study. *J. Clin. Endocrinol. Metab.* **2010**, *95*, 4227–4234. [CrossRef] [PubMed]
30. Pop, V.J.; Brouwers, E.P.; Vader, H.L.; Vulsma, T.; van Baar, A.L.; de Vijlder, J.J. Maternal hypothyroxinaemia during early pregnancy and subsequent child development: A 3-year follow-up study. *Clin. Endocrinol.* **2003**, *59*, 282–288. [CrossRef]
31. Patel, J.; Landers, K.; Li, H.; Mortimer, R.H.; Richard, K. Thyroid hormones and fetal neurological development. *J. Endocrinol.* **2011**, *209*, 1–8. [CrossRef] [PubMed]

2

Choline and DHA in Maternal and Infant Nutrition: Synergistic Implications in Brain and Eye Health

Jonathan G. Mun *, LeeCole L. Legette, Chioma J. Ikonte and Susan H. Mitmesser

Science & Technology, Pharmavite LLC, West Hills, CA 91304, USA; llegette@pharmavite.net (L.L.L.); cikonte@pharmavite.net (C.J.I.); smitmesser@pharmavite.net (S.H.M.)

* Correspondence: jmun@pharmavite.net

Abstract: The aim of this review is to highlight current insights into the roles of choline and docosahexaenoic acid (DHA) in maternal and infant nutrition, with special emphasis on dietary recommendations, gaps in dietary intake, and synergistic implications of both nutrients in infant brain and eye development. Adequate choline and DHA intakes are not being met by the vast majority of US adults, and even more so by women of child-bearing age. Choline and DHA play a significant role in infant brain and eye development, with inadequate intakes leading to visual and neurocognitive deficits. Emerging findings illustrate synergistic interactions between choline and DHA, indicating that insufficient intakes of one or both could have lifelong deleterious impacts on both maternal and infant health.

Keywords: choline; pregnancy; infant nutrition; brain health; docosahexaenoic acid; DHA; eye function

1. Introduction

Pregnancy is an important time for both mother and baby and a long-standing strategy in supporting healthy pregnancies involves adequate prenatal care. Health care during pregnancy is one of the most frequently used wellness services in the US, with more than 18 million prenatal visits in 2015 [1]. Increasing the percentage of pregnant women who receive early and adequate prenatal care is a key objective for the US Healthy People 2020 public health initiative [2]. As part of adequate prenatal health consciousness and self-care, optimal nutrition plays a key role in maternal and infant health, prior to, during, and after pregnancy. Leading health organizations including the American Congress of Obstetricians and Gynecologists (ACOG), American Academy of Pediatrics (AAP), Europe Food Safety Authority (EFSA), and the World Health Organization (WHO) have highlighted several key nutrients as vital during pregnancy, including choline and DHA. The 2018 AAP policy statement emphasized the role of nutrition in the first 1000 days of life. The AAP recognized choline and long-chain polyunsaturated fatty acids (LC-PUFAs) as key nutrients in supporting early neurodevelopment and lifelong mental health [3]. Both docosahexaenoic acid (DHA) and arachidonic acid (ARA) are common LC-PUFAs that accumulate in tissues and are known for their importance in brain function and development [4,5]. Docosahexaenoic acid and ARA are synthesized from precursor essential fatty acids, omega-3 α-linolenic acid (ALA) and omega-6 linoleic acid (LA), respectively [6]. Endogenous synthesis of choline and DHA is insufficient to meet nutrient demands, reinforcing the need for adequate daily intake. While general dietary intake of omega-6s meets daily recommendations, omega-3 intake is low in the American diet [7]. National survey data in the US population indicates inadequate dietary intakes of choline and DHA. Over 90% of the US population does not meet adequate intake for choline (550 mg/day for men, 425 mg/day for women) [8]. Among US adults, pregnant and lactating women are at increased risk for choline insufficiency as their requirements increase to 450 and 550 mg, respectively, during these life stages [9]. Dietary intakes of DHA are also low in American diet, with general recommendations of 7–8 oz of fish and seafood weekly to equate to 250 mg EPA + DHA omega-3 fatty acids daily. However, the majority of US adults fail to consume adequate amounts of seafood, with averages of 0.43 oz seafood (63 mg DHA) daily [10]. Docosahexaenoic acid recommendations for pregnant and lactating women are slightly higher, with the 2015 US Department of Agriculture Dietary Guidelines advising weekly consumption of 8–12 oz of low-mercury content seafood, noting that DHA is associated with improved infant health outcomes [11]. However, nearly all US women of child-bearing age and pregnant women (95%) have low seafood consumption and do not meet recommended daily intakes of 250 mg total of eicosapentaenoic acid (EPA) and DHA [12]. While supplement use has increased DHA and EPA intakes over time, current intakes are still low, suggesting a need for more effective nutrition education programs to address nutrient shortfalls [12], especially during pregnancy and lactation. Choline and DHA, as a LC-PUFA, are essential nutrients for normal brain development as they are integral structural components of neurological systems, and deficits during early life can have long-term impacts on brain function [3]. Both are also utilized in retinal development and lack of adequate amounts could adversely impact eye health. The main objective of this review is to critically evaluate the roles of choline and DHA in infant and maternal nutrition, to elucidate possible synergistic implications of both nutrients in brain and eye health and increase the awareness of this public health concern.

2. Role of Choline in Maternal and Infant Nutrition

2.1. Essential Functions

Discovered as a component of lecithin from heated pig and ox bile in the 1860s, choline was named from the Greek word for bile, "chole" [13]. Lecithin was later characterized as being largely comprised of phosphatidylcholine, a major constituent of biological membranes. As researchers began to study how nerves communicated with each other in the 1920s, a substance secreted from a stimulated vagus nerve was identified (acetylcholine) and found to be the same molecule as a choline-containing molecule derived from fungi that could activate nerves when applied to organs. This discovery was awarded a Nobel Prize to Otto Loewi and Henry Dale in 1936.

For decades following this work, choline was recognized as being a critical component of the two biologically relevant molecules, phosphatidylcholine and acetylcholine, and yet its requirement in the human diet was substantially underappreciated. In animal models, pancreatectomized dogs developed fatty degeneration of the liver, which could be reversed by feeding raw pancreas or lecithin [14], a consequence later understood to be due to the impaired lipid packaging into lipoproteins for export from the liver. Choline deficiencies were documented in a number of other animal species, including perosis in poultry (deforming leg weakness), atherosclerosis in rodents, and related conditions in rabbit, cattle, and baboon. In addition, choline-deficient animals were found to develop liver cancer, which uncovered yet another a role of choline, as a betaine precursor in the methylation process and DNA repair [15]. Supporting these observations in animal species, human patients fed total parenteral nutrition solutions lacking choline had low circulating levels of choline, coupled with impaired liver function and fatty liver [16–18].

Today, choline is recognized by the National Academy of Medicine (formerly the Institute of Medicine) as an essential nutrient that must be acquired from the diet, as de novo biosynthesis is insufficient to meet human requirements [9]. We now know that choline plays a key role in lipid transport (as phosphatidylcholine in lipoprotein assembly and secretion), cell membrane structural support (as phosphatidylcholine and sphingomyelin), neurotransmission (as acetylcholine), and as a source of methyl groups (as a precursor of betaine).

2.2. Choline: Role in Maternal Health

In addition to the role of choline in general physiology, choline is critically important during pregnancy. Lower serum choline levels are associated with increased risk of neural tube defects [19], suggesting that choline intakes should be increased prior to pregnancy, as closing of the neural tube occurs by the fourth week of pregnancy (28 days after conception) [20]. As pregnancy progresses, the demand for choline significantly increases, as membrane biosynthesis is needed for placental development, increased workload by maternal organs, and to support exponential fetal organ growth. The growing need for choline by the developing fetus is facilitated by elevated maternal plasma free choline, placental accumulation (approximately 50 times higher concentration than maternal blood), and elevated plasma free choline levels that are three times higher than adult concentrations. Consequences of low choline status during pregnancy have major implications not only for fetal development, but also for maternal health. Acute fatty liver of pregnancy, while uncommon, is a potentially fatal complication that occurs in the third trimester or early postpartum period and shares symptoms with more common conditions like pre-eclampsia and cholestasis [21]. Furthermore, increased choline supplementation during pregnancy has demonstrated downregulation of antiangiogenic factor and preeclampsia risk marker, fms-like tyrosine kinase-1 (sFLT1) in in human placental tissues [22]. Simulating decreased placental efficiency in preeclampsia and intrauterine growth restriction, the *Dlx*3+/− mouse model has been used to show that dietary choline drives placental betaine concentration, which downregulates inflammatory gene expression [23] and improves fetal growth patterns [24].

Common genetic variants in choline-metabolizing enzymes are known to alter the metabolic fate of dietary choline, thereby increasing choline intake requirements in some individuals [25]. For instance, choline contributes to phosphatidylcholine synthesis by way of two metabolic pathways—through phosphorylation via the cytidine diphosphate-choline (CDP-choline) pathway or sequential methylation of phosphatidylethanolamine by the phosphatidylethanolamine N-methyltransferase (PEMT) pathway. The latter pathway is critically important in that it enables phosphatidylcholine synthesis even in the absence of dietary choline intake. Activity of PEMT is greater in pre-menopausal women, due to its upregulation by estrogen, but is considered inadequate to support endogenous production alone, necessitating a dietary choline requirement to prevent deficiency. Variations in single-base pairs (single-nucleotide polymorphisms or SNPs) in the *Pemt* gene are known to impact endogenous choline production, thereby influencing interindividual choline requirements and risk for choline deficiency [26,27].

Despite choline's importance in maternal health, many do not meet the daily recommendation. Approximately 90–95% of pregnant women are consuming less than the adequate intake (AI) [28]. Experts note that choline is not found in most prenatal supplements [29,30], suggesting that increased awareness of choline's place in infant and maternal health is needed to improve intakes through consumption of choline-rich foods and/or dietary supplementation.

2.3. Choline: Role in Infant Health

In the late 1970s, Steven Zeisel [31], a pediatric resident and graduate student, observed that blood choline concentrations were much higher in human newborns than in adults. Collaborator, Jan Blusztajn [32], observed that endogenous synthesis of phosphatidylcholine was increased in the brain and liver of rodent pups, demonstrating an increased metabolic demand for choline in newborns. In addition, mechanistic studies in rodents also showed that hepatic choline pools are depleted during pregnancy when fed a normal diet [33–35]. Soon after, choline was found to concentrate across the placenta, raising fetal tissue concentrations of choline [36]. Zeisel's research group and colleagues subsequently discovered that mammary glands accumulate and export choline in milk, providing substantial dietary choline to the developing infant postpartum [37]. Adequate intake recommendations (AI) are 125 mg choline/day for infants 0–6 months and 150 mg choline/day for infants 7–12 months; these AIs are based on choline concentrations in human milk (160 mg/L) and mean volume output of human milk (0.78 L/day) for infants 0–6 months with a reference body weight of 7 kg (approximately 18 mg/kg), and extrapolation for reference body weight at ages 7–12 months [9].

The increased availability of choline for the brain led to the hypothesis that acetylcholine concentrations impact neurological processes and cognitive function. Testing this hypothesis, researchers Christina Williams and Warren Meck [38] found that prenatal and postnatal choline supplementation of developing rat pups improved performance as adults on the 12- and 18-arm radial maze task, a test of spatial memory. Several potential roles that maternal dietary choline play on fetal brain biochemistry that impart lifelong behavioral changes have been suggested. Amongst this is the observation that choline alters timing of neuronal differentiation in the septum and the hippocampus, two brain regions known to be involved in learning and memory [39,40]. Others have confirmed these findings, showing that prenatal choline modulated rates of adult hippocampal neurogenesis, increased hippocampal brain-derived neurotrophic factor, improved cognitive performance on memory tasks as adults [41,42], accelerated hippocampal maturation [43], and decreased the threshold for induction of long-term potentiation (an indication of synapse strength) [44,45]. These findings are especially significant, given that rates of hippocampal neurogenesis decline with age and that nutritional intervention produced a marked change in behavioral output. These impacts of dietary choline on neurogenesis extend beyond the hippocampal development, showing increased neurogenesis in the cerebral cortex [46,47] and increased levels of nerve growth factor (NGF) in both the hippocampus and cortical areas [48]. This is further supported by the observation that maternal choline status influences brain gray and white matter development in piglet brains using magnetic resonance spectroscopy neuroimaging, which is consistent with choline's role in myelin components, phospholipids, and sphingomyelin, and emphasizes the role of choline in early brain development [49]. In humans, the role of choline in cognition have also been observed, with higher choline intakes during pregnancy associated with higher performance on memory tasks in their 7-year-old children [50]. As in brain development, emerging research by Zeisel and colleagues [51] suggests that fetal eye development may also be dependent on choline intakes, with low maternal choline intakes resulting in fewer retinal stem cells and worse eyesight in animal models. Together, the accumulating evidence underscores the long-term significance of choline in prenatal nutrition.

Beyond prenatal brain development, choline plays a significant role in continued growth of the brain and in cognitive measures. In animal models, inadequate choline intakes have demonstrated reductions in maternal plasma and milk concentrations of choline metabolites, and therefore nutrient availability for neonatal development [52]. Observational studies have shown that higher choline intakes during pregnancy have been associated with modestly better visual memory in children at age seven [50]. In a sample of 15-year-old children (n = 324), the sum of school grades in 17 major subjects were used as an outcome measure for academic achievement. Researchers showed that plasma choline level was significantly and positively associated with academic achievement, independent of socioeconomic status (SES) factors, and folate intake [53]. In randomized, double-blind, controlled feeding studies, maternal choline supplementation did not improve measures of infant memory or language development [54], but did improve infant information processing speed [55], bolstering support for prenatal choline supplementation. Recent evidence suggests that postnatal choline supplementation should also be considered, especially in preterm infants, when a choline deficiency may contribute to impaired lean body mass growth and neurocognitive development, despite adequate macronutrient intake and weight gain [56].

3. Role of DHA in Maternal and Infant Nutrition

3.1. Essential Functions

While proteins and carbohydrates were widely regarded as indispensable dietary constituents by the early 20th century, there were still conflicting views on the role of dietary fats in nutrition with initial findings on essential fatty acids not emerging until the late 1920s and early 1930s [57]. Between

1929 and 1932, George O. Burr and colleagues [57–60] conducted animal studies which demonstrated that exclusion of dietary fat led to a deficiency disease in rats. Results from Burr's work also showed that dietary fat, in particular fatty acids, was required to stimulate growth and prevent disease leading Burr to be the first to propose LA as an essential fatty acid in 1930 [58,59]. In 1931, Wesson and Burr also noted that similarly to LA, ALA is not synthesized by rats and can stimulate weight gain in rats consuming an essential fatty acid-deficient diet, which led them to conclude that ALA is also an essential fatty acid [61]. Animal work continued until 1960s to elucidate physiological actions of ALA and LA, including roles as precursors for ARA and DHA fatty acids. Key findings in 1950s led to purification of DHA and determination of its structure from animal brain phosphatides. In 1960, Klerk et al. [62] determined the metabolic pathway for conversion of DHA from ALA. Subsequent work in the 1960s and 1970s illustrated a functional role of DHA in brain and eye health, as DHA was shown to be abundant in both retinal [63,64] and synaptic membrane [65] phospholipids. Clinical research in the 1970s and 80s provided definitive findings on ALA and LA as essential fatty acids for human nutrition. Case reports and clinical studies of infants with essential fatty acid deficiency showed that it is resolved with administration of LA and/or ALA [66–70]. Presently, the National Academy of Medicine (formerly the Institute of Medicine) recognizes LA and ALA as essential fatty acids, recommends amounts for adequate daily intakes (AI), and state the main role of omega-3 fatty acids as structural membrane lipids, particularly in nerve tissue and retina [6]. After establishment of LA and ALA as essential fatty acids, majority of fatty acid research focused on physiological roles of common omega-3s (DHA and EPA) and omega-6 (ARA) synthesized from ALA and LA precursors, respectively. Specifically, observational findings in the 1980s and 1990s on EPA content in plasma phospholipids as well as fish oil/fish consumption (major EPA and DHA) dietary source and associations with heart health parameters led to greater understanding of the role of omega-3s in vascular biology and heart health [57]. Concurrently, omega-6 research focused on the role of ARA in eicosanoid production and downstream impact on inflammation and immune system, rather than its abundance and role in brain gray matter phospholipids. Beginning in the 1990s, focus shifted from omega-3s and heart health to role of DHA specifically in brain and eye health due to its presence in brain and retinal tissues. It is prevalent in structures that underlie cognitive abilities, including the eyes and brain (cerebellum, frontal, and occipital lobe).

The brain is largely comprised of lipids. The predominant LC-PUFAs in the brain are ARA omega-6 fatty acid and DHA omega-3 fatty acid [5,71,72]. Both ARA and DHA can be provided in diet or synthesized via desaturation and elongation pathways from LA and ALA precursors. Findings show DHA affects brain function by modulating neurogenesis [73,74], influencing neurotransmission [75], and promoting synaptic activity [76]. Additionally, DHA exerts other important actions that affect overall health including playing a key role in cell signaling, lipid metabolism, cell membrane function, and eye development and function. Docosahexaenoic acid (DHA) acts as a precursor for autocoid signaling molecules as well as an activator of several gene transcription factors including peroxisome proliferator activated receptors [77], which modulate metabolic processes, cholesterol homeostasis, and inflammation [78]. It also impacts cell membrane properties by increasing membrane permeability [79–83] and facilitating membrane fluidity [84–87]. Docosahexaenoic acid contributes to eye development and function through its signaling [88] and structural [89] effects on retinal photoreceptor cells. Low levels of plasma DHA have been observed in individuals with genetic retinal disorders such as retinitis pigmentosa leading some to theorize that DHA deficiencies could lead to defects in central retinal cones adversely impacting eye health [90]. In all, the totality of scientific literature strongly suggests a role of dietary DHA in various aspects of health including neonatal neurodevelopment.

3.2. DHA: Role in Maternal Health

Pregnancy is a time when higher nutrient demands can impact maternal health and pregnancy outcomes. Maternal DHA intake, endogenous synthesis, and body stores help meet DHA needs for mother and fetus through pregnancy [86,91]. Various genetic and lifestyle factors can influence maternal DHA stores including nutrition as well as pre-pregnancy health conditions, which may alter DHA utilization. Impaired fatty acid metabolism, due to the various single nucleotide polymorphisms (SNPs), can affect DHA status, and consequently, alter DHA requirements [92]. Researchers assessed several SNPs for genes encoding for key enzymes involved in LC-PUFA production—fatty acid desaturase (FADS) and elongase (ELOVL)—and found that *FADS1* and *FADS2* variants impacted mainly omega-6 fatty acid levels, whereas *ELOVL* genetic variants affected omega-3 fatty acid levels [93]. Investigators also observed normal weight women with *FADS1* SNPs had significantly lower levels of ARA and overweight/obese women with ELOVL2 SNPs had an association with lower DHA levels [93]. Gonzalez-Casanova et al. [94] examined the impact of 15 different FADS SNPs along with prenatal DHA supplementation on birth weight in the Mexican population based on earlier observations of high prevalence of SNPs associated with slow LC-PUFA conversion in Hispanic populations. Results showed differential response to prenatal supplementation due to the FADS genotype. Women with *FADS2* SNP that received supplementation had higher birth weight children than those who received the placebo. This led the authors to propose that mixed findings on DHA supplementation's effects on birth weight could be attributed to differential responses due to genetic variance [94]. Xie and Innis [95] found that genetic variation in *FADS1* and *FADS2* influenced maternal plasma and erythrocyte levels of both omega-3 (DHA) and omega-6 (ARA) fatty acids during pregnancy and lipids levels in breast milk during lactation. Overall maternal health status can also impact the role of DHA during pregnancy. A recent study showed pre-pregnancy obesity is associated with higher inflammation and attenuated response to DHA supplementation [96]. In general, the DHA needs of the fetus rise during pregnancy, peaking towards the end of the third trimester (after week 32), a time of great growth and development as well as significant accretion of DHA in fetal brain tissue [97–100]. Kuipers et al. [100] evaluated DHA fetal content at 25, 35, and 40 weeks of gestation. At term (40 weeks), 21% of DHA was present in skeletal muscle, 23% in brain tissue, and most of the DHA residing in fetal adipose tissue (50%), leading researchers to suggest fetal DHA adipose content serves as a reservoir for DHA that can be utilized in infant development. Higher maternal DHA intakes may be required in the late stage of pregnancy to help meet elevating needs. With advancing gestation, there is increased transfer of DHA to the developing fetus which may lead to depleted maternal DHA levels [101]. Low levels of DHA have been associated with increased incidence of various diseases during perinatal period, including postpartum depression [101]. Maternal DHA supplementation (600 mg daily) starting in the last half of gestation (week 20 to birth) resulted in greater gestational duration and infant birth size [102]. Observational and clinical research shows maternal DHA dietary intakes during pregnancy impact blood DHA status of newborns [103]. Maternal and fetal DHA is associated with several brain and eye health outcomes in infants [77,103,104].

3.3. DHA: Role in Infant Health

Maternal DHA status during fetal development can have lasting impacts on brain and eye health throughout life as evident by key recommendations for DHA intakes during the first 1000 days of life [3]. Docosahexaenoic acid is essential for normal vision and brain development. There is rapid DHA accretion in utero during the last weeks of the third trimester to support growth [77,97–100,105,106] and DHA is a major structural lipid in both the brain and retina. It reaches levels of about 4 g in the brain and represents 50% of the fatty acids present in retinal rod and cone components [106]. During pregnancy, DHA insufficiency was noticed to be associated with lower infant neurodevelopment scores up to 18 months old; however, this finding was not detected at later follow up (5 years of age) [107]. Maternal DHA intake, particularly in the last 5 weeks of pregnancy, influences visual acuity development up towards the end of the first year of life [108].

Recent studies have observed an effect of maternal and fetal DHA status on general health including various brain and eye health outcomes well into early and mid-childhood. Researchers found associations with umbilical cord plasma DHA levels and metabolic measures in early childhood

(3 years of age) [109]. Specifically, higher cord plasma DHA was associated with lower body mass index (BMI) scores, waist circumference, and leptin levels. This association was stronger when infant–mother pairs experienced hyperglycemia during pregnancy [109]. Prenatal DHA status may also contribute to improved sustained attention in preschool children [110]. In contrast, some findings have not shown an impact of maternal DHA on brain health measures in childhood. Crozier et al. [111] found neither maternal ARA or DHA levels during pregnancy were associated with cognitive performance in 4- and 6-year-old children. Investigators speculated that diet quality, which was positively associated with neurodevelopment at four years of age may compensate for maternal DHA insufficiencies during pregnancy [111], indicating an effect of postnatal nutrition on health as well. Daily postnatal DHA supplementation, via DHA enriched solid baby food from 6–12 months old, led to improved visual acuity [112]. Some early communicative development benefits were also observed with DHA supplementation during early infancy [113]. However, other neurodevelopment outcomes were not significantly changed in the study [113]. Current findings indicate various factors affect the overall impact of DHA in infant brain and eye health including both pre-pregnancy maternal health status as well as prenatal and postnatal nutritional status of mother and child.

4. Synergistic Relationship between Choline and DHA

4.1. Proposed Mechanisms: Insights from Preclinical Studies

Choline and DHA are two important lipid-based nutrients needed for growth and development. Findings from in vitro studies highlight potential interactions between both nutrients and effects on metabolism. For example, DHA supplementation significantly increased cellular choline uptake in human retinal cells compared to cultured cells without supplemental DHA [114], which demonstrates how DHA may impact choline status. This finding is consistent with an earlier report demonstrating that the high unsaturated fatty acid content of human retinoblastoma cell membranes facilitated the capacity of the high-affinity choline uptake system to transport low concentrations of choline [114,115]. Docosahexaenoic acid has been shown to stimulate choline acetyltransferase (ChAT) enzymatic activity as well as support growth and function in neural cell culture studies [116,117]. The interaction of DHA and choline status has also been demonstrated in vivo, in the *Pemt−/−* mouse model. Discussed in Section 2.2, the PEMT enzyme facilitates endogenous hepatic synthesis of phosphatidylcholine from phosphatidylethanolamine. Deficiency of PEMT in *Pemt* gene knockout (*Pemt−/−*) mice yields disrupted fetal hippocampal development that can be reversed through maternal dietary DHA supplementation compared to control diets [118]. Maternal DHA supplementation not only increased fetal brain *Pemt−/−* phospholipid-DHA levels to wild-type levels, and eliminated differences in neural progenitor cell proliferation and apoptosis differences, but the DHA supplementation also halved the rate of neural apoptosis in wild type [118], affirming roles of DHA and choline in developmental neurogenesis. This observation is consistent with the specificity of PEMT in synthesizing polyunsaturated-phosphatidylcholine species [119] and highlights the coordinated roles of choline and DHA in neural lipid metabolism. Recent work in evaluating aspects of neural development processes revealed that specific nutrient combinations have a beneficial impact on brain function. Both in vitro and in vivo studies illustrate the role of nutrient combinations in neurodevelopment, particularly the presence of both DHA and choline. van Deijk et al. [120] showed that a medical food with DHA and choline, as well as other micronutrients, positively affected synaptic function in neuronal cells. When assessing aspects of neuroinflammation, investigators observed that administration of a DHA-containing choline phospholipid led to decreased lipopolysaccharide (LPS)-induced neuroinflammation in both cell culture and animal models [121]. Similar to its anti-inflammatory effects, supplementing with choline and DHA also attenuated brain oxidative stress in a perinatal maternal separation stress rodent model [122]. Favorable effects of nutrient combinations were also seen when supplementing during pregnancy. Results from several studies indicate a valuable impact of prenatal choline and DHA supplementation on offspring brain function in rats [123,124], dogs [125], and pigs [126]. In a study of choline, DHA, or saline control supplementation of pregnant rat dams and pups from choline or DHA supplemented groups showed significantly increased numbers of CA1 hippocampal neurons compared to both untreated and saline control group pups ($p < 0.05$). The combined supplementation of choline and DHA during pregnancy further enhanced neurodevelopment of the fetal hippocampus in rats compared to control ($p < 0.001$), with these effects proving better than supplementing with choline ($p < 0.05$) or DHA ($p < 0.05$) alone [124]. These results are supported by work by van Wijk et al. [123], who showed that supplementation of DHA in rats significantly increased DHA levels in plasma and red blood cells compared to control, and supplementation of choline from lecithin significantly increased plasma free choline, but did not affect DHA levels. However, combined supplementation of DHA and lecithin increased DHA to levels significantly greater than DHA supplementation alone ($p < 0.025$), which indicated that the impact of combined choline and DHA supplementation on circulating DHA levels were greater than an additive effect [123]. Advantageous effects of nutrient combinations could be due to the role of choline in placental nutrient transport. Kwan et al. [127] found that maternal choline supplementation modulates placental nutrient metabolism in a late gestational mouse pregnancy model, which may be attributed to its influence on vascular development. Furthermore, maternal choline supplementation increased placental transcript abundance of DHA, choline, and acetylcholine transporters [127]. Collectively, the evidence presented in this section supports the hypothesis that supplementation of choline or DHA alone yield complementary outcomes on choline and DHA metabolism, and that supplementation in combination produce benefits that must be greater than additive effects. Current in vivo and in vitro evidence supports co-supplementation of choline and DHA, particularly during pregnancy to support brain and eye development of offspring, and while the literature to date provides novel leads on how choline and DHA function in synergy, additional work is needed to clarify its mechanism of action.

4.2. Proposed Mechanisms: Insights from Clinical Findings

In this review, we have thus far discussed the roles of choline and DHA independently on infant brain and eye development, and synergistic relationships from preclinical models. From a clinical standpoint, the roles of choline and DHA on infant development may be best observed in premature birth, a circumstance wherein nutrient availability is interrupted, when levels would otherwise remain high *in utero*. Furthermore, human brain and eye development is known to begin *in utero*, and continue postnatally, with choline and LC-PUFAs (DHA, ARA) supplied together postpartum from human milk or supplemental infant formula. Human milk choline content from mothers of preterm infants have also been reported to be lower than from mothers following full-term delivery [128]. Preterm births in the US occurred in about 1 in 10 babies from 2007 to 2014, with an estimated associated cost of $26.2 billion USD annually, equating to approximately $51,600 per infant born preterm [129,130]. More importantly, premature births are associated with increased health problems, longer hospital stays, and learning and behavioral problems through childhood. To highlight the mechanistic synergy of choline and DHA, Bernhard and colleagues [131] demonstrated through a randomized, controlled trial that in preterm infants supplemented with choline, DHA, both, or neither, choline alone did not significantly increase phosphatidylcholine-DHA (PC-DHA), DHA alone increased PC-DHA content by only 35% ($p < 0.05$), but the combined treatment increased PC-DHA by 63% compared to control ($p < 0.001$). Additionally, supplementation with choline increased plasma choline concentrations in preterm infants to near-fetal concentrations and improved DHA status [131]. Since phosphatidylcholine is the major transport form of DHA in plasma, these findings provide strong support for the hypothesis that actions of each nutrient are metabolically linked through phosphatidylcholine and that their actions cannot be mutually exclusive.

To better understand the role(s) choline and DHA play in unison in infant brain and eye health, researchers have studied how choline intakes influence phosphatidylcholine-DHA enrichment [132]. West and colleagues [133] showed that phosphatidylcholine-DHA levels were greater in pregnant women than non-pregnant women, suggesting a greater demand for methyl donors and increased

PEMT activity. Additionally, they showed that when choline and DHA were both supplemented in non-pregnant women, higher choline intakes resulted in greater PC-DHA enrichment, suggesting that higher choline intakes may increase PEMT activity [132,134]. These findings suggest a metabolic synergy between choline and DHA, and are further supported by research that demonstrated consumption of n-3 fatty acid-enriched eggs increased plasma free choline and betaine compared to non-enriched eggs [133]. Consistent with these findings, McNamara et al. [135] showed that low DHA status is associated with lower cortical metabolism of choline using proton magnetic resonance spectroscopy. To explore the relationship between infant nutrition and subsequent cognitive performance, Cheatham et al. [136] collected and analyzed human milk samples at 3–4 months postpartum and tested recognition memory ability in infants at 6-months old. Through this work, Cheatham demonstrated that brain electrical activity expressed as event-related potential latency scores from the frontal, central, and midline areas were predicted by the DHA and choline interaction and that higher choline and DHA content was related to better recognition memory [136]. Together, these clinical findings provide evidence that choline and DHA function is synergistic in infant neurocognitive development.

5. Conclusions and Future Directions

The evidence presented in this review of cell culture, animal model, and human clinical trials provide compelling support for choline and DHA in maternal and infant nutrition. The interactions between choline and DHA support roles in brain and eye health, and the findings that supplementation with one augments the other points to synergy between the two nutrients. Dietary intakes of choline and DHA in the US population are lower than recommended levels, and vulnerable populations may require additional supplementation, particularly women during pregnancy and lactation. Infants receiving nutrition from breastmilk are provided with choline and LC-PUFAs (inclusive of ARA, LA, and DHA) from the maternal intake, but those who are not breastfed will require formula that contains choline and LC-PUFAs for proper growth and development.

Ensuring optimal nutrition during pregnancy requires a multi-faceted approach. Effective strategies are needed to determine nutrient status, address key nutrient gaps, and gain a deeper understanding of nutrient interactions during pregnancy. Prenatal testing for DHA status has been proposed [137] and should also include choline to inform on nutrient adequacy and guide strategy for obtaining optimal intake levels. Moreover, commercial tools for screening of common SNPs may enable personalized tailoring of dietary recommendations. With a greater understanding of maternal nutrient needs and how genetic and lifestyle factors impact metabolism, we are empowered to improve nutritional approaches to prenatal care.

Author Contributions: J.G.M. and L.L.L. conceptualized and drafted the manuscript; C.J.I. and S.H.M. contributed, reviewed, and edited the manuscript. All authors read and approved the final manuscript.

References

1. Rui, O.T.P. National Ambulatory Medical Care Survey: 2015 State and National Summary Tables. Available online: https://www.cdc.gov/nchs/data/ahcd/namcs_summary/2015_namcs_web_tables.pdf (accessed on 20 February 2019).
2. US Department of Health and Human Services. Healthy People 2020: Maternal, Infant, and Child Health Objectives. Available online: https://www.healthypeople.gov/2020/topics-objectives/topic/maternal-infant-and-child-health/objectives (accessed on 20 February 2020).
3. Schwarzenberg, S.J.; Georgieff, M.K.; Committee on Nutrition. Advocacy for Improving Nutrition in the First 1000 Days to Support Childhood Development and Adult Health. *Pediatrics* **2018**, 141. [CrossRef]
4. Koletzko, B.; Carlson, S.E.; van Goudoever, J.B. Should Infant Formula Provide Both Omega-3 DHA and Omega-6 Arachidonic Acid? *Ann. Nutr. Metab.* **2015**, *66*, 137–138. [CrossRef] [PubMed]

5. Martinez, M. Tissue levels of polyunsaturated fatty acids during early human development. *J. Pediatr.* **1992**, *120*, S129–S138. [CrossRef]
6. Institute of Medicine (US). Dietary Fat: Total Fat and Fatty Acids. In *Dietary References Intakes: The Essential Guide to Nutrient Requirements*; National Academies Press: Washington, DC, USA, 2006.
7. US Department of Agriculture—Agricultural Research Service. Nutrient Intakes from Food: Mean Amounts Consumed per Individual, by Gender and Age. Available online: https://www.ars.usda.gov/ARSUserFiles/80400530/pdf/1516/Table_1_NIN_GEN_15.pdf (accessed on 22 April 2019).
8. Wallace, T.C.; Fulgoni, V.L., 3rd. Assessment of Total Choline Intakes in the United States. *J. Am. Coll. Nutr.* **2016**, *35*, 108–112. [CrossRef] [PubMed]
9. IoM (US). Choline. In *Dietary Reference Intakes for Thiamin, Riboflavin, Niacin, Vitamin B_6, Folate, Vitamin B_{12}, Pantothenic Acid, Biotin, and Choline*; National Academies Press: Washington, DC, USA, 1998. [CrossRef]
10. Papanikolaou, Y.; Brooks, J.; Reider, C.; Fulgoni, V.L. US adults are not meeting recommended levels for fish and omega-3 fatty acid intake: Results of an analysis using observational data from NHANES 2003–2008. *Nutr. J.* **2014**, *13*, 31. [CrossRef]
11. US Department of Health and Human Services. 2015–2020 Dietary Guidelines for Americans. Available online: https://health.gov/dietaryguidelines/2015/resources/2015-2020_Dietary_Guidelines.pdf (accessed on 4 March 2019).
12. Zhang, Z.; Fulgoni, V.L.; Kris-Etherton, P.M.; Mitmesser, S.H. Dietary Intakes of EPA and DHA Omega-3 Fatty Acids among US Childbearing-Age and Pregnant Women: An Analysis of NHANES 2001–2014. *Nutrients* **2018**, *10*, 416. [CrossRef]
13. Zeisel, S.H. A brief history of choline. *Ann. Nutr. Metab.* **2012**, *61*, 254–258. [CrossRef]
14. Hershey, J.M.; Soskin, S. Substitution of "lecithin" for raw pancreas in the diet of the depancreatized dog. *Am. J. Physiol.-Leg. Content* **1931**, *98*, 74–85. [CrossRef]
15. Mehedint, M.G.; Zeisel, S.H. Choline's role in maintaining liver function: New evidence for epigenetic mechanisms. *Curr. Opin. Clin. Nutr. Metab. Care* **2013**, *16*, 339–345. [CrossRef] [PubMed]
16. Chawla, R.K.; Berry, C.J.; Kutner, M.H.; Rudman, D. Plasma concentrations of transsulfuration pathway products during nasoenteral and intravenous hyperalimentation of malnourished patients. *Am. J. Clin. Nutr.* **1985**, *42*, 577–584. [CrossRef]
17. Sheard, N.F.; Tayek, J.A.; Bistrian, B.R.; Blackburn, G.L.; Zeisel, S.H. Plasma choline concentration in humans fed parenterally. *Am. J. Clin. Nutr.* **1986**, *43*, 219–224. [CrossRef]
18. Tayek, J.A.; Bistrian, B.; Sheard, N.F.; Zeisel, S.H.; Blackburn, G.L. Abnormal liver function in malnourished patients receiving total parenteral nutrition: A prospective randomized study. *J. Am. Coll. Nutr.* **1990**, *9*, 76–83. [CrossRef] [PubMed]
19. Shaw, G.M.; Finnell, R.H.; Blom, H.J.; Carmichael, S.L.; Vollset, S.E.; Yang, W.; Ueland, P.M. Choline and risk of neural tube defects in a folate-fortified population. *Epidemiology* **2009**, *20*, 714–719. [CrossRef]
20. Cavalli, P. Prevention of Neural Tube Defects and proper folate periconceptional supplementation. *J. Prenat. Med.* **2008**, *2*, 40–41. [PubMed]
21. Ko, H.; Yoshida, E.M. Acute fatty liver of pregnancy. *Can. J. Gastroenterol. J. Can. Gastroenterol.* **2006**, *20*, 25–30. [CrossRef]
22. Jiang, X.; Bar, H.Y.; Yan, J.; Jones, S.; Brannon, P.M.; West, A.A.; Perry, C.A.; Ganti, A.; Pressman, E.; Devapatla, S.; et al. A higher maternal choline intake among third-trimester pregnant women lowers placental and circulating concentrations of the antiangiogenic factor fms-like tyrosine kinase-1 (sFLT1). *FASEB J.* **2013**, *27*, 1245–1253. [CrossRef]
23. King, J.H.; Kwan, S.T.; Yan, J.; Jiang, X.; Fomin, V.G.; Roberson, M.S.; Caudill, M.A. Maternal Choline Supplementation Modulates Maternal and Fetal Choline Metabolism and Downregulates Inflammatory Gene Expression in a Mouse Model of Placental Insufficiency. *FASEB J.* **2016**, *30*, 272.1. [CrossRef]
24. King, J.H.; Kwan, S.T.C.; Yan, J.; Klatt, K.C.; Jiang, X.; Roberson, M.S.; Caudill, M.A. Maternal Choline Supplementation Alters Fetal Growth Patterns in a Mouse Model of Placental Insufficiency. *Nutrients* **2017**, *9*, 765. [CrossRef] [PubMed]
25. Ganz, A.B.; Cohen, V.V.; Swersky, C.C.; Stover, J.; Vitiello, G.A.; Lovesky, J.; Chuang, J.C.; Shields, K.; Fomin, V.G.; Lopez, Y.S.; et al. Genetic Variation in Choline-Metabolizing Enzymes Alters Choline Metabolism in Young Women Consuming Choline Intakes Meeting Current Recommendations. *Int. J. Mol. Sci.* **2017**, *18*, 252. [CrossRef]

26. da Costa, K.A.; Kozyreva, O.G.; Song, J.; Galanko, J.A.; Fischer, L.M.; Zeisel, S.H. Common genetic polymorphisms affect the human requirement for the nutrient choline. *FASEB J.* **2006**, *20*, 1336–1344. [CrossRef]
27. Resseguie, M.E.; da Costa, K.-A.; Galanko, J.A.; Patel, M.; Davis, I.J.; Zeisel, S.H. Aberrant Estrogen Regulation of PEMT Results in Choline Deficiency-associated Liver Dysfunction. *J. Biol. Chem.* **2011**, *286*, 1649–1658. [CrossRef]
28. Brunst, K.J.; Wright, R.O.; DiGioia, K.; Enlow, M.B.; Fernandez, H.; Wright, R.J.; Kannan, S. Racial/ethnic and sociodemographic factors associated with micronutrient intakes and inadequacies among pregnant women in an urban US population. *Public Health Nutr.* **2014**, *17*, 1960–1970. [CrossRef]
29. Bell, C.; Aujla, J. Prenatal vitamins deficient in recommended Choline intake for pregnant women. *J. Fam. Med. Dis. Prev.* **2016**, *2*, 048. [CrossRef]
30. Caudill, M.A. Pre- and postnatal health: Evidence of increased choline needs. *J. Am. Diet. Assoc.* **2010**, *110*, 1198–1206. [CrossRef]
31. Zeisel, S.H.; Epstein, M.F.; Wurtman, R.J. Elevated choline concentration in neonatal plasma. *Life Sci.* **1980**, *26*, 1827–1831. [CrossRef]
32. Blusztajn, J.K.; Zeisel, S.H.; Wurtman, R.J. Synthesis of lecithin (phosphatidylcholine) from phosphatidylethanolamine in bovine brain. *Brain Res.* **1979**, *179*, 319–327. [CrossRef]
33. Gwee, M.C.; Sim, M.K. Free choline concentration and cephalin-N-methyltransferase activity in the maternal and foetal liver and placenta of pregnant rats. *Clin. Exp. Pharmacol. Physiol.* **1978**, *5*, 649–653. [CrossRef]
34. Gwee, M.C.; Sim, M.K. Changes in the concentration of free choline and cephalin-N-methyltransferase activity of the rat material and foetal liver and placeta during gestation and of the maternal and neonatal liver in the early postpartum period. *Clin. Exp. Pharmacol. Physiol.* **1979**, *6*, 259–265. [CrossRef]
35. Zeisel, S.H.; Mar, M.H.; Zhou, Z.; da Costa, K.A. Pregnancy and lactation are associated with diminished concentrations of choline and its metabolites in rat liver. *J. Nutr.* **1995**, *125*, 3049–3054. [CrossRef]
36. Sweiry, J.H.; Page, K.R.; Dacke, C.G.; Abramovich, D.R.; Yudilevich, D.L. Evidence of saturable uptake mechanisms at maternal and fetal sides of the perfused human placenta by rapid paired-tracer dilution: Studies with calcium and choline. *J. Dev. Physiol.* **1986**, *8*, 435–445.
37. Chao, C.K.; Pomfret, E.A.; Zeisel, S.H. Uptake of choline by rat mammary-gland epithelial cells. *Biochem. J.* **1988**, *254*, 33–38. [CrossRef]
38. Meck, W.H.; Smith, R.A.; Williams, C.L. Pre- and postnatal choline supplementation produces long-term facilitation of spatial memory. *Dev. Psychobiol.* **1988**, *21*, 339–353. [CrossRef]
39. Albright, C.D.; Friedrich, C.B.; Brown, E.C.; Mar, M.H.; Zeisel, S.H. Maternal dietary choline availability alters mitosis, apoptosis and the localization of TOAD-64 protein in the developing fetal rat septum. *Brain Res. Dev. Brain Res.* **1999**, *115*, 123–129. [CrossRef]
40. Craciunescu, C.N.; Albright, C.D.; Mar, M.H.; Song, J.; Zeisel, S.H. Choline availability during embryonic development alters progenitor cell mitosis in developing mouse hippocampus. *J. Nutr.* **2003**, *133*, 3614–3618. [CrossRef]
41. Glenn, M.J.; Gibson, E.M.; Kirby, E.D.; Mellott, T.J.; Blusztajn, J.K.; Williams, C.L. Prenatal choline availability modulates hippocampal neurogenesis and neurogenic responses to enriching experiences in adult female rats. *Eur. J. Neurosci.* **2007**, *25*, 2473–2482. [CrossRef]
42. Tees, R.C.; Mohammadi, E. The effects of neonatal choline dietary supplementation on adult spatial and configural learning and memory in rats. *Dev. Psychobiol.* **1999**, *35*, 226–240. [CrossRef]
43. Mellott, T.J.; Williams, C.L.; Meck, W.H.; Blusztajn, J.K. Prenatal choline supplementation advances hippocampal development and enhances MAPK and CREB activation. *FASEB J.* **2004**, *18*, 545–547. [CrossRef]
44. Pyapali, G.K.; Turner, D.A.; Williams, C.L.; Meck, W.H.; Swartzwelder, H.S. Prenatal dietary choline supplementation decreases the threshold for induction of long-term potentiation in young adult rats. *J. Neurophysiol.* **1998**, *79*, 1790–1796. [CrossRef]
45. Jones, J.P.; Meck, W.H.; Williams, C.L.; Wilson, W.A.; Swartzwelder, H.S. Choline availability to the developing rat fetus alters adult hippocampal long-term potentiation. *Brain Res. Dev. Brain Res.* **1999**, *118*, 159–167. [CrossRef]
46. Trujillo-Gonzalez, I.; Wang, Y.; Friday, W.B.; Vickers, K.C.; Toth, C.L.; Molina-Torres, L.; Surzenko, N.; Zeisel, S.H. microRNA-129-5p is regulated by choline availability and controls EGF receptor synthesis and neurogenesis in the cerebral cortex. *FASEB J.* **2018**. [CrossRef]

47. Wang, Y.; Surzenko, N.; Friday, W.B.; Zeisel, S.H. Maternal dietary intake of choline in mice regulates development of the cerebral cortex in the offspring. *FASEB J.* **2016**, *30*, 1566–1578. [CrossRef]
48. Sandstrom, N.J.; Loy, R.; Williams, C.L. Prenatal choline supplementation increases NGF levels in the hippocampus and frontal cortex of young and adult rats. *Brain Res.* **2002**, *947*, 9–16. [CrossRef]
49. Mudd, A.T.; Getty, C.M.; Dilger, R.N. Maternal Dietary Choline Status Influences Brain Gray and White Matter Development in Young Pigs. *Curr. Dev. Nutr.* **2018**, *2*, nzy015. [CrossRef]
50. Boeke, C.E.; Gillman, M.W.; Hughes, M.D.; Rifas-Shiman, S.L.; Villamor, E.; Oken, E. Choline intake during pregnancy and child cognition at age 7 years. *Am. J. Epidemiol.* **2013**, *177*, 1338–1347. [CrossRef]
51. Surzenko, N.; Trujillo-González, I.; Zeisel, S.H. Low Intake of Choline During Pregnancy Leads to Aberrant Retinal Architecture and Poor Visual Function in the Offspring. *FASEB J.* **2016**, *30*, 679. [CrossRef]
52. Mudd, A.T.; Alexander, L.S.; Johnson, S.K.; Getty, C.M.; Malysheva, O.V.; Caudill, M.A.; Dilger, R.N. Perinatal Dietary Choline Deficiency in Sows Influences Concentrations of Choline Metabolites, Fatty Acids, and Amino Acids in Milk throughout Lactation. *J. Nutr.* **2016**, *146*, 2216–2223. [CrossRef]
53. Nilsson, T.K.; Hurtig-Wennlof, A.; Sjostrom, M.; Herrmann, W.; Obeid, R.; Owen, J.R.; Zeisel, S. Plasma 1-carbon metabolites and academic achievement in 15-yr-old adolescents. *FASEB J.* **2016**, *30*, 1683–1688. [CrossRef]
54. Cheatham, C.L.; Goldman, B.D.; Fischer, L.M.; da Costa, K.A.; Reznick, J.S.; Zeisel, S.H. Phosphatidylcholine supplementation in pregnant women consuming moderate-choline diets does not enhance infant cognitive function: A randomized, double-blind, placebo-controlled trial. *Am. J. Clin. Nutr.* **2012**, *96*, 1465–1472. [CrossRef]
55. Caudill, M.A.; Strupp, B.J.; Muscalu, L.; Nevins, J.E.H.; Canfield, R.L. Maternal choline supplementation during the third trimester of pregnancy improves infant information processing speed: A randomized, double-blind, controlled feeding study. *FASEB J.* **2018**, *32*, 2172–2180. [CrossRef]
56. Bernhard, W.; Poets, C.F.; Franz, A.R. Choline and choline-related nutrients in regular and preterm infant growth. *Eur. J. Nutr.* **2018**. [CrossRef]
57. Spector, A.A.; Kim, H.Y. Discovery of essential fatty acids. *J. Lipid Res.* **2015**, *56*, 11–21. [CrossRef]
58. Burr, G.O.; Burr, M.M. A new deficiency disease produced by the rigid exclusion of fat from the diet. *J. Biol. Chem.* **1929**, *82*, 345–367. [CrossRef]
59. Burr, G.O.; Burr, M.M. On the nature and role of the fatty acids essential in nutrition. *J. Biol. Chem.* **1930**, *86*, 587–621. [CrossRef]
60. Burr, G.O.; Burr, M.M.; Miller, E.S. On the fatty acids essential in nutrition. III. *J. Biol. Chem.* **1932**, *97*, 1–9.
61. Wesson, L.G.; Burr, G.O. The metabolic rate and respiratory quotients of rats on a fat-deficient diet. *J. Biol. Chem.* **1931**, *91*, 525–539.
62. Klenk, E.; Mohrhauer, H. Studies on the metabolism of polyenoic fatty acids in the rat. *Hoppe Seylers Z. Physiol. Chem.* **1960**, *320*, 218–232. [CrossRef] [PubMed]
63. Anderson, R.E.; Benolken, R.M.; Dudley, P.A.; Landis, D.J.; Wheeler, T.G. Proceedings: Polyunsaturated fatty acids of photoreceptor membranes. *Exp. Eye Res.* **1974**, *18*, 205–213. [CrossRef]
64. Benolken, R.M.; Anderson, R.E.; Wheeler, T.G. Membrane fatty acids associated with the electrical response in visual excitation. *Science* **1973**, *182*, 1253–1254. [CrossRef]
65. Cotman, C.; Blank, M.L.; Moehl, A.; Snyder, F. Lipid composition of synaptic plasma membranes isolated from rat brain by zonal centrifugation. *Biochemistry* **1969**, *8*, 4606–4612. [CrossRef]
66. Caldwell, M.D.; Jonsson, H.T.; Othersen, H.B., Jr. Essential fatty acid deficiency in an infant receiving prolonged parenteral alimentation. *J. Pediatr.* **1972**, *81*, 894–898. [CrossRef]
67. Collins, F.D.; Sinclair, A.J.; Royle, J.P.; Coats, D.A.; Maynard, A.T.; Leonard, R.F. Plasma lipids in human linoleic acid deficiency. *Nutr. Metab.* **1971**, *13*, 150–167. [CrossRef]
68. Holman, R.T.; Johnson, S.B.; Hatch, T.F. A case of human linolenic acid deficiency involving neurological abnormalities. *Am. J. Clin. Nutr.* **1982**, *35*, 617–623. [CrossRef]
69. Postuma, R.; Pease, P.W.; Watts, R.; Taylor, S.; McEvoy, F.A. Essential fatty acid deficiency in infants receiving parenteral nutrition. *J. Pediatr. Surg.* **1978**, *13*, 393–398. [CrossRef]
70. Tashiro, T.; Ogata, H.; Yokoyama, H.; Mashima, Y.; Itoh, K. The effect of fat emulsion (Intralipid) on essential fatty acid deficiency in infants receiving intravenous alimentation. *J. Pediatr. Surg.* **1976**, *11*, 505–515. [CrossRef]
71. Carlson, S.E.; Colombo, J. Docosahexaenoic Acid and Arachidonic Acid Nutrition in Early Development. *Adv. Pediatr.* **2016**, *63*, 453–471. [CrossRef]

72. Svennerholm, L.; Vanier, M.T. The distribution of lipids in the human nervous system. 3. Fatty acid composition of phosphoglycerides of human foetal and infant brain. *Brain Res.* **1973**, *50*, 341–351. [CrossRef]
73. Dyall, S.C.; Michael, G.J.; Michael-Titus, A.T. Omega-3 fatty acids reverse age-related decreases in nuclear receptors and increase neurogenesis in old rats. *J. Neurosci. Res.* **2010**, *88*, 2091–2102. [CrossRef]
74. Janssen, C.I.; Zerbi, V.; Mutsaers, M.P.; de Jong, B.S.; Wiesmann, M.; Arnoldussen, I.A.; Geenen, B.; Heerschap, A.; Muskiet, F.A.; Jouni, Z.E.; et al. Impact of dietary n-3 polyunsaturated fatty acids on cognition, motor skills and hippocampal neurogenesis in developing C57BL/6J mice. *J. Nutr. Biochem.* **2015**, *26*, 24–35. [CrossRef]
75. Kodas, E.; Galineau, L.; Bodard, S.; Vancassel, S.; Guilloteau, D.; Besnard, J.C.; Chalon, S. Serotoninergic neurotransmission is affected by n-3 polyunsaturated fatty acids in the rat. *J. Neurochem.* **2004**, *89*, 695–702. [CrossRef]
76. Cao, D.; Kevala, K.; Kim, J.; Moon, H.S.; Jun, S.B.; Lovinger, D.; Kim, H.Y. Docosahexaenoic acid promotes hippocampal neuronal development and synaptic function. *J. Neurochem.* **2009**, *111*, 510–521. [CrossRef]
77. Lauritzen, L.; Brambilla, P.; Mazzocchi, A.; Harslof, L.B.; Ciappolino, V.; Agostoni, C. DHA Effects in Brain Development and Function. *Nutrients* **2016**, *8*, 6. [CrossRef]
78. Muskiet, F.A.; Fokkema, M.R.; Schaafsma, A.; Boersma, E.R.; Crawford, M.A. Is Docosahexaenoic Acid (DHA) Essential? Lessons from DHA Status Regulation, Our Ancient Diet, Epidemiology and Randomized Controlled Trials. *J. Nutr.* **2004**, *134*, 183–186. [CrossRef]
79. Ehringer, W.; Belcher, D.; Wassall, S.R.; Stillwell, W. A comparison of the effects of linolenic (18:3 omega 3) and docosahexaenoic (22:6 omega 3) acids on phospholipid bilayers. *Chem. Phys. Lipids* **1990**, *54*, 79–88. [CrossRef]
80. Jenski, L.J.; Sturdevant, L.K.; Ehringer, W.D.; Stillwell, W. Omega-3 fatty acid modification of membrane structure and function. I. Dietary manipulation of tumor cell susceptibility to cell- and complement-mediated lysis. *Nutr. Cancer* **1993**, *19*, 135–146. [CrossRef]
81. Stillwell, W.; Ehringer, W.; Jenski, L.J. Docosahexaenoic acid increases permeability of lipid vesicles and tumor cells. *Lipids* **1993**, *28*, 103–108. [CrossRef]
82. Stillwell, W.; Jenski, L.J.; Crump, F.T.; Ehringer, W. Effect of docosahexaenoic acid on mouse mitochondrial membrane properties. *Lipids* **1997**, *32*, 497–506. [CrossRef]
83. Stillwell, W.; Wassall, S.R. Docosahexaenoic acid: Membrane properties of a unique fatty acid. *Chem. Phys. Lipids* **2003**, *126*, 1–27. [CrossRef]
84. Lee, A.G.; East, J.M.; Froud, R.J. Are essential fatty acids essential for membrane function? *Prog. Lipid Res.* **1986**, *25*, 41–46. [CrossRef]
85. Stubbs, C.D.; Smith, A.D. The modification of mammalian membrane polyunsaturated fatty acid composition in relation to membrane fluidity and function. *Biochim. Biophys. Acta* **1984**, *779*, 89–137. [CrossRef]
86. Uauy, R.; Mena, P.; Rojas, C. Essential fatty acids in early life: Structural and functional role. *Proc. Nutr. Soc.* **2000**, *59*, 3–15. [CrossRef]
87. Wheeler, T.G.; Benolken, R.M.; Anderson, R.E. Visual membranes: Specificity of fatty acid precursors for the electrical response to illumination. *Science* **1975**, *188*, 1312–1314. [CrossRef]
88. Knott, E.J.; Gordon, W.C.; Jun, B.; Do, K.; Bazan, N.G. Retinal Pigment Epithelium and Photoreceptor Preconditioning Protection Requires Docosanoid Signaling. *Cell. Mol. Neurobiol.* **2018**, *38*, 901–917. [CrossRef]
89. Shindou, H.; Koso, H.; Sasaki, J.; Nakanishi, H.; Sagara, H.; Nakagawa, K.M.; Takahashi, Y.; Hishikawa, D.; Iizuka-Hishikawa, Y.; Tokumasu, F.; et al. Docosahexaenoic acid preserves visual function by maintaining correct disc morphology in retinal photoreceptor cells. *J. Biol. Chem.* **2017**, *292*, 12054–12064. [CrossRef]
90. Gong, J.; Rosner, B.; Rees, D.G.; Berson, E.L.; Weigel-DiFranco, C.A.; Schaefer, E.J. Plasma docosahexaenoic acid levels in various genetic forms of retinitis pigmentosa. *Investig. Ophthalmol. Vis. Sci.* **1992**, *33*, 2596–2602.
91. Singh, M. Essential Fatty Acids, DHA and Human Brain. *Indian J. Pediatr.* **2005**, *72*, 239–242. [CrossRef]
92. Minihane, A.M. Impact of Genotype on EPA and DHA Status and Responsiveness to Increased Intakes. *Nutrients* **2016**, *8*, 123. [CrossRef]
93. de la Garza Puentes, A.; Montes Goyanes, R.; Chisaguano Tonato, A.M.; Torres-Espinola, F.J.; Arias Garcia, M.; de Almeida, L.; Bonilla Aguirre, M.; Guerendiain, M.; Castellote Bargallo, A.I.; Segura Moreno, M.; et al. Association of maternal weight with FADS and ELOVL genetic variants and fatty acid levels- The PREOBE follow-up. *PLoS ONE* **2017**, *12*, e0179135. [CrossRef]

94. Gonzalez-Casanova, I.; Rzehak, P.; Stein, A.D.; Garcia Feregrino, R.; Rivera Dommarco, J.A.; Barraza-Villarreal, A.; Demmelmair, H.; Romieu, I.; Villalpando, S.; Martorell, R.; et al. Maternal single nucleotide polymorphisms in the fatty acid desaturase 1 and 2 coding regions modify the impact of prenatal supplementation with DHA on birth weight. *Am. J. Clin. Nutr.* **2016**, *103*, 1171–1178. [CrossRef]
95. Xie, L.; Innis, S.M. Genetic variants of the FADS1 FADS2 gene cluster are associated with altered (n-6) and (n-3) essential fatty acids in plasma and erythrocyte phospholipids in women during pregnancy and in breast milk during lactation. *J. Nutr.* **2008**, *138*, 2222–2228. [CrossRef]
96. Monthe-Dreze, C.; Penfield-Cyr, A.; Smid, M.C.; Sen, S. Maternal Pre-Pregnancy Obesity Attenuates Response to Omega-3 Fatty Acids Supplementation During Pregnancy. *Nutrients* **2018**, *10*, 1908. [CrossRef]
97. Bernhard, W.; Raith, M.; Koch, V.; Maas, C.; Abele, H.; Poets, C.F.; Franz, A.R. Developmental changes in polyunsaturated fetal plasma phospholipids and feto-maternal plasma phospholipid ratios and their association with bronchopulmonary dysplasia. *Eur. J. Nutr.* **2016**, *55*, 2265–2274. [CrossRef]
98. Clandinin, M.T.; Chappell, J.E.; Leong, S.; Heim, T.; Swyer, P.R.; Chance, G.W. Intrauterine fatty acid accretion rates in human brain: Implications for fatty acid requirements. *Early Hum. Dev.* **1980**, *4*, 121–129. [CrossRef]
99. van Houwelingen, A.C.; Foreman-van Drongelen, M.M.; Nicolini, U.; Nicolaides, K.H.; Al, M.D.; Kester, A.D.; Hornstra, G. Essential fatty acid status of fetal plasma phospholipids: Similar to postnatal values obtained at comparable gestational ages. *Early Hum. Dev.* **1996**, *46*, 141–152. [CrossRef]
100. Kuipers, R.S.; Luxwolda, M.F.; Offringa, P.J.; Boersma, E.R.; Dijck-Brouwer, D.A.; Muskiet, F.A. Fetal intrauterine whole body linoleic, arachidonic and docosahexaenoic acid contents and accretion rates. *Prostaglandins Leukot Essent Fat. Acids* **2012**, *86*, 13–20. [CrossRef]
101. Kuipers, R.S.; Luxwolda, M.F.; Sango, W.S.; Kwesigabo, G.; Dijck-Brouwer, D.A.; Muskiet, F.A. Maternal DHA equilibrium during pregnancy and lactation is reached at an erythrocyte DHA content of 8 g/100 g fatty acids. *J. Nutr.* **2011**, *141*, 418–427. [CrossRef]
102. Carlson, S.E.; Colombo, J.; Gajewski, B.J.; Gustafson, K.M.; Mundy, D.; Yeast, J.; Georgieff, M.K.; Markley, L.A.; Kerling, E.H.; Shaddy, D.J. DHA supplementation and pregnancy outcomes. *Am. J. Clin. Nutr.* **2013**, *97*, 808–815. [CrossRef]
103. Guesnet, P.; Alessandri, J.M. Docosahexaenoic acid (DHA) and the developing central nervous system (CNS)—Implications for dietary recommendations. *Biochimie* **2011**, *93*, 7–12. [CrossRef]
104. Rogers, L.K.; Valentine, C.J.; Keim, S.A. DHA supplementation: Current implications in pregnancy and childhood. *Pharm. Res.* **2013**, *70*, 13–19. [CrossRef]
105. Harris, W.S.; Baack, M.L. Beyond building better brains: Bridging the docosahexaenoic acid (DHA) gap of prematurity. *J. Perinatol.* **2015**, *35*, 1–7. [CrossRef]
106. Koletzko, B.; Lien, E.; Agostoni, C.; Bohles, H.; Campoy, C.; Cetin, I.; Decsi, T.; Dudenhausen, J.W.; Dupont, C.; Forsyth, S.; et al. The roles of long-chain polyunsaturated fatty acids in pregnancy, lactation and infancy: Review of current knowledge and consensus recommendations. *J. Perinat. Med.* **2008**, *36*, 5–14. [CrossRef]
107. Mulder, K.A.; Elango, R.; Innis, S.M. Fetal DHA inadequacy and the impact on child neurodevelopment: A follow-up of a randomised trial of maternal DHA supplementation in pregnancy. *Br. J. Nutr.* **2018**, *119*, 271–279. [CrossRef]
108. Rees, A.; Sirois, S.; Wearden, A. Prenatal maternal docosahexaenoic acid intake and infant information processing at 4.5 mo and 9 mo: A longitudinal study. *PLoS ONE* **2019**, *14*, e0210984. [CrossRef]
109. Maslova, E.; Rifas-Shiman, S.L.; Olsen, S.F.; Gillman, M.W.; Oken, E. Prenatal n-3 long-chain fatty acid status and offspring metabolic health in early and mid-childhood: Results from Project Viva. *Nutr. Diabetes* **2018**, *8*, 29. [CrossRef]
110. Ramakrishnan, U.; Gonzalez-Casanova, I.; Schnaas, L.; DiGirolamo, A.; Quezada, A.D.; Pallo, B.C.; Hao, W.; Neufeld, L.M.; Rivera, J.A.; Stein, A.D.; et al. Prenatal supplementation with DHA improves attention at 5 y of age: A randomized controlled trial. *Am. J. Clin. Nutr.* **2016**, *104*, 1075–1082. [CrossRef]
111. Crozier, S.R.; Sibbons, C.M.; Fisk, H.L.; Godfrey, K.M.; Calder, P.C.; Gale, C.R.; Robinson, S.M.; Inskip, H.M.; Baird, J.; Harvey, N.C.; et al. Arachidonic acid and DHA status in pregnant women is not associated with cognitive performance of their children at 4 or 6–7 years. *Br. J. Nutr.* **2018**, *119*, 1400–1407. [CrossRef]
112. Hoffman, D.R.; Theuer, R.C.; Castañeda, Y.S.; Wheaton, D.H.; Bosworth, R.G.; O'Connor, A.R.; Morale, S.E.; Wiedemann, L.E.; Birch, E.E. Maturation of visual acuity is accelerated in breast-fed term infants fed baby food containing DHA-enriched egg yolk. *J. Nutr.* **2004**, *134*, 2307–2313. [CrossRef]

113. Meldrum, S.J.; D'Vaz, N.; Simmer, K.; Dunstan, J.A.; Hird, K.; Prescott, S.L. Effects of high-dose fish oil supplementation during early infancy on neurodevelopment and language: A randomised controlled trial. *Br. J. Nutr.* **2012**, *108*, 1443–1454. [CrossRef]
114. Treen, M.; Uauy, R.D.; Jameson, D.M.; Thomas, V.L.; Hoffman, D.R. Effect of docosahexaenoic acid on membrane fluidity and function in intact cultured Y-79 retinoblastoma cells. *Arch. Biochem. Biophys.* **1992**, *294*, 564–570. [CrossRef]
115. Hyman, B.T.; Spector, A.A. Choline uptake in cultured human Y79 retinoblastoma cells: Effect of polyunsaturated fatty acid compositional modifications. *J. Neurochem.* **1982**, *38*, 650–656. [CrossRef]
116. Machova, E.; Novakova, J.; Lisa, V.; Dolezal, V. Docosahexaenoic acid supports cell growth and expression of choline acetyltransferase and muscarinic receptors in NG108-15 cell line. *J. Mol. Neurosci.* **2006**, *30*, 25–26. [CrossRef]
117. Machova, E.; Malkova, B.; Lisa, V.; Novakova, J.; Dolezal, V. The increase of choline acetyltransferase activity by docosahexaenoic acid in NG108-15 cells grown in serum-free medium is independent of its effect on cell growth. *Neurochem. Res.* **2006**, *31*, 1239–1246. [CrossRef]
118. da Costa, K.-A.; Rai, K.S.; Craciunescu, C.N.; Parikh, K.; Mehedint, M.G.; Sanders, L.M.; McLean-Pottinger, A.; Zeisel, S.H. Dietary Docosahexaenoic Acid Supplementation Modulates Hippocampal Development in the Pemt−/− Mouse. *J. Biol. Chem.* **2010**, *285*, 1008–1015. [CrossRef]
119. Pynn, C.J.; Henderson, N.G.; Clark, H.; Koster, G.; Bernhard, W.; Postle, A.D. Specificity and rate of human and mouse liver and plasma phosphatidylcholine synthesis analyzed in vivo. *J. Lipid Res.* **2011**, *52*, 399–407. [CrossRef]
120. van Deijk, A.F.; Broersen, L.M.; Verkuyl, J.M.; Smit, A.B.; Verheijen, M.H.G. High Content Analysis of Hippocampal Neuron-Astrocyte Co-cultures Shows a Positive Effect of Fortasyn Connect on Neuronal Survival and Postsynaptic Maturation. *Front. Neurosci.* **2017**, *11*, 440. [CrossRef]
121. Fourrier, C.; Remus-Borel, J.; Greenhalgh, A.D.; Guichardant, M.; Bernoud-Hubac, N.; Lagarde, M.; Joffre, C.; Laye, S. Docosahexaenoic acid-containing choline phospholipid modulates LPS-induced neuroinflammation in vivo and in microglia in vitro. *J. Neuroinflam.* **2017**, *14*, 170. [CrossRef]
122. Almeida, P.M.D.; Kamath, S.U.; Shenoy, P.R.; Bernhardt, L.K.; Kishore, A.; Rai, K.S. Persistent attenuation of brain oxidative stress through aging in perinatal maternal separated rat pups supplemented with choline and docosahexaenoic acid or Clitoria ternatea aqueous root extract. *Folia Neuropathol.* **2018**, *56*, 206–214. [CrossRef]
123. van Wijk, N.; Balvers, M.; Cansev, M.; Maher, T.J.; Sijben, J.W.; Broersen, L.M. Dietary Crude Lecithin Increases Systemic Availability of Dietary Docosahexaenoic Acid with Combined Intake in Rats. *Lipids* **2016**, *51*, 833–846. [CrossRef]
124. Rajarethnem, H.T.; Megur Ramakrishna Bhat, K.; Jc, M.; Kumar Gopalkrishnan, S.; Mugundhu Gopalram, R.B.; Rai, K.S. Combined Supplementation of Choline and Docosahexaenoic Acid during Pregnancy Enhances Neurodevelopment of Fetal Hippocampus. *Neurol Res. Int.* **2017**, *2017*, 8748706. [CrossRef]
125. Zicker, S.C.; Jewell, D.E.; Yamka, R.M.; Milgram, N.W. Evaluation of cognitive learning, memory, psychomotor, immunologic, and retinal functions in healthy puppies fed foods fortified with docosahexaenoic acid-rich fish oil from 8 to 52 weeks of age. *J. Am. Vet. Med. Assoc.* **2012**, *241*, 583–594. [CrossRef]
126. Lima, H.K.; Lin, X.; Jacobi, S.K.; Man, C.; Sommer, J.; Flowers, W.; Blikslager, A.; Gonzalez, L.; Odle, J. Supplementation of Maternal Diets with Docosahexaenoic Acid and Methylating Vitamins Impacts Growth and Development of Fetuses from Malnourished Gilts. *Curr. Dev. Nutr.* **2018**, *2*, nzx006. [CrossRef]
127. Kwan, S.T.C.; King, J.H.; Yan, J.; Wang, Z.; Jiang, X.; Hutzler, J.S.; Klein, H.R.; Brenna, J.T.; Roberson, M.S.; Caudill, M.A. Maternal Choline Supplementation Modulates Placental Nutrient Transport and Metabolism in Late Gestation of Mouse Pregnancy. *J. Nutr.* **2017**, *147*, 2083–2092. [CrossRef]
128. Maas, C.; Franz, A.R.; Shunova, A.; Mathes, M.; Bleeker, C.; Poets, C.F.; Schleicher, E.; Bernhard, W. Choline and polyunsaturated fatty acids in preterm infants' maternal milk. *Eur. J. Nutr.* **2017**, *56*, 1733–1742. [CrossRef]
129. Ferre, C.; Callaghan, W.; Olson, C.; Sharma, A.; Barfield, W. Effects of Maternal Age and Age-Specific Preterm Birth Rates on Overall Preterm Birth Rates—United States, 2007 and 2014. *Mmwr. Morb. Mortal. Wkly. Rep.* **2016**, *65*, 1181–1184. [CrossRef]
130. Institute of Medicine Committee on Understanding Premature Birth; Assuring Healthy Outcomes. The National Academies Collection: Reports funded by National Institutes of Health. In *Preterm Birth: Causes,*

Consequences, and Prevention; Behrman, R.E., Butler, A.S., Eds.; National Academies Press (US), National Academy of Sciences: Washington, DC, USA, 2007. [CrossRef]

131. Bernhard, W.; Böckmann, K.; Maas, C.; Mathes, M.; Hovelmann, J.; Shunova, A.; Hund, V.; Schleicher, E.; Poets, C.F.; Franz, A.R. Combined choline and DHA supplementation: A randomized controlled trial. *Eur. J. Nutr.* **2019**. [CrossRef]
132. West, A.A.; Yan, J.; Jiang, X.; Perry, C.A.; Innis, S.M.; Caudill, M.A. Choline intake influences phosphatidylcholine DHA enrichment in nonpregnant women but not in pregnant women in the third trimester. *Am. J. Clin. Nutr.* **2013**, *97*, 718–727. [CrossRef]
133. West, A.A.; Shih, Y.; Wang, W.; Oda, K.; Jaceldo-Siegl, K.; Sabate, J.; Haddad, E.; Rajaram, S.; Caudill, M.A.; Burns-Whitmore, B. Egg n-3 fatty acid composition modulates biomarkers of choline metabolism in free-living lacto-ovo-vegetarian women of reproductive age. *J. Acad. Nutr. Diet.* **2014**, *114*, 1594–1600. [CrossRef]
134. da Costa, K.A.; Sanders, L.M.; Fischer, L.M.; Zeisel, S.H. Docosahexaenoic acid in plasma phosphatidylcholine may be a potential marker for in vivo phosphatidylethanolamine N-methyltransferase activity in humans. *Am. J. Clin. Nutr.* **2011**, *93*, 968–974. [CrossRef]
135. McNamara, R.K.; Jandacek, R.; Tso, P.; Weber, W.; Chu, W.J.; Strakowski, S.M.; Adler, C.M.; Delbello, M.P. Low docosahexaenoic acid status is associated with reduced indices in cortical integrity in the anterior cingulate of healthy male children: A 1H MRS Study. *Nutr. Neurosci.* **2013**, *16*, 183–190. [CrossRef]
136. Cheatham, C.L.; Sheppard, K.W. Synergistic Effects of Human Milk Nutrients in the Support of Infant Recognition Memory: An Observational Study. *Nutrients* **2015**, *7*, 9079–9095. [CrossRef]
137. Jackson, K.H.; Harris, W.S. A Prenatal DHA Test to Help Identify Women at Increased Risk for Early Preterm Birth: A Proposal. *Nutrients* **2018**, *10*, 1933. [CrossRef]

3

Maternal Fatty Fish Intake Prior to and during Pregnancy and Risks of Adverse Birth Outcomes: Findings from a British Cohort

Camilla Nykjaer [1,2,*], Charlotte Higgs [3], Darren C. Greenwood [4], Nigel A.B. Simpson [3], Janet E. Cade [1] and Nisreen A. Alwan [5,6]

1 Nutritional Epidemiology Group, School of Food Science and Nutrition, University of Leeds, Leeds LS2 9JT, UK; J.E.Cade@leeds.ac.uk
2 School of Biomedical Sciences, Faculty of Biological Sciences, University of Leeds, Leeds LS2 9JT, UK
3 Department of Obstetrics and Gynaecology, University of Leeds, Leeds LS2 9JT, UK; charlotte.higgs@nhs.net (C.H.); N.A.B.Simpson@leeds.ac.uk (N.A.B.S.)
4 Division of Biostatistics, Centre for Epidemiology and Biostatistics, University of Leeds, Leeds LS2 9JT, UK; D.C.Greenwood@leeds.ac.uk
5 School of Primary Care and Population Sciences, Faculty of Medicine, University of Southampton, Southampton General Hospital, Southampton SO16 6YD, UK; N.A.Alwan@soton.ac.uk
6 NIHR Southampton Biomedical Research Centre, University of Southampton and University Hospital Southampton NHS Foundation Trust, Southampton SO16 6YD, UK
* Correspondence: c.nykjaer@leeds.ac.uk

Abstract: Fish is an important source of the essential fatty acids contributing to foetal growth and development, but the evidence linking maternal fatty fish consumption with birth outcomes is inconsistent. In the UK, pregnant women are recommended to consume no more than two 140 g portions of fatty fish per week. This study aimed to investigate the association between fatty fish consumption before and during pregnancy with preterm birth and size at birth in a prospective birth cohort. Dietary intake data were acquired from a cohort of 1208 pregnant women in Leeds, UK (CARE Study) to assess preconception and trimester-specific fatty fish consumption using questionnaires. Multiple 24-h recalls during pregnancy were used to estimate an average fatty fish portion size. Intake was classified as ≤2, >2 portions/week and no fish categories. Following the exclusion of women taking cod liver oil and/or omega-3 supplements, the associations between fatty fish intake with size at birth and preterm delivery (<37 weeks gestation) were examined in multivariable regression models adjusting for confounders including salivary cotinine as a biomarker of smoking status. The proportion of women reporting any fatty fish intake decreased throughout pregnancy, with the lowest proportion observed in trimester 3 (43%). Mean intakes amongst consumers were considerably lower than that recommended, with the lowest intake amongst consumers observed in the 1st trimester (106 g/week, 95% CI: 99, 113). This was partly due to small portion sizes when consumed, with the mean portion size of fatty fish being 101 g. After adjusting for confounders, no association was observed between fatty fish intake before or during pregnancy with size at birth and preterm delivery.

Keywords: fatty fish; essential fatty acids; omega-3; pregnancy; birth weight; foetal growth; preterm birth

1. Introduction

Preterm birth (<37 weeks gestation) and low birth weight (LBW) are important determinants of neonatal mortality and morbidity. They are also linked with higher risks of metabolic, neurological and cardiovascular disease in adult life [1–3]. Maternal nutrition during pregnancy has been postulated to play a role in the prevention of these adverse birth outcomes [4,5].

Recent research has focused on the role of fatty acids, in particular the omega-6 and omega-3 long chain polyunsaturated fatty acids (LCPUFA), which are derived from their respective precursors, linoleic (LA) and linolenic (LNA) acids. These are vital for the development of cell membranes and new tissues [6–8] and are classified as essential fatty acids (EFA) as they can only be derived from the maternal diet. During pregnancy the most biologically active LCPUFAs, docosahexaenoic acid (DHA) and arachidonic acid (AA) have been shown to have beneficial effects [9], particularly on the development of the foetal brain and retina [8]. These EFA cannot be synthesised in the human body [6,7,10] and the conversion rate of precursor to LCPUFA derivative within the foetus is limited [11]. Consequently, the foetus is heavily dependent on the maternal diet for EFA through transport across the placenta [11–13]. Additionally, as the EFA status of the mother has been found to decline during pregnancy [6,14], a dietary source is paramount for meeting the demand for maternal-foetal exchange.

Fish are an important source of essential LCPUFAs, particularly the n-3 PUFAs. However, the extent to which fish intake plays a role in shaping pregnancy outcomes is unclear, as evidence regarding maternal consumption and birth outcomes is inconclusive. Findings from some birth cohorts suggest a positive association between total fish intake and birth weight [15–19], with women with a high total fish intake being less likely to have low birthweight (LBW) babies [16,19] as well as preterm birth [20,21]. However, negative associations have also been found [15,18,22–24] and in some cases no association with preterm birth [15,17,23–25] nor size at birth [15,24–27] has been evident.

It has been hypothesised that adverse associations may be due to contaminants in fish including mercury and persistent organic pollutants (POPs). Fatty fish is a known source of these contaminants, particularly in larger fish species [22]. However, studies that have focused on differentiating between types of fish consumed including lean, fatty and shellfish in relation to birth outcomes have been inconclusive [15,18,19,24,27] although there may be a trend toward a negative association between fatty fish and foetal growth [18,22].

The current advice in the UK is to consume at least two portions of fish/week (~140 g/portion), one of which should be fatty fish [28]. This recommendation also applies to pregnant women and women trying to conceive but with an upper limit of maximum two portions of fatty fish/week. Pregnant women and women trying to conceive are also advised to avoid consumption of larger species such as marlin, swordfish and shark [28]. Despite the guideline stating that intake of up to two portions of fatty fish/week does not present any harm, many Western pregnant women consume limited amounts of fish [10,29,30] resulting in low intakes of LCPUFA which could be potentially detrimental to foetal development.

Using data from a prospective UK-based birth cohort (the Caffeine and Reproductive Health study (CARE)) [31], this paper aimed to estimate maternal fatty fish intake frequency and portion size before and during pregnancy, and investigate the association between maternal fatty fish intake before and during pregnancy with both preterm birth and size at birth.

2. Materials and Methods

2.1. Participants and Study Design

The CARE study is a British prospective birth cohort with the primary aim of investigating the associations between caffeine in the maternal diet and pregnancy outcomes [31]. Between 2003 and 2006, low risk pregnant women aged 18–45 years were recruited from Leeds Teaching Maternity Hospitals at 8–12 weeks gestation. A total of 5959 women were considered, of whom 4571 met the inclusion criteria. Eligible women were sent detailed information about the study and 1374 consented to participate. All participants gave written, informed consent and the study was conducted in accordance with the Declaration of Helsinki and approved by the Leeds West Local Research Ethics Committee (reference number 03/054).

2.2. *Assessment of Maternal Fatty Fish Intake*

2.2.1. Recall Data

Rather than using the Scientific Advisory Committee on Nutrition (SACN) estimate of 140 grams (g) per portion of fatty fish [28], which is based on data from a non-pregnant population (the National Diet and Nutrition Survey) we derived an estimate of the average portion size of fatty fish from 24 h dietary recalls administered by research midwives at 14–16 and 28 weeks gestation. To get a better picture of usual consumption throughout pregnancy an average portion size of fatty fish was derived for women who consumed fatty fish at both recalls. Participants were asked to record all food and drink consumed in a 24 h period (12 midnight to 12 midnight), including portion size and drink amounts. An example recall was provided as guidance. Reported canned tuna intake was removed from the analysis as it is not considered a fatty fish due the majority of the fat content being removed during the canning process [28].

2.2.2. Self-Reported Questionnaires

Fatty fish consumption was ascertained prior to and throughout pregnancy using a frequency type self-reported questionnaire adapted from the UK Women's Cohort Study [32] and administered at enrolment (12–18 weeks gestation), assessing consumption in the 4 weeks leading up to pregnancy and trimester 1; week 28, assessing trimester 2 consumption and postpartum (weeks 46–50) assessing trimester 3 consumption. Participants were asked how often (never; less than once/month; 1–3 times/month; once/week; 2–4 times/week; 5–6 times/week; once/day; 2–3 times/day; 4–5 times/day and >6 times/day) they consumed fatty fish (examples given were: salmon, tuna (fresh only), herring, kipper, mackerel, pilchards, sprats and swordfish). No examples of what constitutes a portion were given in the questionnaire. Frequency of fish consumption derived from the questionnaires was converted to times per week, which was then multiplied by the portion estimate of fish obtained from the recall data (see above) in order to get weekly consumption in grams for each of the trimesters.

2.3. *Assessment of Pregnancy Outcomes*

Information regarding pregnancy outcomes was collected from hospital maternity records. The two primary outcomes assessed were preterm birth (defined as <37 weeks gestation) and small for gestational age (SGA), defined as <10th individualised birth centile taking into account gestational age, maternal height, weight, ethnicity, parity, child sex and birth weight [33]. Actual birth weight was also analysed as a secondary measurement and expressed as a continuous variable in grams and a binary variable LBW defined as <2500 g. Duration of gestation was calculated from the date of the last menstrual period, and confirmed by ultrasound scans dating at around 12 and 20 weeks gestation.

2.4. *Assessment of Participant Characteristics*

Maternal characteristics including age, ethnicity, pre-pregnancy weight, height, parity, education (university degree versus no degree) were self-reported in the preliminary administered questionnaire. Caffeine intake (mg/day) and alcohol consumption (units/day) were assessed throughout pregnancy using the same frequency type questionnaire used to assess fatty fish intake. Smoking status was objectively measured using salivary cotinine levels at enrolment. Participants were classified based on cotinine concentrations as active smokers (>5 ng/mL), passive smokers (1–5 ng/mL) or non-smokers (<1 ng/mL). Daily total energy intake was derived from the 1st 24 h of food recall data.

2.5. *Statistical Power Calculation*

Comparing mothers consuming > 2 portions/week to non-consumers, the study had 80% power to detect an odds ratio of approximately 0.4 for SGA. The equivalent test for linear trend including the intermediate category half way between these extremes would have 90% power. Similarly, comparing the birth weight of babies born to mothers consuming > 2 portions of fish/week with non-consumers, assuming the SD to be approximately 500 g, this study had 85% power to detect a difference of 150 g in birth weight at $p < 0.05$.

2.6. *Statistical Analysis*

Analysis was conducted using the continuous weekly fish variable assigned into three categories of intake based on the current UK guidelines of no more than 2 portions of fatty fish per week [28] with the addition of a "no fish" category which was used as the referent group: no fish, ≤2 portions/week and >2 portions/week.

Univariable analyses were performed using one-way ANOVA for normally distributed variables, Kruskal-Wallis for non-parametric variables and chi-squared test for categorical outcomes. Multivariable linear and logistic regression models were used to assess the association between maternal fatty fish intake and continuous and dichotomous birth outcomes respectively. Maternal pre-pregnancy weight, height, ethnicity, parity, gestation and neonatal sex were accounted for when calculating the SGA variable and were adjusted for in the preterm delivery (omitting gestation) and birth weight models. Covariates adjusted for in all models were selected based on *a priori* knowledge from the literature and included maternal age, salivary cotinine levels, self-reported caffeine intake and alcohol consumption and university degree status as a marker for socioeconomic status.

In order to separate the effect of fatty fish from supplements as opposed to dietary sources on birth outcomes, women taking any cod liver oil and/or omega-3 supplements were removed from the analysis. Women with extreme values for energy intake (highest 1% and lowest 1%), obtained from the 24 h recall data, were excluded due to possible bias with self-reported dietary intake, as proposed by Meltzer et al. [34].

Sensitivity analyses were conducted taking into account previous high-risk pregnancies (including a previous LBW baby, previous gestational diabetes (GDM) and previous gestational hypertension (GHT)) and total energy intake during pregnancy. Sensitivity analyses were also done by excluding women who developed GHT and GDM during their current pregnancy (3rd trimester only). All analyses were performed using the Stata 14 software (Stata, College Station, TX, USA).

3. Results

Of the 1374 mothers who consented, 1303 agreed to participate and were enrolled into the CARE study. Of these, nine were lost to follow-up, five terminated pregnancies and others were excluded due to stillbirth ($n = 6$), neonatal death ($n = 3$) and late miscarriage ($n = 10$). Following exclusions of women taking cod liver oil and/or omega-3 supplements ($n = 37$) as well as those with extreme energy intakes ($n = 25$) left 1208 mothers with data available on birth outcomes.

3.1. *Estimation of Portion Size and Types of Fatty Fish Consumed (24-h Recall)*

A total of 1276 women reported dietary information by recall at weeks 14–16, and 601 women at week 28. Of these women, 162/1276 (13%) and 70/601 (12%) reported intakes of any fatty fish at the 1st and 2nd recall respectively. Combining both sets of recall data together, a total of 106 women reported fatty fish intake during the 1st and 2nd recall. The amount of fish consumed in grams at each meal was used to obtain an average portion size of 101 g (min: 10 g, max: 300 g).

Of the 106 women consuming fatty fish in the 24 h recall data (14–28 weeks gestation), 52 (49%) women ate salmon, 25 (24%) ate raw tuna and 14 (13%) ate mackerel. Other types of fatty fish included anchovies (5%), sardines (7%), trout (6%) and orange roughy (0.9%). Fatty fish consumption accounted for 4.8% of the total energy intake.

3.2. *Frequency of Fatty Fish Consumption (Questionnaire)*

Of the 1208 women with birth outcome data, 1116 (92%) women had information available on frequency of fatty fish intake before pregnancy, 1114 (92%) in the 1st trimester, 812 (67.2%) in the 2nd trimester and 409 (34%) in the 3rd trimester (Table 1). For those women who reported consuming any fatty fish, intake before pregnancy (123.5 g/week) was significantly higher ($p < 0.0001$) than trimester 1 & 2 (106.4 and 107.4 g/week respectively) but slightly lower than the mean intake in the 3rd trimester (136.5 g/week). The proportion of women reporting any fatty fish intake, however, decreased throughout pregnancy with the lowest proportion observed in trimester 3 (43%).The prevalence of women consuming within the recommended guidelines of no more than 2 portions of fatty fish per week was highest in trimester 1 (47%) and in the 2nd trimester (49%), with mean intakes for women reaching 64.3 g (95% CI 61.0 to 67.7) and 71.3 g (95% CI 66.6 to 75.7) per week, respectively.

Table 1. Self-reported fatty fish intake across pregnancy.

	n (%)	Mean (g)	95% CI
Fish intake (g/week) (consumers only):			
4 weeks before pregnancy ($n = 1116$)	648 (58.1)	123.5	115.1, 131.9
First trimester ($n = 1114$)	652 (58.5)	106.4	98.9, 112.9
Second trimester ($n = 812$)	466 (57.4)	107.4	98.2, 116.6
Third trimester ($n = 409$)	177 (43.3)	136.5	118.8, 154.1
Categories of intake 4 weeks before pregnancy *			
No fish	468 (41.9)	0	0
≤2 portions/week	491 (44.0)	67.6	64.8, 70.5
>2 portions/week	157(14.1)	298.1	286.7, 309.6
Categories of intake trimester 1			
No fish	462 (41.47)	0	0
≤2 portions/week	524 (47.0)	64.3	61.0, 67.7
>2 portions/week	128 (11.5)	278.9	267.1, 290.7
Categories of intake trimester 2			
No fish	346 (42.6)	0	0
≤2 portions/week	396 (48.8)	71.3	66.6, 75.7
>2 portions/week	70 (8.6)	311.8	291.9, 331.7
Categories of intake trimester 3			
No fish	232 (56.7)	0	0
≤2 portions/week	131 (32.0)	75.4	70.4, 80.4
>2 portions/week	46 (11.3)	310.5	279.0, 341.9

* Categories based on the UK recommendations of no more than 2 portions of fatty fish/week [28]. One portion of fish is 101 g.

3.3. *Maternal Characteristics According to Categories of Fish Intake*

Table 2 shows characteristics of participants according to maternal fatty fish intake in trimester 1. Women who consumed fatty fish during pregnancy were more likely to be older, have a university degree, to consume alcohol, were less likely to smoke and less likely to live in an area within the most deprived Index of Multiple Deprivation (IMD) quartile. These characteristics were consistent across all trimesters and the four weeks leading up to pregnancy. Women consuming fish in trimester 1 & 2 were also more likely to have a lower BMI, and those consuming fish in trimester 1 were shown to have a lower caffeine intake than non-fish consumers.

Table 2. Characteristics of mothers by fatty fish intake in the 1st trimester of pregnancy (n = 1114).

	No Fatty Fish	**≤2 Portions/Week**	**>2 Portions/Week**	p *
	(n = 462)	**(n = 524)**	**(n = 128)**	
Age (years) mean (SD)	28.5 (5.6)	30.8 (4.4)	31.7 (4.6)	0.0001
Pre-pregnancy BMI (kg/m^2) mean (SD)	25.1 (5.3)	24.4 (4.3)	23.9 (5.3)	0.01
Total energy intake (kcal) mean (SD)	2109.4 (595.6)	2111.5 (614.3)	2183.5 (670.8)	0.8
Caffeine intake (mg/day) mean (SD)	223.3 (225.4)	159.9 (151.3)	190.6 (177.6)	0.0001
Alcohol intake: % non-drinkers (n)	28.3 (127)	16.4 (84)	20.0 (24)	0.0001
Smoker at 12 weeks % (n) **	26.8 (117)	9.1 (461)	10.6 (13)	0.0001
IMD most deprived quartile % (n)	41.1 (182)	21.7 (109)	19.1 (24)	0.0001
University degree % (n)	24.5 (113)	50.4 (264)	56.3 (72)	<0.0001
European origin % (n)	94.8 (437)	93.5 (489)	94.5 (121)	0.7
Primigravida % (n)	45.3 (209)	51.1 (267)	40.9 (52)	0.06
Baby's gender: % male (n)	52.6 (243)	49.1 (257)	43.8 (56)	0.2
Gestational hypertension % (n)	1.1 (5)	1.9 (10)	1.6 (2)	0.6
Gestational diabetes % (n)	0.2 (1)	0.4 (2)	0 (0)	0.7
Past history of miscarriage % (n)	22.4 (102)	22.9 (119)	27.8 (35)	0.4

* p-Value using one-way ANOVA and Kruskal-Wallis for normally and non-normally distributed continuous variables respectively, and χ^2-test & Fisher's exact test for categorical variables. Significant difference at $p < 0.05$. ** Smoking status based on salivary cotinine concentrations: non-smoker < 1 ng/mL, passive smoker 1–5 ng/mL, current smoker > 5 ng/mL. Where numbers do not add up it is due to a small proportion of missing data. SD, standard deviation; BMI, body mass index; IMD, Index of Multiple Deprivation.

3.4. Pregnancy Outcomes

Of the 1208 women with information on birth outcomes, 44 babies (4%) were delivered preterm (<37 weeks gestation) with a mean gestational age of 34.29 weeks (SD = 2.99). A further 153 (13%) babies were born SGA (<10th centile) and 46 (4%) were LBW (<2500 g); the latter of which 27 (56%) were born preterm. The mean birth weight of the total sample was 3446 g (SD = 537 g).

3.5. Relationship between Fish Intake before Pregnancy and Birth Outcomes

There was no evidence of an association between fatty fish intake before pregnancy and preterm birth nor size at birth (Table 3).

3.6. Relationship between Fish Intake during Pregnancy and Preterm Birth

Compared to mothers consuming no fish in trimester 1, in unadjusted analysis mothers consuming up to 2 portions and >2 portions of fatty fish/week were less likely to have babies born preterm (OR: 0.5, 95% CI: 0.3, 1.0 & OR: 0.3, 95% CI: 0.1, 1.1 respectively; $p_{trend} = 0.05$) (Table 4). After adjustment for potential confounders, these estimates were largely unchanged, though no longer statistically significant (OR: 0.6, 95% CI: 0.3, 1.3 & OR: 0.3, 95% CI: 0.1, 1.3 respectively, $p_{trend} = 0.2$). A similar trend could be observed in trimester 2 for mothers consuming ≤2 portions of fatty fish/week compared to non-consumers (OR: 0.4, 95% CI: 0.2, 0.9; $p_{trend} = 0.06$), becoming non-significant after adjustment (OR: 0.5, 95% CI: 0.2, 1.2, $p_{trend} = 0.2$). There was no association between fatty fish intake in the 3rd trimester and preterm birth.

Table 3. The relationship between maternal fatty fish intake 4 weeks before pregnancy and size at birth & preterm delivery.

		Unadjusted Change (95% CI)	p *		Adjusted Change ** (95% CI)	p *
Birth weight (g)	*n*			*n*		
No fatty fish	468	0	0.3	426	0	0.7
≤2 portions/week	491	45.8 (−23.3, 115.0)		459	−17.9 (−75.3, 39.5)	
>2 portions/week	157	71.6 (−27.1, 170.3)		144	−35.7 (−115.6, 44.1)	
		Unadjusted OR (95% CI)	**p ***		**Adjusted OR ** (95% CI)**	**p ***
SGA (<10th centile) ***	**cases/*n***			**cases/*n***		
No fatty fish	70/468	1	0.3	67/444	1	0.6
≤2 portions/week	57/491	0.7 (0.5, 1.1)		55/473	1.0 (0.6, 1.5)	
>2 portions/week	23/157	1.0 (0.6, 1.6)		23/150	1.3 (0.8, 2.3)	
Low birth weight (≤2500 g)						
No fatty fish	21/468	1	0.8	19/426	1	0.3
≤2 portions/week	20/491	0.9 (0.5, 1.7)		19/459	1.9 (0.7, 5.3)	
>2 portions/week	5/157	0.7 (0.3, 1.9)		5/144	3.1 (0.8, 12.7)	
Preterm birth (<37 weeks gestation)						
No fatty fish	24/468	1	0.2	23/426	1	0.4
≤2 portions/week	17/491	0.7 (0.4, 1.3)		17/459	0.8 (0.4, 1.6)	
>2 portions/week	3/157	0.4 (0.1, 1.2)		3/144	0.4 (0.1, 1.5)	

* *p* for trend for categories of fish intake ** Adjusted for maternal pre-pregnancy weight, height, age, parity, ethnicity, salivary cotinine levels, caffeine intake, alcohol intake, education, gestation and baby's sex in multivariable linear regression for continuous outcome and multivariable logistic regression for categorical outcomes. *** Takes into account maternal pre-pregnancy weight, height, parity, ethnicity, gestation and baby's sex.

3.7. Relationship between Fish Intake during Pregnancy and Size at Birth

When comparing babies born to mothers consuming no fatty fish in trimester 1, mothers consuming up to two portions of fatty fish/week had babies weighing 58.4 g less (95% CI: −115.1, −1.5) although there was no linear trend (p_{trend} = 0.1). There was no evidence of any relationship between fish intake in the second or third trimester and size at birth expressed as birth weight (g), SGA (<10th centile) or low birth weight (Table 4).

3.8. Sensitivity Analysis

Adding total energy intake to the regression models did not affect the results. Similarly, including an indicator for high risk pregnancies as a possible moderator (n = 175) did not significantly alter findings nor did excluding women who developed GDM (n = 3) or GHT (n = 19).

Table 4. The relationship between maternal fatty fish intake during pregnancy and size at birth & preterm delivery.

	Trimester 1						Trimester 2						Trimester 3					
		Unadjusted Change (95% CI)	p *		Adjusted Change ** (95% CI)	p *		Unadjusted Change (95% CI)	p *		Adjusted Change ** (95% CI)	p *		Unadjusted Change (95% CI)	p *		Adjusted Change ** (95% CI)	p *
Birth weight (g)	n			n			n			n			n			n		
No fatty fish	462	0	0.3	422	0	0.1	346	0	0.2	316	0	0.3	232	0	0.3	218	0	0.8
≤2 portions/week	524	30.4 (−37.9, 98.7)		488	−58.4 (−115.1, −1.7)		396	75.3 (−6.5, 157.1)		371	−47.3 (−113.0, 18.4)		131	109.6 (−25.4, 244.6)		126	−35.6 (−139.9, 68.7)	
>2 portions/week	128	87.7 (−19.2, 194.6)		118	−64.0 (−151.1, 23.1)		70	42.3 (−103.4, 188.1)		64	−71.4 (−185.8, 43.13)		46	52.6 (−146.8, 251.9)		43	−21.8 (−169.0, 125.4)	
		Unadjusted OR (95% CI)	p *		Adjusted OR ** (95% CI)	p *		Unadjusted OR (95% CI)	p *		Adjusted OR ** (95% CI)	p *		Unadjusted OR (95% CI)	p *		Adjusted OR ** (95% CI)	p *
SGA (<10th centile) * **	**cases/n**			**cases/n**			**cases/n**			**cases/n**			**cases/n**			**cases/n**		
No fatty fish	69/462	1	0.2	65/436	1	0.3	60/346	1	0.6	56/328	1	0.6	74/232	1	0.9	24/218	1	0.8
≤2 portions/week	69/524	0.9 (0.6, 1.2)		68/506	1.2 (0.8, 1.8)		58/396	0.8 (0.6, 1.2)		58/385	1.1 (0.4, 1.7)		40/131	0.9 (0.6, 1.5)		10/126	1.1 (0.7, 1.9)	
>2 portions/week	11/128	0.5 (0.3, 1.0)		11/123	0.7 (0.4, 1.5)		12/70	1.0 (0.5, 1.9)		12/67	1.5 (0.7, 3.0)		5/46	1.0 (0.5, 2.0)		5/43	1.2 (0.6, 2.5)	
Low birth weight (≤2500 g)	**cases/n**			**cases/n**			**cases/n**			**cases/n**			**cases/n**			**cases/n**		
No fatty fish	23/462	1	0.3	21/422	1	0.4	23/346	1	0.3	21/316	1	0.2	26/232	1	0.5	69/220	1	0.2
≤2 portions/week	21/524	0.8 (0.4, 1.5)		20/488	2.0 (0.7, 5.6)		17/396	0.6 (0.3, 1.2)		17/371	3.0 (0.9, 9.7)		10/131	0.7 (0.3, 1.4)		40/129	2.4 (0.6, 9.7)	
>2 portions/week	2/128	0.3 (0.1, 1.3)		2/118	1.2 (0.2, 7.4)		3/70	0.6 (0.2, 2.2)		3/64	1.5 (0.3, 8.1)		5/46	1.0 (0.4, 2.7)		15/45	5.5 (0.9, 31.9)	
Preterm birth (<37 weeks gestation)	**cases/n**			**cases/n**			**cases/n**			**cases/n**			**cases/n**			**cases/n**		
No fatty fish	26/462	1	0.05	25/422	1	0.2	21/346	1	0.06	21/316	1	0.2	18/232	1	0.3	18/218	1	0.6
≤2 portions/week	16/524	0.5 (0.3, 1.0)		16/488	0.6 (0.3, 1.3)		10/396	0.4 (0.2, 0.9)		10/371	0.5 (0.2, 1.2)		5/131	0.5 (0.2, 1.3)		5/126	0.6 (0.2, 1.7)	
>2 portions/week	2/128	0.3 (0.1, 1.1)		2/118	0.3 (0.1, 1.3)		4/70	0.9 (0.3, 2.8)		4/64	1.1 (0.4, 3.6)		3/46	0.8 (0.2, 2.9)		3/43	0.7 (0.2, 2.8)	

* p for trend for categories of maternal fish intake in linear and logistic regression models for continuous and dichotomous outcomes respectively. ** Adjusted for maternal pre-pregnancy weight, height, age, parity, ethnicity, salivary cotinine levels, caffeine intake, alcohol intake, education, gestation and baby's sex in multivariable linear regression for continuous outcome and multivariable logistic regression for categorical outcomes. *** Takes into account maternal pre-pregnancy weight, height, parity, ethnicity, gestation and baby's sex. LBW, low birth weight; n, number; OR, odds ratio; SGA, small for gestation age.

4. Discussion

As far as we are aware this is the only British prospective birth cohort study assessing maternal fatty fish intake prior to and throughout each of the trimesters separately in relation to pregnancy outcomes.

The results showed the majority of pregnant women were consuming considerably less than two portions of fatty fish per week prior to and throughout pregnancy and a trend towards a decreased fatty fish consumption with the progression of pregnancy. Within this study there was no evidence of a statistically significant association between maternal fatty fish intake and gestational length and size at birth, when taking known confounders into account.

4.1. Fish Intake and Maternal Characteristics

The proportion of mothers reporting any fatty fish consumption decreased as pregnancy progressed. Among consumers, mean weekly intakes were highest for the period leading up to pregnancy and the 3rd trimester (124 g and 137 g/week respectively) but still considerably lower than the mean of 190 g of fatty fish/week reported in a UK national survey of women (non-pregnant women aged 19–64) carried out around the same time [35] and noticeably lower than the UK guidelines of up to two portions of 140 g fatty fish/week.

The proportion of women in our study not consuming any fatty fish in the 3rd trimester (56.7%) was slightly higher compared to results from the Avon Longitudinal Study of Parents and Children (ALSPAC) which showed in their study of fish intake in pregnancy and birth weight that 42.6% of pregnant women (n = 11,511) reported never or rarely consumed any fatty fish in the 3rd trimester [17]. Compared to other non UK studies assessing fatty fish intakes in Western pregnant women, the proportion not consuming any fatty fish were 33% during the 1st trimester in a Dutch birth cohort (n = 3380) [25], 11% during the 2nd trimester in a large Norwegian birth cohort (n = 62,099) [19] and 24% reported consuming <0.2 portions of fatty fish/month before pregnancy in a US cohort [27], all lower than that observed in our cohort. Results from the Danish National Birth Cohort (DNBC) however (n = 44,824) reported a similar proportion of 54% of non-consumers from their assessment of fatty fish intake in the 2nd trimester [22]. Similarly, results from a Spanish cohort of pregnant women (INMA) showed 41% of women reporting consuming <1 portion of fatty fish/month [18]. Results from a meta-analysis by Leventakou et al., (2014) of 19 European cohorts (some of which are mentioned above) showed a considerable variation in fatty fish intake between countries; with Italian, Spanish and Portuguese mothers consuming fatty fish more than twice as often as Irish & French mothers. It is however impossible to tell how much more fatty fish the Spanish mothers ate than the Irish mothers, for instance, because the researchers had data only on frequency, not quantity [36].

Although it is probable that some women simply do not like fish, reasons for low consumption are likely to include perceptions about cost, access to stores that sell fish, and uncertainty about preparation and cooking methods. Furthermore, some women may abstain from eating fish out of a worry that they and their babies will be harmed by contaminants present in some types of fish, a concern which is highlighted in the current UK guidelines but may actually result in a lack of consumption rather than a lowered intake of fatty fish. The characteristics of the mothers in our study across categories of increased fatty fish consumption are consistent with those observed in other studies where slightly older women, those consuming alcohol and women of higher socioeconomic status and higher education tended to consume higher levels of fish and were less likely to be smokers [16,17,19,22,23,25,26].

4.2. Interpretation of Main Findings

We did not find any evidence of an association between maternal fatty fish intake before and during pregnancy with gestational age or size at birth.

In another British birth cohort (ALSPAC), Rogers et al., (2004) used n-3 fatty acids as a marker of fish consumption and found no association with preterm birth, LBW or intrauterine growth retardation once they adjusted for confounders [17]. Despite having data on type of fish consumed they did not relate this to birth outcomes but focused instead on n-3 fatty acid intake from fish as well as frequency of total fish consumption making it impossible to make direct comparisons to our study. Other studies have reported a similar lack of association between maternal fatty fish intake and birth outcomes [18,19,24,27]. In their meta-analysis Leventakou et al. (2014) in addition to assessing total fish intake, also assessed types of fish (fatty, lean and seafood) in relation to birth outcomes and similarly to our results, they found no association between fatty fish and gestational age or LBW. Where lean fish and shellfish had no significant associations with any birth outcomes, they did observe a positive association between fatty fish and birth weight, albeit a small one at 2.38 g (95% CI: 0.51, 4.25) for every 1 unit (times/week) increment. The authors stipulated that the n-3 LCPUFA content in fatty fish could be the contributing factor behind the overall positive association they found between total fish intake and birth weight [36]. Contrary to this, Halldorson et al. (2007) reported a reduction of 27.5 g in birthweight of babies born to mothers consuming fatty fish more than four times/month compared to non-consumers as well as an increased risk of having babies born SGA [22].

Differences in findings are partly due to heterogeneity between studies. In particular what constitutes a portion of fish varies from study to study and has been shown to range from 85 g to 200 g depending on the type of fish as well as the country of the study [15,27,36]. In addition, categories of intake differ from study to study with some choosing very high or low categories of intake. We chose to assess intake from a more public health relevant context, but this resulted in very small numbers in the high consumption category (>2 portions/week), which limited the power to detect a true association. Furthermore, it is unclear whether the timing of exposure has any effect on outcomes and to our knowledge; no study to date has looked at all trimester specific fatty fish intakes in relation to birth outcomes. Of the studies which have assessed intake in more than one trimester and/or prior to pregnancy [16,20,23,26], one found a positive association with size at birth in overweight women for intakes before pregnancy but not in the final period of pregnancy [26]. Another found an increased risk of LBW babies in women reporting no fish consumption in the 3rd trimester, but not in trimester 1 [16]. Results from a Danish study showed a decreased risk of preterm birth with increasing total fish consumption in both trimester 1 and 2 [20]. Finally one study found a negative association with size at birth and fish intake reported in the 1st trimester but not in the 2nd trimester [23]. None of these studies however looked at types of fish consumed. Moreover, the choice of confounders tends to be inconsistent across studies and since not only in the present study, but also in other studies, high fish consumption has been shown to be strongly related to a higher education level and more healthy lifestyle habits, any positive associations between fish consumption and birth outcomes may be partly due to residual confounding by lifestyle-related characteristics if studies have failed to take these into account in their analysis. Additionally, discrepancies in findings between countries may be a reflection of differences in dietary patterns. This heterogeneity makes it hard to compare results.

4.3. Strengths

As a unique feature of this study we had two sources of dietary intake available which allowed us to derive a study specific estimation of a portion of fatty fish rather than using the SACN estimation of 140 g/portion [28]. This may have given a truer picture of actual intake of fatty fish within a cohort of British pregnant women. Fatty fish intake was averaged to weekly consumption and then divided into categories. This was done so as to better reflect the current UK guidelines on fatty fish consumption for pregnant women and women trying to conceive, and to make the results more applicable in a public health context.

We assessed maternal fish intake at three time points covering a wide window of exposure and taking into account variations across trimesters. Furthermore, only self-reported fatty fish intake was accounted for in the questionnaire. Therefore, the relationship with fatty fish could be assessed, as previous studies have combined type of fish such as lean fish, shellfish and molluscs in their overall analysis, biasing the true effect. Halldorsson et al. (2007) found a negative association with size at birth [22] and Ramon et al. (2009) found that consumption of larger fatty fish $\geq$ twice/week (such as swordfish) compared to <once/month was associated with a higher risk of SGA, however the P for trend across categories of intake was not significant [18]. Other studies have not specifically identified fatty fish within their analysis and therefore findings cannot be explicitly compared.

In our study information was available for a wide range of confounders. The objective measurement of salivary cotinine samples meant that smoking, a significant confounder in relation to maternal fish intake and birth outcomes, was assessed accurately with a biomarker.

4.4. Limitations

The questionnaires used in this study were originally designed to assess caffeine intake in pregnancy and not dietary fatty fish consumption. However, the questionnaire was validated with reference to caffeine intake in pregnant women [37]; and other food related questions were comparable to other methods used in the assessment of fish. Despite intakes being self-reported and thus presenting the issue of possible under-reporting, fatty fish consumption was assessed prospectively in trimesters 1 and 2, reducing the potential for differential measurement (recall) bias.

An explanation for non-statistically significant findings with fatty fish intake and birth outcomes could be due to the number of women included in the analysis (n = 1208) compared to other large well known cohorts [15,17,20,22,23] as well as the low consumption of fatty fish reported in our cohort. We had limited power to detect small associations due to the low numbers in the high consumption category, especially in trimester 3 (n = 409). The original study of caffeine and birth outcomes planned to follow up women several weeks after delivery to investigate whether their caffeine metabolism had returned to normal, using a caffeine challenge. This proposed data collection was expensive. To reduce costs without introducing selection bias, all cases (SGA and LBW infants) were recruited for postpartum follow-up, but only a sample of controls were taken to be the next two births that were not SGA or LBW. However, previous studies with smaller cohorts have detected associations in relation to fatty fish intake [18,24], although these women consumed high intakes of fish due to their Mediterranean diets.

In this analysis, fresh tuna was considered a fatty fish and was therefore included in the estimation of fatty fish intake and portion size. UK guidance has recently changed to exclude fresh tuna from being considered a type of fatty fish [38,39]. However, our analysis included fresh tuna as a fatty fish, to facilitate comparison with previous studies. With the low intake of fatty fish within this cohort and the relatively low proportion of consumers reporting fresh tuna intake (n = 25) this is unlikely to have influenced results. Canned tuna was excluded in the estimation of fatty fish intake as it is not considered a fatty fish in the UK. However, it is important to acknowledge that canned tuna still contains levels of EPA and DHA, and with tuna being the second most consumed type of fish in our cohort, it could still be a contributor to total EPA and DHA intake. Nevertheless, the few studies that have looked at fish subtypes such as canned tuna in relation to birth outcomes have been inconclusive making it hard to elucidate the potential impact excluding it could have on our findings. Mendez et al. (2010) found in their Spanish cohort of 657 pregnant women that maternal consumption of canned tuna (more than 1 portion per week) was associated with a significantly increased risk of SGA (adjusted OR: 2.49, 95% CI: 1.04 to 5.97). However, another Spanish study [18] similar in size found that mothers consuming more than or equal to 2 portions per week of canned tuna had a lower risk of having infants who were SGA (adjusted OR: 0.3, 95% CI: 0.1, 0.8) compared to mothers in the lower consumption categories.

Finally, a major weakness within this cohort was the lack of objective measurement of self-reported fish consumption. This could have been validated using a biomarker, such as erythrocytes concentrations of n-3 fatty acids, to indicate accurate fish intake during pregnancy, which has been addressed in previous studies [18,19,22–24].

5. Conclusions

Within this UK cohort of low risk pregnant women there was a low prevalence of fatty fish consumption and no evidence of an association between fatty fish intake prior to or throughout pregnancy with size at birth or preterm birth after adjusting for confounding.

Ideally, large cohort studies focusing on types of fish as well as timing of exposure, with a particular focus on the preconception period, are needed to help improve the understanding of the relationship between maternal fish intake during pregnancy and birth outcomes.

Author Contributions: The CARE study was designed by and carried out under the leadership of J.E.C. and N.A.B.S. N.A.A., N.A.B.S. and C.H. conceptualised the research questions. C.N. & C.H. conducted the statistical analysis with guidance from D.C.G. and N.A.A. and led the drafting of the manuscript. All authors contributed to subsequent drafts of the manuscript and have read and approved the final manuscript.

Acknowledgments: We would like to acknowledge the women participating in this study and the research midwives for their invaluable contribution, Sinead Boylan for recruitment and data collection, Susan Shires, Alastair Kay & Kay White for laboratory analysis of cotinine and caffeine levels and James Thomas & Neil Hancock for database management.

References

1. Barker, D. Fetal origins of coronary heart disease. *BMJ* **1995**, *311*, 171–174. [CrossRef] [PubMed]
2. Osmond, C.; Barker, D.J. Fetal, infant and childhood growth are predictors of coronary heart disease, diabetes, and hypertension in adult men and women. *Environ. Health Perspect.* **2000**, *108*, 545–553. [PubMed]
3. NICE. *Scope Guideline—Preterm Labour and Birth*; National Collaborating Centre for Women's and Children's Health: London, UK, 2013.
4. Wu, G.; Bazer, F.W.; Cudd, T.A.; Meininger, C.J.; Spencer, T.E. Maternal nutrition and fetal development. *J. Nutr.* **2004**, *134*, 2169–2172. [CrossRef] [PubMed]
5. Burdge, G.C.; Hanson, M.A.; Slater-Jefferies, J.L.; Lillycrop, K.A. Epigenetic regulation of transciption: A mechanism of inducing variations in phenotype (fetal programming) by differences in nutrition during early life? *Br. J. Nutr.* **2007**, *97*, 1036–1046. [CrossRef] [PubMed]
6. Hornstra, G. Essential fatty acids in mothers and their neonates. *Am. J. Clin. Nutr.* **2000**, *71*, 1262–1269. [CrossRef] [PubMed]
7. McGregor, J.A.; Allen, K.G.; Harris, M.A.; Reece, M.; Wheeler, M.; French, J.I.; Morrison, J. The omega-3 story: Nutritional prevention of preterm birth and other adverse pregnancy outcomes. *Obstet. Gynecol. Surv.* **2001**, *56*, S1–S13. [CrossRef]
8. Simopoulos, A.P.; Leaf, A.; Salem, N., Jr. Essentiality of and recommended dietary intakes for omega-6 and omega-3 fatty acids. *Ann. Nutr. Metab.* **1999**, *43*, 127–130. [CrossRef]
9. Coletta, J.M.; Bell, S.J.; Roman, A.S. Omega-3 fatty acids and pregnancy. *Rev. Obstretrics Gynaecol.* **2010**, *3*, 163–171.
10. Oken, E.; Belfort, M.B. Fish, fish oil, and pregnancy. *JAMA J. Am. Med. Assoc.* **2010**, *304*, 1717–1718. [CrossRef]
11. Makrides, M.; Neumann, M.; Simmer, K.; Gibson, R.; Pater, J. Are long-chain polyunsaturated fatty acids essential nutrients in infancy? *Lancet* **1995**, *345*, 1463–1468. [CrossRef]
12. Williamson, C. Nutrition in pregnancy. *Br. Nutr. Found. Nutr. Bull.* **2006**, *31*, 28–59. [CrossRef]
13. Hanebutt, F.L.; Demmelmair, H.; Schiessl, B.; Larqué, E.; Koletzko, B. Long-chain polyunsaturated fatty acid (lc-pufa) transfer across the placenta. *Clin. Nutr.* **2008**, *27*, 685–693. [CrossRef] [PubMed]
14. Makrides, M.; Gibson, R.A. Long-chain polyunsaturated fatty acid requirements during pregnancy and lactation. *Am. J. Clin. Nutr.* **2000**, *71*, S307–S311. [CrossRef] [PubMed]
15. Guldner, L.; Monfort, C.; Rouget, F.; Garlantezec, R.; Cordier, S. Maternal fish and shellfish intake and pregnancy outcomes: A prospective cohort study in brittany, france. *Environ. Health* **2007**, *6*, 33. [CrossRef] [PubMed]
16. Muthayya, S.; Dwarkanath, P.; Thomas, T.; Ramprakash, S.; Mehra, R.; Mhaskar, A.; Mhaskar, R.; Thomas, A.; Bhat, S.; Vaz, M.; et al. The effect of fish and n-3 lcpufa intake on low birth weight in indian pregnancy women. *Eur. J. Clin. Nutr.* **2009**, *63*, 340–346. [CrossRef]

17. Rogers, I.; Emmett, P.; Ness, A.; Golding, J. ALSPAC Study Team. Maternal fish intake in late pregnancy and the frequency of low birth weight and intrauterine growth retardation in a cohort of british infants. *J. Epidemiol. Community Health* **2004**, *58*, 486–492. [CrossRef] [PubMed]
18. Ramon, R.; Ballester, F.; Aguinagalde, X.; Amurrio, A.; Vioque, J.; Lacasana, M.; Rebagliato, M.; Murcia, M.; Iniguez, C. Fish consumption during pregnancy, prenatal mercury exposure, and anthropometric measures at birth in a prospective mother-infant cohort in spain. *Am. J. Clin. Nutr.* **2009**, *90*, 1047–1055. [CrossRef] [PubMed]
19. Brantsaeter, A.L.; Birgisdottir, B.E.; Meltzer, H.M.; Kvalem, H.E.; Alexander, J.; Magnus, P.; Haugen, M. Maternal seafood consumption and infant birth weight, length and head circumference in the norwegian mother and child cohort study. *Br. J. Nutr.* **2012**, *107*, 436–444. [CrossRef]
20. Olsen, S.F.; Østerdal, M.L.; Salvig, J.D.; Kesmodel, U.; Henriksen, T.B.; Hedegaard, M.; Secher, N.J. Duration of pregnancy in relation to seafood intake during early and mid pregnancy: Prospective cohort. *Perinat. Epidemol.* **2006**, *21*, 749–758. [CrossRef] [PubMed]
21. Haugen, M.; Margrete Meltzer, H.; Lise Brantsæter, A.; Mikkelsen, T.; Louise Østerdal, M.; Alexander, J.; Olsen, S.F.; Bakketeig, L. Mediterranean-type diet and risk of preterm birth among women in the norwegian mother and child cohort study (moba): A prospective cohort study. *Acta Obstet. Gynecol. Scand.* **2008**, *87*, 319–324. [CrossRef] [PubMed]
22. Halldorsson, T.I.; Meltzer, H.M.; Thorsdottir, I.; Knudsen, V.; Olsen, S.F. Is high consumption of fatty fish during pregnancy a risk factor for fetal growth retardation? A study of 44824 danish pregnant women. *Am. J. Epidemiol.* **2007**, *166*, 687–696. [CrossRef]
23. Oken, E.; Kleinman, K.P.; Olsen, S.F.; Rich-Edwards, J.W.; Gillman, M.W. Associations of seafood and elongated n-3 fatty acid intake with fetal growth and length of gestation: Results from a us pregnancy cohort. *Am. J. Epidemiol.* **2004**, *160*, 774–783. [CrossRef] [PubMed]
24. Mendez, M.A.; Plana, E.; Guxens, M.; Morillo, C.M.F.; Albareda, R.M.; Garcia-Esteban, R.; Goñi, F.; Kogevinas, M.; Sunyer, J. Seafood consumption in pregnancy and infant size at birthl results from a prospective spanish cohort. *J. Epidemiol. Community Health* **2010**, *64*, 216–222. [CrossRef]
25. Heppe, D.H.; Steegers, E.A.; Timmermans, S.; Breeijen, H.; Tiemeier, H.; Hofman, A.; Jaddoe, V.W. Maternal fish consumption, fetal growth and the risks of neonatal complications: The generation r study. *Br. J. Nutr.* **2011**, *105*, 938–949. [CrossRef]
26. Drouillet, P.; Kaminski, M.; De Lauzon-Guillain, B.; Forhan, A.; Ducimetiere, P.; Schweitzer, M.; Magnin, G.; Goua, V.; Thiebaugeorges, O.; Charles, M.A. Association between maternal seafood consumption before pregnancy and fetal growth: Evidence for an association in overweight women. The eden mother-child cohort. *Paediatr. Perinat. Epidemiol.* **2009**, *23*, 76–86. [CrossRef] [PubMed]
27. Mohanty, A.F.; Thompson, M.L.; Burbacher, T.M.; Siscovick, D.S.; Williams, M.A.; Enquobahrie, D.A. Periconceptional seafood intake and fetal growth. *Paediatr. Perinat. Epidemiol.* **2015**, *29*, 376–387. [CrossRef]
28. SACN. *Advice on Fish Consumption: Benefits & Risks*; SACN: London, UK, 2004.
29. Cetin, I.; Koletzko, B. Long-chain omega-3 fatty acid supply in pregnancy and lactation. *Curr. Opin. Clin. Nutr. Metab. Care* **2008**, *11*, 297–302. [CrossRef] [PubMed]
30. Bloomingdale, A.; Guthrie, L.B.; Price, S.; Wright, R.O.; Platek, D.; Haines, J.; Oken, E. A qualitative study of fish consumption during pregnancy. *Am. J. Clin. Nutr.* **2010**, *92*, 1234–1240. [CrossRef]
31. CARE Study Group. Maternal caffeine intake during pregnancy and risk of fetal growth restriction: A large prospective observational study. *BMJ* **2008**, *337*, a2332. [CrossRef]
32. Cade, J.E.; Burley, V.J.; Greenwood, D.C.; UK Women's Cohort Study Steering Group. The UK women's cohort study: Comparison of vegetarians, fish-eaters and meat-eaters. *Public Health Nutr.* **2004**, *7*, 871–878. [CrossRef]
33. Gardosi, J. New definition of small for gestational age based on fetal growth potential. *Horm. Res.* **2006**, *65*, 15–18. [CrossRef] [PubMed]
34. Meltzer, H.M.; Brantsæter, A.L.; Ydersbond, T.A.; Alexander, J.; Haugen, M.; MoBa Dietary Support Group. Methodological challenges when monitoring the diet of pregnant women in a large study: Experiences from the norwegian mother and child cohort study (MoBa). *Matern. Child Nutr.* **2008**, *4*, 14–27. [CrossRef] [PubMed]

35. Henderson, L.; Gregory, J.; Swan, G. *The National Diet and Nutrition Survey: Adults Aged 19 to 64 Years. Volume 1: Types and Quantities of Foods Consumed*; The Stationery Office: London, UK, 2002.
36. Leventakou, V.; Roumeliotaki, T.; Martinez, D.; Barros, H.; Brantsaeter, A.L.; Casas, M.; Charles, M.A.; Cordier, S.; Eggesbo, M.; van Eijsden, M.; et al. Fish intake during pregnancy, fetal growth, and gestational length in 19 european birth cohort studies. *Am. J. Clin. Nutr.* **2014**, *99*, 506–516. [CrossRef]
37. Boylan, S.M.; Cade, J.E.; Kirk, S.F.; Greenwood, D.C.; White, K.L.; Shires, S.; Simpson, N.A.; Wild, C.P.; Hay, A.W. Assessing caffeine exposure in pregnant women. *Br. J. Nutr.* **2008**, *100*, 875–882. [CrossRef] [PubMed]
38. Roe, M.; Pinchen, H.; Finglas, P. *Nutrient Analysis of Fish and Fish Products*; Department of Health: London, UK, 2018.
39. Clark, R. In the News: Fresh Tuna no Longer Counts as an Oily Fish. Available online: https://www.wcrf-uk.org/informed/articles/news-fresh-tuna-no-longer-counts-oily-fish (accessed on 21 January 2019).

4

Higher Maternal Diet Quality during Pregnancy and Lactation Is Associated with Lower Infant Weight-For-Length, Body Fat Percent and Fat Mass in Early Postnatal Life

Muna J. Tahir [1,*], Jacob L. Haapala [1], Laurie P. Foster [1], Katy M. Duncan [2], April M. Teague [2], Elyse O. Kharbanda [3], Patricia M. McGovern [4], Kara M. Whitaker [5,6], Kathleen M. Rasmussen [7], David A. Fields [2], David R. Jacobs Jr. [1], Lisa J. Harnack [1] and Ellen W. Demerath [1]

1 Division of Epidemiology and Community Health, University of Minnesota, Minneapolis, MN 55454, USA; haap0016@umn.edu (J.L.H.); fost0112@umn.edu (L.P.F.); jacob004@umn.edu (D.R.J.J.); harna001@umn.edu (L.J.H.); ewd@umn.edu (E.W.D.)
2 Department of Pediatrics, University of Oklahoma Health Sciences Center, Oklahoma City, OK 73104, USA; Katy-Duncan@ouhsc.edu (K.M.D.); April-Teague@ouhsc.edu (A.M.T.); David-Fields@ouhsc.edu (D.A.F.)
3 HealthPartners Institute, Minneapolis, MN 55425, USA; elyse.o.kharbanda@healthpartners.com
4 Division of Environmental Health Sciences, University of Minnesota, Minneapolis, MN 55455, USA; pmcg@umn.edu
5 Department of Health and Human Physiology, University of Iowa, Iowa City, IA 52242, USA; kara-whitaker@uiowa.edu
6 Department of Epidemiology, University of Iowa, Iowa City, IA 52246, USA
7 Division of Nutritional Sciences, Cornell University, Ithaca, NY 14850, USA; kathleen.rasmussen@cornell.edu
* Correspondence: mtahir@umn.edu

Abstract: Maternal pregnancy nutrition influences fetal growth. Evidence is limited, however, on the relationship of maternal diet during pregnancy and lactation on infant postnatal growth and adiposity. Our purpose was to examine associations between maternal diet quality during pregnancy and lactation with offspring growth and body composition from birth to six months. Maternal diet quality was serially assessed in pregnancy and at one and three months postpartum, using the Healthy Eating Index–2015 in a cohort of 354 fully breastfeeding mother–infant dyads. Infant length-for-age (LAZ), weight-for-age (WAZ), and weight-for-length (WLZ) Z-scores were assessed at birth, one, three, and six months. Infant body fat percent (BF%), fat mass (FM), and fat-free mass (FFM) were measured at six months using dual-energy X-ray absorptiometry. Higher maternal diet quality from pregnancy through three months postpartum was associated with lower infant WLZ from birth to six months ($p = 0.02$) and BF% at six months ($p \leq 0.05$). Higher maternal diet quality at one and three months postpartum was also associated with lower infant FM at six months ($p < 0.01$). In summary, maternal diet quality during pregnancy and lactation was inversely associated with infant relative weight and adiposity in early postnatal life. Additional research is needed to explore whether associations persist across the life course.

Keywords: maternal diet quality; pregnancy; lactation; infancy; growth; body composition

---

1. Introduction

The in utero environment is known to play an important role in fetal programming and subsequent offspring growth and development [1]. Intrauterine nutritional and environmental exposures may have adverse effects on lifelong organ structure and function, which ultimately influence offspring health and disease risk [1,2]. Within this context, research has shown that maternal pre-pregnancy body mass index (BMI) [3], gestational weight gain [3,4], and lifestyle during pregnancy [5] may influence offspring obesity. These effects may appear immediately in the form of macrosomia and birth weight large-for-gestational age, or may be latent, with adiposity appearing later in life [3]. The role of maternal diet during this window of vulnerability is of particular interest for obesity prevention [6]. Although maternal obesity is the strongest predictor of offspring obesity [3], the modifiability of maternal diet is potentially a crucial tool in combating obesity in offspring.

Accruing animal and human evidence also indicates that maternal nutrition beyond the pregnancy period may play a role in early life infant health and subsequent obesity and chronic disease risk [7–9]. For example, exclusive breastfeeding is recommended by the American Academy of Pediatrics and other as the optimal nutritional source for infants and is currently initiated by the majority of United States mothers [10,11]. It is possible that maternal diet influences breast milk composition, providing a pathway by which maternal diet may directly influence offspring growth [12]. It is known, for instance, that the composition of breast milk may alter epigenetic programming [13] and the infant gut microbiome and later health and obesity risk [14]. Maternal diet preferences also indirectly influence the general nutritional environment the infant is exposed to in the household through her purchasing and child feeding patterns [15].

Studies exploring the associations of maternal diet during pregnancy and lactation with offspring anthropometry or body composition have often focused on specific dietary components and the macronutrient composition of diet with inconsistent findings [8,16–18]. Dietary intake as measured by "single nutrients" is difficult to interpret given the interrelationships of most nutrients and biologically active components within and among foods and the associations of overall food-intake patterns with health [19]. Indices of diet quality, rather than specific nutrient intakes, may better reflect broader food-intake patterns, intakes of combinations of foods, nutrient-nutrient interactions, and may be more generalizable across populations [19]. A number of such indicators of diet quality have been developed and are increasingly used in health outcomes research [20].

There is a paucity of research assessing the relationship of maternal diet quality across the entire perinatal period (including both pregnancy and lactation) with offspring growth and body composition in early life [21–25]. Most studies have focused on anthropometry at birth [21,22] or in childhood [24], with few evaluating repeated measures of growth during infancy, a period of rapid change with potential effects extending across the lifespan [26]. Furthermore, limited research has examined the impact of maternal diet quality during pregnancy and lactation on measures of offspring body composition [23,25], which may provide different insights into growth trajectories and chronic disease risk [27].

The purpose of the present study is to evaluate associations of maternal diet quality during pregnancy and lactation with measures of infant growth (length-for-age (LAZ), weight-for-age (WAZ), and weight-for-length (WLZ) Z-scores from birth to six six months of age) and body composition (body fat percent (BF%)), fat mass (FM), and fat-free mass (FFM) at six months of age). We hypothesized that higher maternal diet quality (as measured by higher Healthy Eating Index–2015 (HEI–2015) total scores) would be associated with higher infant LAZ and lower infant WAZ and WLZ from birth to six months. We further hypothesized that higher maternal diet quality would be related to lower infant BF% and FM and higher infant FFM at six months of age.

2. Materials and Methods

2.1. Study Population

Mother–infant dyads included in these analyses were enrolled in the Mothers and Infants LinKed for Health (MILK) study, an ongoing prospective cohort study [28]. Mothers and their infants were recruited from Minneapolis, MN, and Oklahoma City, OK. A total of 367 pregnant women aged 21–45 years, with a pre-pregnancy BMI of 18.5–40.0 kg/m^2, an intention to exclusively breastfeed for at least 3 months, a healthy delivery (defined as <3 days in the hospital for vaginal deliveries and <5 days in the hospital for caesarean section deliveries), and who delivered singleton infants born at-term with a birth weight of ≥2500–≤4500 g were recruited into the study. Exclusion criteria for the study were as follows: (1) mothers consumed tobacco or >1 alcoholic drink per week during pregnancy/lactation; (2) mothers had a history of Type 1 or Type 2 diabetes or current gestational diabetes; (3) mothers had a congenital illness affecting infant feeding or growth; and/or (4) mothers were unable to speak or understand English. The final analytic sample included 354 mother–infant dyads who had maternal dietary data and infant growth measures on at least one of the time points when these items were measured.

The MILK study protocols were approved by the institutional review boards of the University of Minnesota, HealthPartners Institute and the University of Oklahoma Health Sciences Center. All women provided written informed consent at baseline and compensation was provided after each measurement visit.

2.2. Maternal Diet

Maternal dietary intake data was collected during the third trimester of pregnancy and at one and three months postpartum using the Diet History Questionnaire II (DHQ II), a food frequency questionnaire (FFQ) designed to assess frequency of intake and portion sizes for 134 food and beverage items and 8 dietary supplement items over the previous month [29]. A prior version of the DHQ II (DHQ I) with minimal modifications to food lists and nutrient databases has been evaluated for validity in prior research [29–31]. While one study showed that the DHQ I performed better than the Willett FFQ and Block FFQ at estimating energy and absolute nutrient intake [29], others showed that men and women under-reported energy and protein intakes on the DHQ I [30] which may lead to attenuation of estimated disease relative risks for these nutrients [31]. The DHQ II was analyzed using Diet Calc (National Cancer Institute, Bethesda, MD, USA), and food and nutrient values were generated using the United States Department of Agriculture (USDA) Food Patterns Equivalent Database and the Food and Nutrient Database for Dietary Studies.

Maternal diet quality during pregnancy and lactation was estimated using the HEI–2015, a scoring system designed to measure adherence to the 2015–2020 Dietary Guidelines for Americans (2015–2020 DGA) [32]. The psychometric properties of the HEI–2015 were evaluated using data from exemplary menus, a nationally representative sample and a prospective cohort study, with evidence supporting construct validity and reliability and criterion validity [33]. Previous studies have assessed the validity of prior HEI versions among pregnant women and showed that the index was useful in providing a composite dietary intake measure [34].

The HEI–2015 total score is the sum of 13 subcomponent scores that measure adequacy (Total Fruits, Whole Fruits, Total Vegetables, Greens and Beans, Whole Grains, Dairy Products, Total Protein Foods, Seafood and Plant Proteins, and Unsaturated:Saturated fats) and moderation (Refined Grains, Sodium, Added Sugars, and Saturated Fats). All subcomponents are scored from 0–5 or 0–10 based on intake between the minimum and maximum standards. Moderation components are reverse scored such that higher scores reflect lower intake. To account for variation in caloric intake between participants, all HEI–2015 components are standardized to 1000 kilocalories, except for the ratio of unsaturated to saturated fats. A higher HEI–2015 total score (out of 100) represents greater consistency of the diet with the 2015–2020 DGA (32). The code used to calculate the HEI–2015 scores was developed by the Division of Cancer Control and Population Sciences in the National Cancer Institute [35].

2.3. Infant Growth and Body Composition

At birth, one, three, and six months, infant length was measured with the infant undressed, but diapered using the Seca 416 infantometer (Seca, Birmingham, UK). Infant naked weight was measured using the high sensitivity scale embedded in the PEA POD (COSMED USA, Inc., Concord, CA, USA). Age and sex-specific LAZ, WAZ, and WLZ were subsequently calculated using the World

Health Organization Z-score classification system for term infants [36]. At six months, infant BF%, FM, and FFM were assessed utilizing dual X-ray energy absorptiometry (DXA), with the infant in a supine position wearing only a disposable diaper and swaddled in a light cotton blanket [37]. All measurements were obtained using standardized protocols and after cross-training of study staff [38].

2.4. Statistical Analyses

To provide a comprehensive description of the mother–infant dyads, demographic and clinical characteristics are presented as means ± standard deviations (SD) for continuous variables, and frequencies for categorical variables by tertiles of maternal HEI–2015 total scores during pregnancy. Differences in participant characteristics by maternal diet quality during pregnancy were evaluated using one-way ANOVAs and chi-square tests for continuous and categorical variables, respectively. Differences in participant characteristics among dyads who had complete dietary data during pregnancy and infant WLZ at birth ($N = 319$) versus those who had complete dietary data at three months postpartum and infant WLZ at six months ($N = 257$) were compared using t-tests and chi-square tests for continuous and categorical variables, respectively. Pearson correlations were calculated to test correlations between maternal HEI–2015 total scores during pregnancy and at one and three months postpartum.

Linear mixed effects models (PROC MIXED) were then used to evaluate the associations of repeated measures of maternal diet quality (HEI–2015 total scores) from pregnancy through three months postpartum with within-subject measures of infant LAZ, WAZ, and WLZ from birth to six months. The exposures were analyzed as continuous variables owing to the relatively limited sample size and after studying goodness of linear fit using scatter plots. The data were first adjusted for study site (Minneapolis, Oklahoma), maternal age (years), race (white, other), education (high school/GED/associates degree, Bachelor's degree, graduate degree), household income (<\$60,000, \$60,000–90,000, >\$90,000), and total energy intake (time-dependent; kilocalories) (Model 1). The full models (Model 2) were additionally adjusted for the following potential confounders: pre-pregnancy BMI (kg/m^2), gestational weight gain (kilograms), parity (0, $\geq$1), mode of delivery (vaginal, cesarean section), duration of exclusive breastfeeding (one, three, six months), infant gestational age (weeks), and infant sex (male, female). The main exposures and all confounders were included as main effects, but interactions with time were only retained if the corresponding p-value estimates were significant at <0.05.

Next, linear regression models (PROC GLM) were run to examine separately the associations of maternal diet quality during pregnancy, one and three months postpartum with infant BF%, FM, and FFM at six months of age. The models were similarly adjusted for all aforementioned potential confounders (Models 1 and 2), with the addition of infant WLZ at birth and infant exact age at six months (Model 2). Given that infant fat mass index (FMI) and fat-free mass index (FFMI) scale to length (fat mass or fat-free mass/length^2) and have been proposed as more precise indicators of adiposity and nutrition status [39], we also tested the associations of maternal perinatal diet quality with these indices. We further explored associations of maternal diet during pregnancy and lactation with compartment specific fat mass (trunk, arm, and leg) to detect changes in the relative distribution of fat within the body in sub-analyses.

Lastly, in sensitivity analyses to examine if the relationship of maternal diet with infant growth and/or body composition is modified by exclusivity of breastfeeding, the full models for both infant growth and body composition were re-run to include only infants who were fully breastfed to six months. All statistical analyses were performed using SAS 9.4 (SAS Institute Inc., Cary, NC, USA).

3. Results

3.1. Participant Characteristics

The mothers included in the present study were mostly highly educated, white, multiparous, fully breastfeeding at six months with average gestational weight gain, and above average HEI–2015 scores during pregnancy and lactation (Table 1). Maternal education, parity, HEI–2015 scores at one and three months postpartum, and infant gestational age differed significantly by tertiles of maternal HEI–2015 scores during the third trimester of pregnancy, whereby mothers with higher pregnancy HEI–2015 scores were on average more educated, nulliparous, had higher postpartum HEI–2015 scores and delivered their infants later ($p < 0.05$). No significant differences were observed between characteristics of the mother–infant dyads who had complete dietary data during pregnancy/infant WLZ at birth and complete dietary data at three months postpartum/infant WLZ at six months postpartum ($p >$ 0.05; data not shown). Maternal HEI–2015 scores during pregnancy were correlated with scores at one and three months postpartum ($r = 0.60$ and $r = 0.65$; $p < 0.001$, respectively). HEI–2015 scores at one and three months postpartum were also correlated with one another ($r = 0.63$, $p < 0.001$).

Table 1. Participant demographic and clinical characteristics by tertiles of maternal HEI–2015 total scores during the third trimester of pregnancy (n = 329).

Participant Characteristics	HEI–2015 Tertiles (T) [a]				
	Total	T1 (n = 109)	T2 (n = 110)	T3 (n = 110)	
	N (%) or Mean ± SD				p-Value
Study site					
Minnesota	233 (66)	69 (63)	72 (65)	78 (71)	0.47
Oklahoma	121 (34)	40 (37)	38 (35)	32 (29)	
Age, years	30.9 ± 4.1	30.2 ± 4.3	30.7 ± 4.4	31.4 ± 3.7	0.1
Race					
White	299 (86)	92 (85)	93 (87)	97 (89)	0.71
Other	49 (14)	16 (15)	14 (13)	12 (11)	
Education					
High school/GED/Associates degree	80 (24)	37 (36)	26 (24)	11 (11)	<0.001 *
Bachelor's degree	136 (40)	42 (41)	38 (36)	48 (46)	
Graduate degree	121 (36)	24 (23)	42 (40)	45 (43)	
Household income					
<$60,000	105 (31)	37 (36)	34 (32)	25 (24)	0.19
$60,000–90,000	85 (25)	30 (29)	24 (23)	27 (26)	
>90,000	147 (44)	36 (35)	48 (45)	52 (50)	
Parity					
0	146 (42)	33 (31)	54 (50)	52 (47)	0.01 *
≥1	204 (58)	74 (69)	55 (50)	58 (53)	
Pre-pregnancy BMI, kg/m^2	26.4 ± 5.4	27.2 ± 6.2	26.4 ± 4.9	25.5 ± 5.0	0.06
Gestational weight gain					
Below or within IOM guidelines	200 (57)	54 (501)	67 (62)	63 (57)	0.23
Exceeding IOM guidelines	149 (43)	53 (50)	41 (38)	47 (43)	
Energy intake during pregnancy	1827 ± 530	1747 ± 550	1876 ± 535	1859 ± 498	0.15
Mode of delivery					
Vaginal	278 (80)	90 (83)	82 (76)	87 (81)	0.39
Caesarean section	70 (20)	18 (17)	26 (24)	21 (19)	
HEI–2015 score during third trimester of pregnancy	67.2 ± 8.7	57.5 ± 5.8	67.8 ± 2.1	76.1 ± 4.0	<0.001 *
HEI–2015 score at one month postpartum	65.9 ± 8.4	60.6 ± 7.5	65.2 ± 7.0	71.2 ± 7.6	<0.001 *
HEI–2015 score at three months postpartum	66.1 ± 8.7	60.5 ± 7.9	65.3 ± 7.2	71.5 ± 7.4	<0.001 *

Table 1. *Cont.*

Participant Characteristics	HEI–2015 Tertiles (T) [a]				
	Total	T1 (n = 109)	T2 (n = 110)	T3 (n = 110)	
	N (%) or Mean ± SD				p-Value
Duration of exclusive breastfeeding					
one month	21 (7)	7 (7)	10 (10)	2 (2)	0.16
three months	58 (18)	20 (22)	16 (16)	20 (19)	
six months	235 (75)	65 (71)	74 (74)	81 (79)	
Infant gestational age, weeks	39.8 ± 1.1	39.7 ± 1.0	39.6 ± 1.1	40.0 ± 1.1	0.04 *
Infant sex					
Male	178 (50)	53 (49)	57 (52)	53 (48)	0.84
Female	176 (50)	56 (51)	53 (48)	57 (52)	

Abbreviations: HEI = Healthy Eating Index; BMI = Body Mass Index; IOM = Institute of Medicine. [a] HEI–2015 T1: ≤63.9; T2: 64.0–70.9; T3: ≥70.9. * $p < 0.05$ for tests of differences in participant characteristics by tertiles of maternal HEI–2015 total scores during pregnancy using chi-square and one-way ANOVAs for categorical and continuous variables, respectively. Data are presented as mean ± SD or column percentages.

As expected, higher intake of all adequacy components (except Dairy Products) and lower intake of all moderation components were seen among mothers in the highest versus lowest tertile of HEI–2015 total scores (Supplementary file Table S1). Higher (better) scores for Whole and Total Fruits, Total Vegetables, Greens and Beans, Seafood and Plant Proteins, Total Protein Foods, Refined Grains, and Added Sugars appeared to drive higher average HEI–2015 total scores. HEI–2015 total scores were normally distributed at all time points and average scores were highest during the third trimester of pregnancy (Supplementary file Figure S1).

Among infants, on average, LAZ decreased from birth to six months, whereas WAZ and WLZ decreased from birth to three months, followed by a subsequent increase after three months (Table 2). The mean fat mass among infants at six months was approximately 2.8 kg (34% of total body weight), with most of the fat distributed in the legs (1.08 kg) and trunk (0.92 kg).

3.2. Maternal Diet Quality and Infant Growth

Maternal diet quality through pregnancy and lactation was inversely and significantly associated with WLZ, such that a 10-unit increase in the HEI–2015 total score from pregnancy through three months postpartum was associated with an approximately 0.12 lower infant WLZ from birth to six months in the fully-adjusted model ($\beta = -0.12$, $p = 0.02$) (Table 3). There was no significant interaction between maternal diet quality from pregnancy through three months postpartum and time, suggesting no difference between prenatal and postnatal exposure on these outcomes. No associations of maternal diet quality from pregnancy through three months postpartum with infant LAZ or WAZ were observed. In sensitivity analyses, findings for infant LAZ, WAZ, and WLZ were comparable when models were restricted to the 75% of study infants who were fully breastfed to six months.

3.3. Maternal Diet Quality and Infant Body Composition

Maternal diet quality during pregnancy and lactation was also inversely associated with infant adiposity (Table 4). Specifically, a 10-unit increase in HEI–2015 total scores during pregnancy was associated with an approximately 0.6% lower infant BF% at six months ($\beta = -0.58$, $p = 0.05$). A 10-unit increase in HEI–2015 total score at one month postpartum was associated with more than a 1% lower infant BF% ($\beta = -1.28$, $p < 0.001$) and 0.10 kg lower FM ($\beta = -0.13$, $p = 0.001$) at six months. Likewise, a 10-unit increase in HEI–2015 total score at three months postpartum was associated with an approximately 0.7% lower infant BF% ($\beta = -0.66$, $p = 0.01$) and 0.10 kg lower FM ($\beta = -0.10$, $p = 0.01$) at six months. Findings were similar for associations between maternal diet quality at one and three months postpartum and FMI/FFMI (data not shown). In sub-analyses, a 10-unit increase in HEI–2015 total scores at one and three months postpartum were associated with both lower trunk FM ($\beta = -0.06$,

$p = 0.001$ and $\beta = -0.04$, $p = 0.03$, respectively) and lower leg FM ($\beta = -0.05$, $p = 0.01$ and $\beta = -0.04$, $p = 0.03$, respectively). No other associations between maternal HEI–2015 scores during pregnancy or lactation and infant body composition were found. In sensitivity analyses that restricted the analysis to study infants that were fully breastfeeding at six months of age, associations between maternal HEI–2015 scores and infant body composition were similar to those incorporating all infants, except for associations between maternal HEI–2015 scores at three months postpartum and infant BF% and FM at six months, which were no longer significant ($p < 0.10$).

Table 2. Average infant growth measures from birth to six months and body composition measures at six months.

Infant Characteristics	N	Mean ± SD
Infant Growth from Birth to Six Months		
Weight-for-age, Z-scores		
Birth	350	0.46 ± 0.87
one month	343	0.13 ± 0.87
three months	332	−0.07 ± 0.88
six months	321	0.04 ± 0.96
Length-for-age, Z-scores		
Birth	342	1.17 ± 1.23
one month	346	0.06 ± 1.09
three months	332	−0.03 ± 1.06
six months	321	−0.20 ± 1.09
Weight-for-length, Z-scores		
Birth	341	−0.72 ± 1.40
one month	342	0.12 ± 1.08
three months	332	0.02 ± 0.98
six months	321	0.33 ± 1.07
Infant body composition at six months		
Total body fat, %	317	33.98 ± 3.76
Fat mass, kg	317	2.76 ± 0.48
Fat-free mass, kg	317	5.29 ± 0.67
Trunk fat mass, kg	317	0.92 ± 0.22
Arm fat mass, kg	317	0.38 ± 0.20
Leg fat mass, kg	317	1.08 ± 0.23

Abbreviations: SD = standard deviation.

Table 3. Associations of HEI–2015 total scores from the third trimester of pregnancy through three months postpartum with infant growth measures from birth to six months.

	Model 1				**Model 2**			
Infant Growth Measures from Birth to Six Months	**N**	**β [a]**	**SE**	***p*-Value**	**N**	**β [a]**	**SE**	***p*-Value**
LAZ	330	0.05	0.04	0.25	290	0.02	0.04	0.58
WAZ	330	−0.02	0.03	0.43	290	−0.04	0.03	0.15
WLZ	330	−0.13	0.05	**0.01**	290	−0.12	0.05	**0.02**

Abbreviations: SE = standard error; LAZ = length-for-age Z-score; WAZ = weight-for-age Z-score; WLZ = weight-for-length Z-score. [a] HEI–2015 total score was converted such that a 1-unit increase corresponds to a 10-point increase in HEI–2015 score. Model 1 = adjusted for study site, maternal age, race, education, household income and total energy intake during pregnancy. Model 2 = Model 1 + maternal pre-pregnancy BMI, gestational weight gain, mode of delivery, parity, breastfeeding exclusivity at six months, infant sex, and gestational age. Bolded values are statistically significant at $p < 0.05$.

Table 4. Associations of HEI–2015 total scores during the third trimester of pregnancy and at one and three months postpartum with infant body composition at six months.

	Model 1				Model 2			
Infant Body Composition Measures at Six Months	**N**	**β [a]**	**SE**	***p*-Value**	**N**	**β [a]**	**SE**	***p*-Value**
HEI–2015 total scores during pregnancy								
BF%	281	−0.72	0.28	**0.01**	262	−0.58	0.29	**0.05**
FM	281	−0.06	0.04	0.12	262	−0.03	0.04	0.36
FFM	281	0.002	0.05	0.97	262	−0.001	0.05	0.99
HEI–2015 total scores at one month postpartum								
BF%	254	−1.22	0.30	**<0.001**	235	−1.28	0.30	**<0.001**
FM	254	−0.10	0.04	**0.01**	235	−0.13	0.04	**0.001**
FFM	254	−0.003	0.05	0.94	235	−0.05	0.04	0.28
HEI–2015 total scores at three months postpartum								
BF%	248	−0.69	0.25	**0.01**	229	−0.66	0.26	**0.01**
FM	248	−0.09	0.04	**0.02**	229	−0.10	0.04	**0.01**
FFM	248	−0.04	0.05	0.52	229	−0.05	0.06	0.37

Abbreviations: BF% = body fat percent; FM = fat mass; FFM = fat free mass. [a] HEI–2015 total score was converted such that a 1-unit increase corresponds to a 10-point increase in HEI–2015 score. Model 1 = adjusted for study site, maternal age, race, education, household income, and total energy intake during pregnancy. Model 2 = Model 1 + maternal pre-pregnancy BMI, gestational weight gain, mode of delivery, parity, breastfeeding exclusivity at six months, infant sex, gestational age, weight-for-length Z-score, and exact age at body composition assessment. Bolded values are statistically significant at $p < 0.05$.

4. Discussion

In this prospective cohort study, we examined the associations of maternal diet quality during pregnancy and lactation with infant growth from birth to six months and body composition at six months. We found that higher maternal diet quality (as evidenced by higher HEI–2015 scores) from pregnancy through three months postpartum was inversely associated with infant WLZ from birth to six months and BF% at six months. Similarly, higher maternal diet quality during lactation (one and three months postpartum) was inversely related to infant FM (specifically trunk and leg fat mass) at six months. These associations occurred independently of important confounders, such as pre-pregnancy BMI and gestational weight gain. This research adds to accumulating animal and human evidence that suggests that not only the in utero but also the postnatal nutritional environment influences infant growth and body composition in infants who are breastfed and points to a potentially important role of dietary constituents and quality in shaping offspring future health [6].

Our findings are concordant with those of several other studies assessing mostly maternal prenatal diet quality and offspring growth and/or body composition at birth or later in life [21–25]. In line with our findings, Shapiro et al. [23] showed that maternal HEI–2010 scores of ≤57 (v > 57) measured via repeated 24-h recalls throughout pregnancy were associated with higher infant BF% ($\beta = 0.58$, $p < 0.05$) and FM ($\beta = 20.74$, $p < 0.05$) at birth among mother-offspring pairs in the Healthy Start Study in the United States. Likewise, in a pooled analysis of mother-child pairs from Project Viva (United States) and the Rhea study (Greece) [24], a three-point increase in the Mediterranean diet score during the first—second trimester of pregnancy (evaluated using an FFQ) was associated with lower offspring BMI Z-scores in mid-childhood at a magnitude similar to that found for WLZ in our study ($\beta = -0.14$, 95% CI = −0.15, −0.13).

Conversely, several studies have not found significant associations between maternal prenatal diet and infant growth [8,21,40]. For example, using data from the Infant Feeding Practices Study II, Poon et al. [21] showed that both the alternate Mediterranean diet score and the Alternative Healthy Eating Index for Pregnancy (AHEI-P) diet score (measured using an FFQ during the third trimester of pregnancy) were unrelated to infant birth weight, birth size (large or small for gestational age), birth

WLZ or change in WLZ at 4–6 months. Similarly, Rifas-Shiman et al. [40] reported a non-significant lower risk of giving birth to a small-for-gestational age infant with increasing AHEI-P scores calculated from responses to an FFQ during the first trimester of pregnancy among mother–infant dyads in Project Viva. The literature does not adequately assess the role of maternal postpartum diet on infant growth and/or body composition, which theoretically influences the infant via breast milk or the household nutritional environment. In one study assessing maternal macronutrient intake during the first trimester of pregnancy and at five years postpartum, Murrin et al. [8] demonstrated that higher prenatal sugar intake and both prenatal and postnatal saturated fat intake as measured by an FFQ were associated with a non-significant trend towards higher likelihood of having overweight/obese offspring. Although many diet quality scores were moderately to strongly correlated in various populations [41,42], use of the HEI–2015 as a measure of diet quality during pregnancy and postpartum may explain some discrepancies in findings and may limit our ability to compare findings to other studies using different diet quality scores or prior versions of the HEI.

The HEI–2015 aims to reflect the most recent DGA (2015–2020) and is thus generalizable to other studies using these guidelines [32]. The mean HEI–2015 scores across pregnancy and lactation ranged from 65.9 to 67.2 in our cohort. These scores are higher than the average scores for American adults (~58 out of 100) [43] but may reflect the potential improvement in dietary intake that women may pursue during the perinatal period [44]. Our study population is also more socioeconomically advantaged and healthy relative to pregnant and lactating women in the United States, as evidenced by a higher maternal education level, household income, lower pre-pregnancy BMI, and longer duration of exclusive breastfeeding. Given the dearth of studies that parallel the timing and methods of our exposure and outcome assessment and confounders considered, additional research is warranted to replicate our findings in larger, more diverse cohorts.

It is important to note that, although our findings are qualitatively similar to those of several other studies of maternal perinatal diet with infant growth and/or body composition [23,24], our effect sizes and those of related studies are small relative to the contribution of other maternal factors, such as obesity and gestational weight gain [45]. Even so, it is likely that infant adiposity is multifactorial, with several elements each contributing small effects to overall growth and fat accrual [46]. Recognizing and targeting these immediately modifiable factors, such as maternal diet in holistic interventions, could have a significant influence on offspring obesity throughout the lifespan [47]. For example, within the context of our study, a 10-unit increase in the HEI–2015 score could translate into increasing consumption of fruits from none to $\geq$0.8 cup equivalents to maximize points for this adequacy subcomponent (10 points). Alternatively, mothers could reduce consumption of refined grains from $\geq$4.3 oz equivalents to $\leq$1.8 oz equivalents to maximize points for this moderation subcomponent (10 points).

Maternal perinatal diet quality may impact infant growth and/or body composition through numerous mechanisms. Aside from direct influences on fetal growth, maternal prenatal and postnatal nutrition may lead to epigenetic modifications that affect offspring metabolic function, growth hormone secretion and appetite programming [13,48]. Higher HEI scores were associated with greater intake of fruits, fibers, folate, and vitamin C, higher plasma concentrations of carotenoids and vitamin C, and greater dietary variety in previous research [49]. In our study, we found that mothers in the highest tertile of HEI–2015 had especially high scores (scores that were greater than or equal to 80% of the maximum possible points for index components) on the Whole and Total Fruits, Total Vegetables, Greens and Beans, Seafood and Plant Proteins, Total Protein Foods, Refined Grains, and Added Sugars components. These beneficial characteristics of maternal diet are associated with reduced oxidative stress and inflammation, which may be reflected in the nutritional environment in the household during this critical period of offspring growth and development and throughout the life course [50]. Maternal diet may also alter the fatty acid profile [51] and the hormonal [52] and growth factor [53] content of breast milk the infants in this study were ingesting, which could theoretically influence growth and body composition [54].

Our study has several notable strengths, including the prospective cohort design with repeated measures of maternal diet from pregnancy through postpartum and infant growth from birth to six months. These factors provide a valuable opportunity to assess concurrent and prospective associations of maternal nutrition with offspring growth at a critical period of sensitivity in the life course. Our use of overall diet quality as an exposure (*v* specific macronutrients) may better mirror whole diet, accounting for the synergistic, interactive, and cumulative effects of multiple foods and nutrients, and may be a more practical tool for nutrition communication throughout pregnancy and lactation [19]. We also measured infant body composition at six months of age using DXA, which accurately measures fat mass and soft-tissue body components and serves as a marker of potential developmental programming [55]. We were able to account for the influence of a range of demographic, clinical, and lifestyle factors, which may confound the association of maternal diet and offspring growth and/or body composition.

We acknowledge potential limitations in our study. Maternal dietary intake was self-reported by mothers using the DHQ-II, which is subject to recall bias, measurement error, and exposure misclassification [56,57]. Nonetheless, this FFQ has been evaluated for validity in adult populations [29] and our models adjusted for total energy intake to reduce potential systematic measurement error. Our relatively small sample size and loss of data at later time points may have decreased statistical power. However, mother–infant dyads with complete exposure and outcome data during pregnancy/at birth were similar to those with complete exposure and outcome data at three months postpartum/six months. Our study population comprises predominantly non-Hispanic white women, which may limit generalizability across race/ethnicities. We did not follow-up infants beyond six months of age, which may limit our understanding of the long-term consequences of maternal nutrition on offspring growth, body composition and cardiometabolic diseases across the life course [58,59]. Important confounding variables may have not been controlled for in analyses. Most notably, it is possible that maternal diet is a marker for infant feeding practices that may influence child growth outcomes (including responsive infant feeding and timing of introduction of solid foods). Lastly, given the observational nature of the study, it is not possible to draw causal inferences from observed associations.

5. Conclusions

In conclusion, we found that higher maternal diet quality from pregnancy through three months postpartum was associated with lower infant WLZ from birth to six months and lower infant BF% at six months. Likewise, higher maternal diet quality at one and three months postpartum was associated with lower total body, trunk, and leg FM at six months. These findings point to the importance of focusing on maternal diet quality at critical periods of development, and the appreciable, albeit small, independent influence that maternal nutrition may play in optimal infant growth and fat development. Additional research is needed to determine the interplay between maternal perinatal diet quality, long-term offspring growth/body composition, and later chronic disease risk susceptibility in hopes of aiding current efforts to develop more specific dietary guidelines for pregnant and postpartum women.

Author Contributions: Conceptualization, D.A.F. and E.W.D.; Data curation, J.L.H.; Formal analysis, M.J.T., D.R.J.J., and E.W.D.; Funding acquisition, D.A.F. and E.W.D.; Investigation, L.P.F., K.M.D., and A.M.T.; Supervision, E.W.D.; Writing—original draft, M.J.T.; Writing—review & editing, L.P.F., K.M.D., A.M.T., E.O.K., P.M.M., K.M.W., K.M.R., D.A.F., D.R.J.J., L.J.H., and E.W.D.

Acknowledgments: We would like to gratefully acknowledge and thank the mothers who gave us their time and agreed to participate in the MILK study.

References

1. Calkins, K.; Devaskar, S.U. Fetal origins of adult disease. *Curr. Probl. Pediatr. Adolesc. Health Care* **2011**, *41*, 158–176. [CrossRef] [PubMed]
2. Kwon, E.J.; Kim, Y.J. What is fetal programming?: A lifetime health is under the control of in utero health. *Obstet. Gynecol. Sci.* **2017**, *60*, 506–519. [CrossRef] [PubMed]
3. Williams, C.B.; Mackenzie, K.C.; Gahagan, S. The effect of maternal obesity on the offspring. *Clin. Obstet. Gynecol.* **2014**, *57*, 508–515. [CrossRef]
4. Kaar, J.L.; Crume, T.; Brinton, J.T.; Bischoff, K.J.; McDuffie, R.; Dabelea, D. Maternal obesity, gestational weight gain, and offspring adiposity: The exploring perinatal outcomes among children study. *J. Pediatr.* **2014**, *165*, 509–515. [CrossRef] [PubMed]
5. Mourtakos, S.P.; Tambalis, K.D.; Panagiotakos, D.B.; Antonogeorgos, G.; Arnaoutis, G.; Karteroliotis, K.; Sidossiset, L.S. Maternal lifestyle characteristics during pregnancy, and the risk of obesity in the offspring: A study of 5125 children. *BMC Pregnancy Childbirth* **2015**, *15*, 1–8. [CrossRef] [PubMed]
6. Parlee, S.D.; MacDougald, O.A. Maternal nutrition and risk of obesity in offspring: The Trojan horse of developmental plasticity. *Biochim. Biophys. Acta* **2014**, *1842*, 495–506. [CrossRef]
7. Bayol, S.A.; Farrington, S.J.; Stickland, N.C. A maternal 'junk food' diet in pregnancy and lactation promotes an exacerbated taste for 'junk food' and a greater propensity for obesity in rat offspring. *Br. J. Nutr.* **2007**, *98*, 843–851. [CrossRef] [PubMed]
8. Murrin, C.; Shrivastava, A.; Kelleher, C.C.; Lifeways Cross-Generation Cohort Study Steering Group. Maternal macronutrient intake during pregnancy and 5 years postpartum and associations with child weight status aged five. *Eur. J. Clin. Nutr.* **2013**, *67*, 670–679. [CrossRef] [PubMed]
9. Jackson, C.M.; Alexander, B.T.; Roach, L.; Haggerty, D.; Marbury, D.C.; Hutchens, Z.M.; Flynn, E.R.; Maric-Bilkan, C. Exposure to maternal overnutrition and a high-fat diet during early postnatal development increases susceptibility to renal and metabolic injury later in life. *Am. J. Physiol. Renal Physiol.* **2012**, *302*, F774–F783. [CrossRef] [PubMed]
10. Section on Breastfeeding. Breastfeeding and the use of human milk. *Pediatrics* **2012**, *129*, 827–841. [CrossRef] [PubMed]
11. Centers for Disease Control and Prevention. Breastfeeding Report Card—United States. 2018. Available online: https://www.cdc.gov/breastfeeding/pdf/2018breastfeedingreportcard.pdf (accessed on 8 December 2018).
12. Ballard, O.; Morrow, A.L. Human milk composition: Nutrients and bioactive factors. *Pediatr. Clin. N. Am.* **2013**, *60*, 49–74. [CrossRef] [PubMed]
13. Indrio, F.; Martini, S.; Francavilla, R.; Corvaglia, L.; Cristofori, F.; Mastrolia, S.A.; Neu, J.; Rautava, S.; Spena, G.R.; Raimondi, F.; et al. Epigenetic Matters: The Link between Early Nutrition, Microbiome, and Long-term Health Development. *Front. Pediatr.* **2017**, *5*, 1–14. [CrossRef] [PubMed]
14. Chu, D.M.; Meyer, K.M.; Prince, A.L.; Aagaard, K.M. Impact of maternal nutrition in pregnancy and lactation on offspring gut microbial composition and function. *Gut Microbes* **2016**, *7*, 459–470. [CrossRef] [PubMed]
15. Dhana, K.; Haines, J.; Liu, G.; Zhang, C.; Wang, X.; Field, A.E.; Chavarro, J.E.; Sun, Q. Association between maternal adherence to healthy lifestyle practices and risk of obesity in offspring: Results from two prospective cohort studies of mother-child pairs in the United States. *BMJ* **2018**, *362*, k2486. [CrossRef]
16. Tielemans, M.J.; Steegers, E.A.P.; Voortman, T.; Jaddoe, V.W.V.; Rivadeneira, F.; Franco, O.H.; Kiefte-de Jong, J.C. Protein intake during pregnancy and offspring body composition at 6 years: The Generation R Study. *Eur. J. Nutr.* **2017**, *56*, 2151–2160. [CrossRef] [PubMed]
17. Moon, R.J.; Harvey, N.C.; Robinson, S.M.; Ntani, G.; Davies, J.H.; Inskip, H.M.; Godfrey, K.M.; Dennison, E.M.; Calder, P.C.; Cooper, C.; et al. Maternal plasma polyunsaturated fatty acid status in late pregnancy is associated with offspring body composition in childhood. *J. Clin. Endocrinol. Metab.* **2013**, *98*, 299–307. [CrossRef] [PubMed]
18. Mckenzie, K.M.; Dissanayake, H.U.; McMullan, R.; ICaterson, I.D.; Celermajer, D.S.; Gordon, A.; Hyett, J.; Meroni, A.; Phang, M.; Raynes-Greenow, C.; et al. Quantity and Quality of Carbohydrate Intake during Pregnancy, Newborn Body Fatness and Cardiac Autonomic Control: Conferred Cardiovascular Risk? *Nutrients* **2017**, *9*, 1375. [CrossRef]
19. Tapsell, L.C.; Neale, E.P.; Satija, A.; Hu, F.B. Foods, Nutrients, and Dietary Patterns: Interconnections and Implications for Dietary Guidelines. *Adv. Nutr.* **2016**, *7*, 445–454. [CrossRef]

20. Schwingshackl, L.; Hoffmann, G. Diet quality as assessed by the Healthy Eating Index, the Alternate Healthy Eating Index, the Dietary Approaches to Stop Hypertension score, and health outcomes: A systematic review and meta-analysis of cohort studies. *J. Acad. Nutr. Diet.* **2015**, *115*, 780–800. [CrossRef]
21. Poon, A.K.; Yeung, E.; Boghossian, N.; Albert, P.S.; Zhang, C. Maternal Dietary Patterns during Third Trimester in Association with Birthweight Characteristics and Early Infant Growth. *Scientifica* **2013**, *2013*, 786409. [CrossRef]
22. Rodríguez-Bernal, C.L.; Rebagliato, M.; Iñiguez, C.; Vioque, J.; Navarrete-Muñoz, E.M.; Murcia, M.; Bolumar, F.; Marco, A.; Ballester, F. Diet quality in early pregnancy and its effects on fetal growth outcomes: The Infancia y Medio Ambiente (Childhood and Environment) Mother and Child Cohort Study in Spain. *Am. J. Clin. Nutr.* **2010**, *91*, 1659–1666. [CrossRef]
23. Shapiro, A.L.; Kaar, J.L.; Crume, T.L.; Starling, A.P.; Siega-Riz, A.M.; Ringham, B.M.; Glueck, D.H.; Norris, J.M.; Barbour, L.A.; Friedman, J.E.; et al. Maternal diet quality in pregnancy and neonatal adiposity: The Healthy Start Study. *Int. J. Obes.* **2016**, *40*, 1056–1062. [CrossRef]
24. Chatzi, L.; Rifas-Shiman, S.L.; Georgiou, V.; Joung, K.E.; Koinaki, S.; Chalkiadaki, G.; Margioris, A.; Sarri, K.; Vassilaki, M.; Vafeiadi, M.; et al. Adherence to the Mediterranean diet during pregnancy and offspring adiposity and cardiometabolic traits in childhood. *Pediatr. Obes.* **2017**, *12*, 47–56. [CrossRef] [PubMed]
25. Van den Broek, M.; Leermakers, E.T.; Jaddoe, V.W.; Steegers, E.A.; Rivadeneira, F.; Raat, H.; Hofman, A.; Franco, O.H.; Kiefte-de Jong, J.C. Maternal dietary patterns during pregnancy and body composition of the child at age 6 y: The Generation R Study. *Am. J. Clin. Nutr.* **2015**, *102*, 873–880. [CrossRef] [PubMed]
26. Gillman, M.W. Early infancy as a critical period for development of obesity and related conditions. In *Importance of Growth for Health and Development*; Nestec Ltd.: Vevey, Switzerland; S. Karger AG: Basel, Switzerland, 2010; Volume 65, pp. 13–20.
27. Rolland-Cachera, M.F.; Péneau, S. Growth trajectories associated with adult obesity. *World Rev. Nutr. Diet.* **2013**, *106*, 127–134. [PubMed]
28. Whitaker, K.M.; Marino, R.C.; Haapala, J.L.; Foster, L.; Smith, K.D.; Teague, A.M.; Jacobs, D.R., Jr.; Fontaine, P.L.; McGovern, P.M.; Schoenfuss, T.C.; et al. Associations of Maternal Weight Status Before, During, and After Pregnancy with Inflammatory Markers in Breast Milk. *Obesity* **2017**, *25*, 2092–2099. [CrossRef] [PubMed]
29. Subar, A.F.; Thompson, F.E.; Kipnis, V.; Midthune, D.; Hurwitz, P.; McNutt, S.; McIntosh, A.; Rosenfeld, S. Comparative validation of the Block, Willett, and National Cancer Institute food frequency questionnaires: The Eating at America's Table Study. *Am. J. Epidemiol.* **2001**, *154*, 1089–1099. [CrossRef] [PubMed]
30. Subar, A.F.; Kipnis, V.; Troiano, R.P.; Midthune, D.; Schoeller, D.A.; Bingham, S.; Sharbaugh, C.O.; Trabulsi, J.; Runswick, S.; Ballard-Barbash, R.; et al. Using intake biomarkers to evaluate the extent of dietary misreporting in a large sample of adults: The OPEN study. *Am. J. Epidemiol.* **2003**, *158*, 1–13. [CrossRef] [PubMed]
31. Kipnis, V.; Subar, A.F.; Midthune, D.; Midthune, D.; Schoeller, D.A.; Bingham, S.; Sharbaugh, C.O.; Trabulsi, J.; Runswick, S.; Ballard-Barbash, R.; et al. Structure of dietary measurement error: Results of the OPEN biomarker study. *Am. J. Epidemiol.* **2003**, *158*, 14–21. [CrossRef] [PubMed]
32. Krebs-Smith, S.M.; Pannucci, T.E.; Subar, A.F.; Kirkpatrick, S.I.; Lerman, J.L.; Tooze, J.A.; Wilson, M.M.; Reedy, J. Update of the Healthy Eating Index: HEI-2015. *J. Acad. Nutr. Diet.* **2018**, *118*, 1591–1602. [CrossRef]
33. Reedy, J.; Lerman, J.L.; Krebs-Smith, S.M.; Kirkpatrick, S.I.; Pannucci, T.E.; Wilson, M.M.; Subar, A.F.; Kahle, L.L.; Tooze, J.A. Evaluation of the Healthy Eating Index-2015. *J. Acad. Nutr. Diet.* **2018**, *118*, 1622–1633. [CrossRef]
34. Pick, M.E.; Edwards, M.; Moreau, D.; Ryan, E.A. Assessment of diet quality in pregnant women using the Healthy Eating Index. *J. Am. Diet. Assoc.* **2005**, *105*, 240–246. [CrossRef] [PubMed]
35. National Cancer Institute. SAS Code. US Department of Health and Human Services. 2018. Available online: https://epi.grants.cancer.gov/hei/sas-code.html (accessed on 22 January 2019).
36. WHO Multicentre Growth Reference Study Group. WHO Child Growth Standards based on length/height, weight and age. *Acta Paediatr. Suppl.* **2006**, *450*, 76–85.
37. Mazess, R.B.; Barden, H.S.; Bisek, J.P.; Hanson, J. Dual-energy X-ray absorptiometry for total-body and regional bone-mineral and soft-tissue composition. *Am. J. Clin. Nutr.* **1990**, *51*, 1106–1112. [CrossRef] [PubMed]

38. Lohman, T.M.R.; Roche, A.F. *Anthropometric Standardization Reference Manual*; Human Kinetics Books: Champaign, IL, USA, 2011.
39. Weber, D.R.; Leonard, M.B.; Zemel, B.S. Body composition analysis in the pediatric population. *Pediatr. Endocrinol. Rev.* **2012**, *10*, 130–139. [PubMed]
40. Rifas-Shiman, S.L.; Rich-Edwards, J.W.; Kleinman, K.P.; Oken, E.; Gillman, M.W. Dietary quality during pregnancy varies by maternal characteristics in Project Viva: A US cohort. *J. Am. Diet. Assoc.* **2009**, *109*, 1004–1011. [CrossRef]
41. George, S.M.; Ballard-Barbash, R.; Manson, J.E.; Reedy, J.; Shikany, J.M.; Subar, A.F.; Tinker, L.F.; Vitolins, M.; Neuhouser, M.L. Comparing indices of diet quality with chronic disease mortality risk in postmenopausal women in the Women's Health Initiative Observational Study: Evidence to inform national dietary guidance. *Am. J. Epidemiol.* **2014**, *180*, 616–625. [CrossRef]
42. Fallaize, R.; Livingstone, K.M.; Celis-Morales, C.; Macready, A.L.; San-Cristobal, R.; Navas-Carretero, S.; Marsaux, C.F.; O'Donovan, C.B.; Kolossa, S.; Moschonis, G.; et al. Association between Diet-Quality Scores, Adiposity, Total Cholesterol and Markers of Nutritional Status in European Adults: Findings from the Food4Me Study. *Nutrients* **2018**, *10*, 49. [CrossRef]
43. United States Department of Agriculture. The Center for Nutrition Policy and Promotion. HEI Scores for Americans. Available online: https://www.cnpp.usda.gov/hei-scores-americans (accessed on 22 January 2019).
44. Forbes, L.E.; Graham, J.E.; Berglund, C.; Bell, R.C. Dietary Change during Pregnancy and Women's Reasons for Change. *Nutrients* **2018**, *10*, 1032. [CrossRef]
45. Black, M.H.; Sacks, D.A.; Xiang, A.H.; Lawrence, J.M. The relative contribution of prepregnancy overweight and obesity, gestational weight gain, and IADPSG-defined gestational diabetes mellitus to fetal overgrowth. *Diabetes Care* **2013**, *36*, 56–62. [CrossRef] [PubMed]
46. Hruby, A.; Hu, F.B. The Epidemiology of Obesity: A Big Picture. *Pharmacoeconomics* **2015**, *33*, 673–689. [CrossRef] [PubMed]
47. Haire-Joshu, D.; Tabak, R. Preventing Obesity Across Generations: Evidence for Early Life Intervention. *Annu. Rev. Public Health* **2016**, *37*, 253–271. [CrossRef]
48. Mühlhäusler, B.S.; Adam, C.L.; McMillen, I.C. Maternal nutrition and the programming of obesity: The brain. *Organogenesis* **2008**, *4*, 144–152. [CrossRef]
49. Hann, C.S.; Rock, C.L.; King, I.; Drewnowski, A. Validation of the Healthy Eating Index with use of plasma biomarkers in a clinical sample of women. *Am. J. Clin. Nutr.* **2001**, *74*, 479–486. [CrossRef] [PubMed]
50. Shrivastava, A.; Murrin, C.; Sweeney, M.R.; Heavey, P.; Kelleher, C.C.; Lifeways Cross-generation Cohort Study Steering Group. Familial intergenerational and maternal aggregation patterns in nutrient intakes in the Lifeways Cross-Generation Cohort Study. *Public Health Nutr.* **2013**, *16*, 1476–1486. [CrossRef] [PubMed]
51. Bravi, F.; Wiens, F.; Decarli, A.; Dal Pont, A.; Agostoni, C.; Ferraroni, M. Impact of maternal nutrition on breast-milk composition: A systematic review. *Am. J. Clin. Nutr.* **2016**, *104*, 646–662. [CrossRef] [PubMed]
52. Kocaadam, B.; Köksal, E.; Türkyılmaz, C. Are breast milk adipokines affected by maternal dietary factors? *J. Pediatr. Endocrinol. Metab.* **2018**, *31*, 1099–1104. [CrossRef] [PubMed]
53. Lu, M.; Jiang, J.; Wu, K.; Li, D. Epidermal growth factor and transforming growth factor-α in human milk of different lactation stages and different regions and their relationship with maternal diet. *Food Funct.* **2018**, *9*, 1199–1204. [CrossRef]
54. Lind, M.V.; Larnkjær, A.; Mølgaard, C.; Michaelsen, K.F. Breastfeeding, Breast Milk Composition, and Growth Outcomes. In *Recent Research in Nutrition and Growth*; Nestlé Nutrition Institute: Vevey, Switzerland; S. Karger AG: Basel, Switzerland, 2018; Volume 89, pp. 63–77.
55. Demerath, E.W.; Fields, D.A. Body composition assessment in the infant. *Am. J. Hum. Biol.* **2014**, *26*, 291–304. [CrossRef]
56. Naska, A.; Lagiou, A.; Lagiou, P. Dietary assessment methods in epidemiological research: Current state of the art and future prospects. *F1000Research* **2017**, *6*, 1–8. [CrossRef]
57. Shim, J.S.; Oh, K.; Kim, H.C. Dietary assessment methods in epidemiologic studies. *Epidemiol. Health* **2014**, *36*, 1–8. [CrossRef] [PubMed]
58. Maslova, E.; Rytter, D.; Bech, B.H.; Henriksen, T.B.; Rasmussen, M.A.; Olsen, S.F.; Halldorsson, T.I. Maternal

protein intake during pregnancy and offspring overweight 20 y later. *Am. J. Clin. Nutr.* **2014**, *100*, 1139–1148. [CrossRef] [PubMed]

59. Maslova, E.; Rytter, D.; Bech, B.H.; Henriksen, T.B.; Olsen, S.F.; Halldorsson, T.I. Maternal intake of fat in pregnancy and offspring metabolic health—A prospective study with 20 years of follow-up. *Clin. Nutr.* **2016**, *35*, 475–483. [CrossRef] [PubMed]

5

Exposure to Vitamin D Fortification Policy in Prenatal Life and the Risk of Childhood Asthma: Results from the D-Tect Study

Fanney Thorsteinsdottir [1,*], Ekaterina Maslova [2,3], Ramune Jacobsen [1,4], Peder Frederiksen [1], Amélie Keller [1], Vibeke Backer [5] and Berit Lilienthal Heitmann [1,6,7]

1 Fanney Thorsteinsdottir, Research Unit for Dietary Studies, The Parker Institute, Bisbebjerg og Frederiksberg Hospital, Nordre Fasanvej 57, 2000 Frederiksberg, Denmark; ramune.jacobsen@sund.ku.dk (R.J.); peder.frederiksen@regionh.dk (P.F.); amelie.cleo.keller@regionh.dk (A.K.); berit.lilienthal.heitmann@egionh.dk (B.L.H.)

2 Department of Primary Care and Public Health, Imperial College London, London W6 8RP, UK; ekaterina.maslova14@imperial.ac.uk

3 Centre for Fetal Programming, Department of Epidemiology Research, Statens Serum Institut, 2300 Copenhagen, Denmark

4 Department of Pharmacy, University of Copenhagen, 2100 Copenhagen, Denmark

5 Department of Respiratory Medicine, Bispebjerg University Hospital, 2400 Copenhagen, Denmark; backer@dadlnet.dk

6 The Boden Institute of Obesity, Nutrition, Exercise & Eating Disorders, University of Sydney, Sydney, NSW 2006, Australia

7 The Department of Public Health, Section for General Practice, University of Copenhagen, 2100 Copenhagen, Denmark

* Correspondence: fanney.thorsteinsdottir@regionh.dk

Abstract: Prenatal vitamin D insufficiency may be associated with an increased risk of developing childhood asthma. Results from epidemiological studies are conflicting and limited by short follow-up and small sample sizes. The objective of this study was to examine if children born to women exposed to the margarine fortification policy with a small dose of extra vitamin D during pregnancy had a reduced risk of developing asthma until age 9 years, compared to children born to unexposed women. The termination of a Danish mandatory vitamin D fortification policy constituted the basis for the study design. We compared the risk of inpatient asthma diagnoses in all Danish children born two years before (n = 106,347, exposed) and two years after (n = 115,900, unexposed) the termination of the policy. The children were followed in the register from 0–9 years of age. Data were analyzed using Cox proportional hazards regression. The Hazard Ratio for the first inpatient asthma admission among exposed versus unexposed children was 0.96 (95%CI: 0.90–1.04). When stratifying by sex and age, 0–3 years old boys exposed to vitamin D fortification showed a lower asthma risk compared to unexposed boys (HR 0.78, 95%CI: 0.67–0.92). Prenatal exposure to margarine fortification policy with extra vitamin D did not affect the overall risk of developing asthma among children aged 0–9 years but seemed to reduce the risk among 0–3 years old boys. Taking aside study design limitations, this could be explained by different sensitivity to vitamin D from different sex-related asthma phenotypes in children with early onset, and sex differences in lung development or immune responses.

Keywords: asthma; fortification; vitamin D; social experiment

1. Introduction

Asthma is one of the most common chronic conditions among children [1]. It is a complex heterogeneous disease that affects both the respiratory and the immune system [2]. It manifests by many phenotypes that vary by sex, age at onset, presence of obesity, as well as the severity of atopy, allergic sensitization, bronchial obstruction, and hyperresponsiveness. Although genetic factors and childhood exposure to environmental triggers, such as tobacco smoke, air pollution, viral infections or aeroallergens play a major role in the development of childhood asthma [3], it has been suggested that environmental exposures during gestation may also be important [4]. Asthma is more prevalent among boys until puberty when a shift towards higher prevalence among girls and women is observed [5,6]. In children, this is thought to be due to sex differences in lung development and inflammatory profile [7].

Vitamin D is a fat-soluble vitamin and a secosteroid hormone playing an important role in both skeletal and non-skeletal functions [8]. It readily crosses the placenta and the fetal supply is totally dependent on the supplies of the mother [9]. Results from animal and human studies have shown that prenatal vitamin D insufficiency may influence both the intrauterine immune system [10] and lung development [11,12], causing permanent changes to these systems. Such changes constitute a plausible biological basis to suggest that vitamin D insufficiency during gestation may have a programming effect contributing to the risk of childhood asthma. This is especially relevant given the high prevalence of vitamin D insufficiency in pregnant women [13]. The research on the association between prenatal vitamin D status and childhood asthma risk in the offspring is quite extensive. Results from several systematic reviews and meta-analyses of observational studies, however, have been inconsistent [14–18]. Two randomized clinical trials (RCT) have recently been conducted; both found non-significant 20% reduced risk of asthma/recurrent wheeze among 0–3 year old children whose mothers were supplemented with vitamin D during pregnancy [19,20], while a combined analysis of the two trials showed a significant reduction in offspring's asthma/recurrent wheeze risk after vitamin D supplementation in pregnancy [21]. Despite sex differences in asthma prevalence and possible sex difference in the effect of vitamin D on asthma development, few observational studies and none of the RCTs have run analyses differentiated by sex. Furthermore, most of the previous studies had limited numbers of participants and short follow-up periods [14–18,21].

In Denmark, between 1937 and 1985, it was mandatory to fortify margarine with 1.25 μg vitamin D per 100 g [22]. The fortification accounted for on average 13% (3–29%) of total vitamin D intake from food in the Danish population [22]. Despite that, the mandatory margarine fortification policy was canceled in June 1985. This study utilized the design of this societal experiment grounded on the distinct in time termination of the Danish margarine vitamin D fortification policy. The objective of the present study was to examine if children born to women exposed to the margarine fortification policy with a small dose of extra vitamin D during pregnancy had a reduced risk of developing asthma until age 9 years compared to children whose mothers were unexposed to the fortification policy during pregnancy. Furthermore, this study examined whether the association between exposure and asthma risk varied by age, sex, and month of birth.

2. Methods

2.1. Study Design

This study is a part of the D-tect project and a detailed study design description has been published elsewhere [23]. Briefly, all individuals born in Denmark during the two years before the termination of the vitamin D policy in 1985 were considered as exposed to vitamin D fortification during prenatal life, and all individuals born during the two years after the termination (excluding a wash-out period), were considered unexposed to vitamin D fortification. The washout period consisted of 9 months for the duration of a full-term pregnancy and an additional 6 months to allow for fortified products to be commercially replaced by non-fortified products (Figure 1).

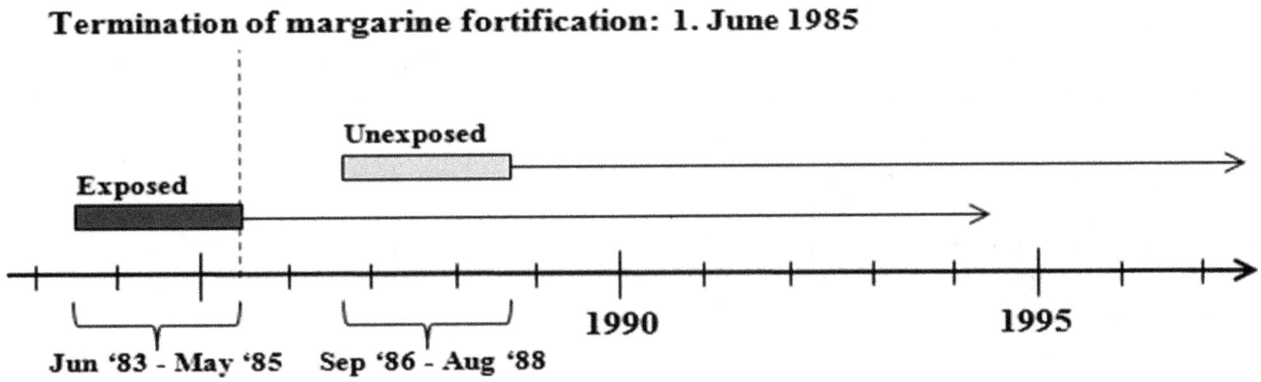

Figure 1. Study design and study population.

All children born alive in Denmark from June 1983–May 1985 and from September 1986–August 1988 were identified using the Danish Civil Registration System (CRS) and included in this study. The CRS was established in 1968 and includes information on all individuals alive and with permanent residence in Denmark at that time, and those who were born in or immigrated to Denmark afterwards [24]. All individuals in Denmark are assigned a unique identification number (CPR number) that can be used to identify the individual in all national registers and databases. From the CRS we retrieved information on the date of birth, date of death (if any), date of emigration or lost to follow up (residence unknown to Danish authorities).

Individuals from our study population were followed in the Danish National Patient Register (DNPR) to identify childhood asthma diagnoses. The DNPR is a national administrative register established in 1977 that contains information on all hospital admissions, including discharge diagnoses, according to the international classification of diseases (ICD) system [25]. Outpatient admissions in DNPR were systematically registered from 1995, and to ensure comparable exposure groups with complete follow-up among both exposed and unexposed individuals we only analyzed inpatient asthma admissions in this study.

According to Danish law, ethical approval is not required for register-based studies. Permission to access data was granted by Forskerservice, Statens Serum Institut (J.no. FSEID-00001369). The Danish Data Protection Agency provided permission to process data (J.no. 2012-41-1156). The study is registered at ClinicalTrials.gov (NCT03330301).

2.2. Definition of Outcome

Childhood asthma was defined as asthma diagnoses from birth to the age of 9 years. We considered puberty as a cut-off for distinguishing childhood asthma from adult asthma, as puberty is the period when there is a sex-based shift in the prevalence of asthma from male predominance to female predominance. In a previous study conducted among Danish children aged 6.0–19.9 years, the mean age for the pre-pubertal stage was 10.88 (SD ± 8.66–13.11) years for girls and 11.83 (SD ± 9.92–13.75) for boys [26], defining the age of 9 as a certain cut-off for pre-pubertal stage.

Asthma was defined based on ICD-8 codes 493.00, 493.01, 493.08 and 493.09; and from 1994 onwards on ICD-10 codes DJ45, DJ45.0, DJ45.1, DJ45.8, DJ45.9, DJ46.0, and DJ46.9. The registry diagnoses of asthma have been previously validated against medical records [27].

2.3. Statistical Analysis

We conducted a time-to-event analysis focusing on the time of first inpatient asthma diagnosis. If asthma was not diagnosed at the age of 9, or if the child became inactive in the CRS (emigrated, lost to follow up or dead) before the age of 9, censoring took place. We used a Cox proportional hazard model with age as the underlying time scale to assess the hazard ratios of first inpatient asthma diagnosis in the group that was exposed to extra vitamin D from fortification during gestation compared to the group that was unexposed to extra vitamin D from fortification. The assumption of proportional hazard was examined using Schoenfeld residuals [28]. Data were presented as the time at risk, incident rate, and hazard ratio (95% confidence interval). Descriptive statistics were presented in frequencies (N) and percentages (%). In multivariable analysis, we adjusted for sex and month of birth. As we included entire birth cohorts of all individuals born in Denmark in adjacent years around the fortification termination, other potential confounders were considered to be equally distributed in both exposure groups, thus adjustment for other confounders was not deemed necessary.

To test our hypothesis that the greatest risk reduction would be observed among those who had most of their prenatal period during the darkest months, we examined if the effect of vitamin D fortification on asthma risk was modified by month of birth by the likelihood ratio test; the statistical tests were two-sided at a 5% significance level. In addition, as decided a priory, we conducted analyses stratified by sex and age at the time of asthma diagnosis hypothesizing potential effect modification by sex and age, since the prevalence of asthma is higher among boys especially in the first few years of life, and both sex and age are important characteristics of different asthma phenotypes [29].

All data management and descriptive statistics were performed using Stata 13 (StataCorp. 2013. Stata Statistical Software: Release 13. College Station, TX, USA, www.stata.com), whereas all statistical analyses were performed using R version 3.3.3 (R Foundation for Statistical Computing, Vienna, Austria, www.R-project.org).

3. Results

Out of 222,247 children included in the study, 106,347 were born to mothers exposed to the margarine fortification policy with extra vitamin D during pregnancy; 115,900 were born to unexposed mothers. Among the exposed children, 1427 (64% boys) had inpatient asthma admission before the age of 9 years; and among unexposed children, 1613 (65% boys) had inpatient asthma admission before the age of 9 years (Figure 2 and Supplementary Table S1).

We did not observe a difference in inpatient asthma admission risk between children exposed and unexposed to the margarine fortification policy with extra vitamin D during the prenatal period (HR 0.96, 95% CI: 0.90–1.03). Furthermore, there was no effect modification by month of birth ($p = 0.28$). The Schoenfeld residuals indicated violation of the proportional hazards assumption with respect to exposure status, and when stratified by age at first diagnoses, we found that among the 0–3 years old, those exposed to extra vitamin D from fortification were less likely to have an inpatient asthma admission (HR 0.86, 95% CI: 0.75–0.98) compared to unexposed ones. Further stratification by sex revealed that reduced risk was confined to the 0–3-year-old boys. Boys of 0–3 years exposed to the margarine fortification policy with extra vitamin D were less likely to have an inpatient asthma admission (HR 0.78, 95% CI: 0.67–0.92) compared to unexposed ones. Adjusting for sex and month of birth gave similar results (Table 1 and Figure 3).

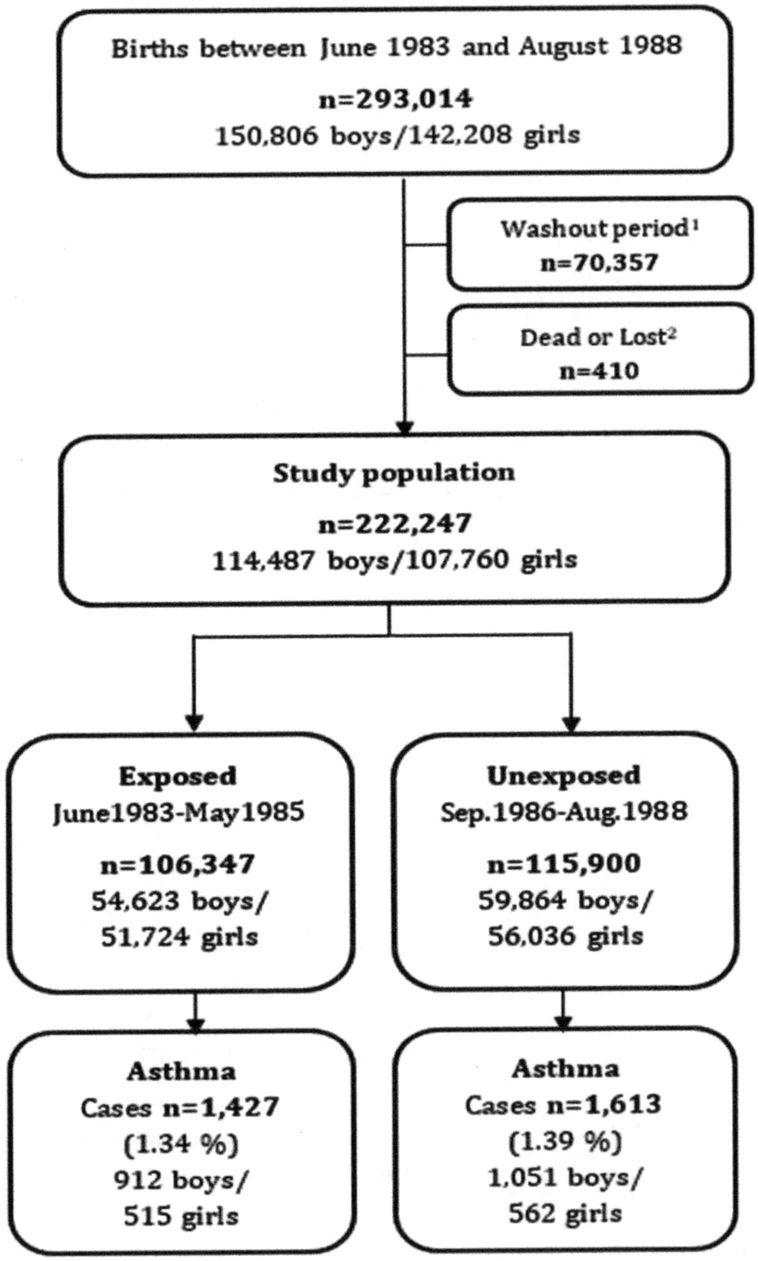

[1] 6 months for fortified products to be commercially replaced, and full 9 month pregnancy after termination of mandatory margarine fortification.

[2] Dead or lost to follow up before birth or on the day of birth.

Figure 2. Flowchart of the study population.

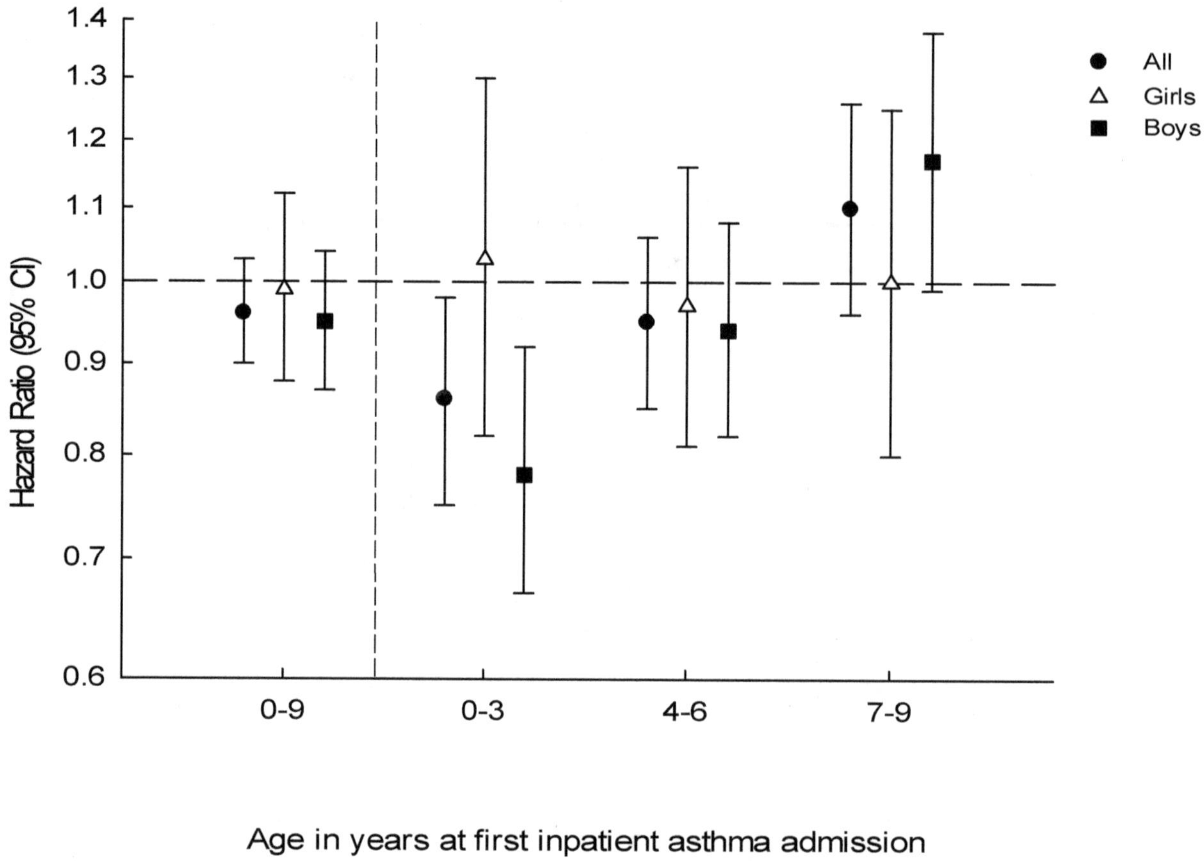

Figure 3. Hazard ratio of childhood asthma among those prenatally exposed to the margarine fortification with vitamin D policy, compared to those unexposed.

Table 1. Incidence, years at risk, rate, and hazard ratio (HR) of childhood asthma among those prenatally exposed to the margarine fortification with vitamin D policy, compared to those unexposed.

	Admissions	Time at Risk (Years)	Rate per 100,000 Years at Risk	Admissions	Time at Risk (Years)	Rate per 100,000 Years at Risk	HR	(95% CI)	Adjusted † HR	(95% CI)	*p* for Interaction with Month of Birth
	Exposed			Unexposed							
All	1427	938,797	152.0	1613	1,022,110	157.8	0.96	(0.90–1.03)	0.96	(0.90–1.04)	0.28
0–3 years	393	315,879	124.4	498	343,928	144.8	0.86	(0.75–0.98)	0.86	(0.75–0.98)	0.63
4–6 years	596	312,640	190.6	682	340,339	200.4	0.95	(0.85–1.06)	0.95	(0.85–1.06)	0.02
7–9 years	438	310,278	141.2	433	337,843	128.2	1.10	(0.96–1.26)	1.10	(0.96–1.26)	0.78
Girls	515	457,866	112.5	562	496,107	113.3	0.99	(0.88–1.12)	0.99	(0.88–1.12)	0.30
0–3 years	146	153,849	94.9	153	166,624	91.8	1.03	(0.82–1.30)	1.03	(0.82–1.30)	0.98
4–6 years	221	152,494	144.9	248	165,223	150.1	0.97	(0.81–1.16)	0.97	(0.81–1.16)	0.14
7–9 years	148	151,523	97.7	161	164,259	98.0	1.00	(0.80–1.25)	1.00	(0.80–1.24)	0.41
Boys	912	480,931	189.6	1,051	526,003	199.8	0.95	(0.87–1.04)	0.95	(0.87–1.04)	0.50
0–3 years	247	177,304	194.6	345	162,030	152.4	0.78	(0.67–0.92)	0.78	(0.67–0.92)	0.24
4–6 years	375	175,116	247.8	434	160,146	234.2	0.94	(0.82–1.08)	0.95	(0.82–1.09)	0.10
7–9 years	290	173,583	156.7	272	158,755	182.7	1.17	(0.99–1.38)	1.16	(0.99–1.37)	0.71

† = adjusted for sex and month of birth, except girls and boys are only adjusted for month of birth.

4. Discussion

Overall, we did not see a difference in the risk of asthma between children of both sexes age 0–9 years born to mothers exposed to the margarine fortification policy with a small extra dose of vitamin D during their entire pregnancy compared to those who were born to mothers who were unexposed. However, our analysis indicated that young children (0–3 years old), and in particular boys born to exposed mothers, had more than 20% lower hazards for developing asthma compared to boys born to unexposed mothers.

Several observational studies have examined the association between prenatal vitamin D and the development of asthma in the offspring, however, the results have been mixed. There are several potential reasons for this inconsistency. The observational studies have differed in study design, number of participants, adjustment for covariates, the time at exposure assessment, the source material for biomarker analysis, the concentration of maternal or cord blood 25(OH)D, and the assay method. Early observational studies looking at vitamin D intake during pregnancy, usually assessed by food frequency questionnaire (FFQ), and later development of asthma and wheezing, tended to find inverse associations [30–32]. Vitamin D may have served as a marker of a healthier diet in general and other dietary-related factors such as differences in the maternal microbiome [33]. The cohort studies examining maternal or cord blood 25(OH)D tended to find no association between 25(OH)D level in pregnancy and offspring asthma [34–36]. This was true across different timing of exposure and outcome assessment as well as geographical settings. Total 25(OH)D level may not be a sufficient indicator of the biologically available vitamin D, as other factors such as level of vitamin D binding protein could influence the metabolism and bioavailability [37,38]. These studies also did not look at the difference in asthma risk between different sex nor stratify according to pre-pregnancy vitamin D status which may be more important for reducing asthma risk than vitamin D status in pregnancy. In two recent randomized trials where mothers were supplemented with daily dose of 60 and 100 μg vitamin D respectively during pregnancy [19–21], inverse associations between 25(OH)D level and asthma/recurrent wheeze were strongest among women with a high 25(OH)D status at baseline (≥75 nmol/L). This could indicate that the programming effect already takes place in early pregnancy or even prior to pregnancy, and therefore, having optimal vitamin D status already at conception might be important for reducing the risk of childhood asthma. This may be supported by the results from observational studies assessing vitamin D intake as women with higher vitamin D intake during pregnancy are likely to have had the same dietary pattern prior to pregnancy and thus have higher vitamin D status at conception. In our study, the mothers were exposed to extra vitamin D from fortification both during a long period prior to pregnancy and during the entire pregnancy. Thus, it is expected that the exposed mothers had a higher vitamin D status pre-pregnancy than unexposed mothers. It is important to stress that the vitamin D dose administered to the subjects in the two trials was substantially higher than what women were exposed to from fortification in our study. We have previously calculated, based on the fortification dose (1.25 μg/100g) and margarine intake statistics, that an average additional 0.4–0.6 μg of vitamin D per day could be provided by the fortified margarine [39]. Compared to vitamin D supplementation in the two trials (i.e. 60 and 100 μg), and in light of the recommended total intake of 10 μg vitamin D per day for skeletal actions [40], the Danish margarine fortification policy provided a very low extra vitamin D dose. However, the optimal vitamin D dose for the prenatal development of the immune system and/or lung development is unknown. Much higher supplementation doses provided in the two previously mentioned trials seemed to be inadequate to reach a level of sufficiency among women during their pregnancy to prevent asthma development in the offspring. In our study, a constant intake of a very low extra dose of vitamin D via fortified foods consumption over entire pregnancy (and before pregnancy), might have been sufficient to reduce the risk in the offspring with the highest risk of developing asthma, the youngest boys [7,41]. Methodological advantages and disadvantages of our societal experiment design study, if compared to clinical trials, are discussed below under strengths and limitations.

Asthma phenotypes are defined based on age at debut, the presence of atopy, allergic sanitization, lung function, responsiveness to steroids, obesity, sex, and inflammatory profile. Many of these different phenotypes vary according to age, making age an important parameter in identifying asthma phenotypes [42]. Therefore, to try to isolate specific phenotypes, we stratified the analysis by age at onset. Our results of a slight reduction in the risk of inpatient asthma admission among 0–3 years old boys born to mothers who were exposed to the margarine fortification policy with extra vitamin D during pregnancy are in accordance with the results from the combined analysis of the two recently published RCTs showing a 26% reduction in the risk of asthma/recurrent wheeze at age 0–3 years among those born to mothers who took vitamin D supplementation during pregnancy [21]. This could indicate that vitamin D has an effect on asthma phenotypes that are prevalent in the youngest children, especially boys, or that the programming effect is relatively weaker than the effect of the risk factors accumulating during childhood. On the other hand, among children younger than 6 years, and particularly those younger than 3 years, the asthma diagnosis is based on symptoms (wheezing, cough, and breathlessness), clinical history of these symptoms, or family history of asthma or atopy, whereas among older children and adults asthma is diagnosed based on symptoms and confirmed with objective measures (spirometry, beta2 agonist reversibility test, bronchial provocation test, and peak flow measurements) [3]. Wheezing is the most common clinical manifestation of asthma onset. As very young children who experience severe and persistent wheezing are more likely to also have asthma in childhood or adulthood [43,44], persistent wheezing in very young children usually is considered to be an asthma indication. At the same time, many young children often experience wheezing due to viral respiratory tract infections (RTI) without having or later developing asthma [44]. Notably, a recent review on the association between maternal vitamin D status and RTI in offspring showed an inverse association between exposure to vitamin D and RTIs (highest vs. lowest 25(OH)D level: OR 0.64, 95% CI: 0.47–0.87), but no association with asthma or wheezing [18]. Hence, it cannot be ruled out that the protective effect observed among the 0–3-year-olds in our study was driven by a proportion of children misdiagnosed with asthma because of wheezing due to viral RTI.

In regard to the sex differences, there are anatomic differences in lung size, maturity, and function between the sexes with boys having larger lungs than girls, however, girls have higher forced expiratory flow rates [7]. The lungs of newborn boys are also less mature than the lungs of newborn girls [45] and thus are more vulnerable to respiratory infection, and consequently, asthma. Moreover, severe allergic asthma, or asthma with multiple sensitizations to allergens, characterized by early onset, high eosinophil count, and a low response to corticosteroid, is more prevalent among boys [29]. Children included in our study were children with asthma diagnosed during hospitalization, thus our outcome measure captured the more severe cases of asthma. It is therefore possible that the protective association observed among the youngest boys in our study was driven by the effects on an allergic type of asthma. Interestingly, despite sex differences in the prevalence of asthma, and different asthma phenotypes in boys and girls [44], very few studies have examined whether the effect of prenatal vitamin D exposure on the development of asthma is sex-specific. We identified only one other study that conducted sex-stratified analyses, and similarly to the results of the present study, the authors found an inverse association between maternal vitamin D and asthma risk at 6 years among boys only [46]. Consequently, vitamin D status in fetal life may contribute differently to the regulation of the immunologic responses in boys and girls.

Based on the present study, we cannot conclude that exposure to the margarine fortification policy with extra vitamin D during the prenatal period influences the risk of offspring asthma. However, our results and those of prior studies may indicate that vitamin D intake, even in small amounts, early in pregnancy or even before conception could influence the risk of asthma development, especially among more vulnerable groups such as very young male children. Future studies of the association between prenatal vitamin D and offspring asthma risk should assess vitamin D status or intervene with vitamin D supplements periconceptually or prior to pregnancy. Furthermore, they should focus on different phenotypes of asthma, using biomarkers shown to have a good prognostic value, and assessment of possible sex differences.

Strengths and Limitations

In this study we utilized a societal experiment of an abrupt abolishment of an obligatory vitamin D fortification, that exposed all individuals living in Denmark to extra vitamin D from fortified margarine during a distinct period of time when the fortification policy was implemented, and not thereafter. A semi-ecological study design has both strengths and limitations.

The strength is that we could include all individuals born in Denmark from entire birth cohorts from the Danish population, capturing all inpatient asthma admissions, which makes our results generalizable for the entire Danish population. This was possible due to the excellent Danish administrative and health registers, extensively used in Danish epidemiological research [47,48]. Additionally, asthma diagnoses in DNPR have been previously validated [27]. Another strength of the design was that potential confounding (i.e., from differences in socioeconomic status, obesity, maternal lifestyle and diet during pregnancy) can be considered to be equally distributed in both the exposed and the unexposed groups as they included all individuals born in adjacent birth cohorts around the time of the policy change. Nevertheless, secular trends in potential confounders during this short period of time between 1983–1988 could have introduced residual confounding. Intake of margarine was remarkably stable during the years around the policy change, and we were not able to identify changes in national recommendations for intake and/or supplementation of vitamin D or in fortification practice. However, a study from Denmark shows that smoking among women, a risk factor for offspring asthma, decreased slightly during this period [49]. This would have attenuated our findings and therefore speaks in favor of a true association between exposure to the margarine fortification policy with extra vitamin D and the development of asthma. Furthermore, we know that overweight and obesity, a risk factor for asthma, has been increasing among women [50], and from 1987–1988 there were changes in fiscal policy in Denmark that caused economic challenges for many households [51,52]. It can be speculated that this economic crisis influenced overall diet quality, such as decreased the intake of fish or fish oil, which is also shown to have a protective effect on asthma development among offspring.

The limitation of this semi-ecological study design is that information on our exposure represents ecological data; we do not have any information on actual vitamin D intake, neither from the fortified margarine nor from other dietary sources and hence cannot make actual intake recommendations. A further limitation of the study is that we only included in-patient discharge diagnoses and not outpatients diagnoses and diagnoses by general practitioners, as the DNPR does not collect this information. Consequently, we have a subgroup of asthmatic children, most likely those with severe or uncontrolled asthma, and can generalize our results only to this group. Another study limitation related to the nature of register data, which does not specify different phenotypes of asthma, nor clinical parameters. To approximate this information, we conducted analyses stratified by age and sex; however, even though the phenotypes differ by age and sex, there are other parameters that are equally important, such as sensitization to allergens, responsiveness to steroids, and inflammatory profile that would also be interesting to examine.

5. Conclusions

Our study, based on the societal experiment concerning margarine fortification with vitamin D in Denmark, suggests that prenatal exposure to a small dose of extra vitamin D from fortification may be associated with a lower risk of childhood asthma among boys aged 0–3 years, but not among older children or the youngest girls. Asthma phenotypes with very early onset that have different vitamin D sensitivity and/or sex differences in lung development or immune responses may explain our findings. However, residual confounding effects due to the semi-ecological design of the study cannot be ruled out.

Author Contributions: B.L.H. designed the study. F.T., B.L.H., E.M. and R.J. formulated the research question. P.F. performed the statistical analysis. F.T. drafted the manuscript. All authors interpreted the results, critically reviewed the manuscript, approved the final version and agreed on the submission of the manuscript.

Acknowledgments: This study was a part of the D-tect study funded by the Danish Agency for Science, Technology and Innovation, the Ministry of Science, Higher Education, under the instrument "Strategic Research Projects" (grant 0603-00453B). The funders had no role in study design, data collection and analysis, decision to publish, or preparation of the manuscript.

References

1. Masoli, M.; Fabian, D.; Holt, S.; Beasley, R. The global burden of asthma: Executive summary of the GINA Dissemination Committee Report. *Allergy* **2004**, *59*, 469–478. [CrossRef] [PubMed]
2. Bush, S.; Kleinert, S.; Pavord, I.D. The asthmas in 2015 and beyond: A Lancet Commission. *Lancet* **2015**, *385*, 1273–1275. [CrossRef]
3. Pedersen, S.E.; Hurd, S.S.; Lemanske, R.F.; Becker, A.; Zar, H.J.; Sly, P.D.; Soto-Quiroz, M.; Wong, G.; Bateman, E.D. Global strategy for the diagnosis and management of asthma in children 5 years and younger. *Pediatr. Pulmonol.* **2011**, *46*, 1–17. [CrossRef] [PubMed]
4. De Luca, G.; Olivieri, F.; Melotti, G.; Aiello, G.; Lubrano, L.; Boner, A.L. Fetal and early postnatal life roots of asthma. *J. Matern. Fetal. Neonatal. Med.* **2010**, *23*, 80–83. [CrossRef] [PubMed]
5. Postma, D.S. Gender Differences in Asthma Development and Progression. *Gend. Med.* **2007**, *4* (Suppl. B), S133–S146. [CrossRef]
6. Almqvist, C.; Worm, M.; Leynaert, B. Impact of gender on asthma in childhood and adolescence: A GA2LEN review. *Allergy* **2008**, *63*, 47–57. [CrossRef]
7. Pignataro, F.S.; Bonini, M.; Forgione, A.; Melandri, S.; Usmani, O.S. Asthma and gender: The female lung. *Pharmacol. Res.* **2017**, *119*, 384–390. [CrossRef]
8. Wimalawansa, S.J. Non-musculoskeletal benefits of vitamin D. *J. Steroid. Biochem. Mol. Biol.* **2018**, *175*, 60–81. [CrossRef]
9. Larque, E.; Morales, E.; Leis, R.; Blanco-Carnerdo, J.E. Maternal and Foetal Health Implications of Vitamin D Status during Pregnancy. *Ann. Nutr. Metab.* **2018**, *72*, 179–192. [CrossRef] [PubMed]
10. Chi, A.; Wildfire, J.; McLoughlin, R.; Wood, R.A.; Bloomberg, G.R.; Kattan, M.; Gregen, P.; Gold, D.R.; Witter, F.; Chen, T.; et al. Umbilical cord plasma 25-hydroxyvitamin D concentration and immune function at birth: The Urban Environment and Childhood Asthma study. *Clin. Exp. Allergy* **2011**, *41*, 842–850. [CrossRef] [PubMed]
11. Chen, L.; Wilson, R.; Bennet, E.; Zosky, R. Identification of vitamin D sensitive pathways during lung development. *Respir Res.* **2016**, *17*, 47. [CrossRef] [PubMed]
12. Kho, A.T.; Sharma, S.; Qiu, W.; Gaedigk, R.; Klanderman, B.; Niu, S.; Anderson, C.; Leeder, J.S.; Weiss, S.T.; Tantisira, K.G. Vitamin D related genes in lung development and asthma pathogenesis. *BMC Med. Genom.* **2013**, *6*, 47. [CrossRef]
13. Hollis, B.; Wagner, C. Nutritional vitamin D status during pregnancy: Reason for concern. *CMAJ* **2006**, *174*, 1287–1290. [CrossRef]
14. Nurmatov, U.; Devereux, G.; Sheikh, A. Nutrients and foods for the primary prevention of asthma and allergy: Systematic review and meta-analysis. *J. Allergy Clin. Immunol.* **2011**, *127*, 724–733. [CrossRef] [PubMed]
15. Beckhaus, A.A.; Garcia-Marcos, L.; Forno, E.; Pacheco-Gonzalez, R.M.; Celedón, J.C.; Castro-Rodriguez, J.A. Maternal nutrition during pregnancy and risk of asthma, wheeze, and atopic diseases during childhood: A systematic review and meta-analysis. *Allergy* **2015**, *70*, 1588–1604. [CrossRef] [PubMed]
16. Feng, H.; Xun, P.; Pike, K.; Wills, A.K.; Chawes, B.L.; Bisgaard, H.; Cai, W.; Wan, Y.; He, K. In utero exposure to 25-hydroxyvitamin D and risk of childhood asthma, wheeze, and respiratory tract infections: A meta-analysis of birth cohort studies. *J. Allergy Clin. Immunol.* **2017**, *139*, 1508–1517. [CrossRef]
17. Song, H.; Yang, L.; Jia, C. Maternal vitamin D status during pregnancy and risk of childhood asthma: A meta-analysis of prospective studies. *Mol. Nutr. Food Res.* **2017**, *61*, 1600657. [CrossRef] [PubMed]

18. Pacheco-Gonzalez, R.M.; Garcia-Marcos, L.; Morales, E. Prenatal vitamin D status and respiratory and allergic outcomes in childhood: A meta-analysis of observational studies. *Pediatr. Allergy Immunol.* **2018**, *29*, 243–253. [CrossRef]
19. Chawes, B.L.; Bønnelykke, K.; Stokholm, J.; Vissing, N.H.; Bjarnadóttir, E.; Schoos, A.M.; Wolsk, H.M.; Pedersen, T.M.; Vinding, R.K.; Thorsteinsdóttir, S.; et al. Effect of vitamin d3 supplementation during pregnancy on risk of persistent wheeze in the offspring: A randomized clinical trial. *JAMA* **2016**, *315*, 353–361. [CrossRef]
20. Litonjua, A.A.; Carey, V.J.; Laranjo, N.; Harshfield, B.J.; McElrath, T.F.; O'Connor, G.T.; Sandel, M.; Iverson, R.E.; Lee-Paritz, A.; Strunk, R.C.; et al. Effect of prenatal supplementation with vitamin d on asthma or recurrent wheezing in offspring by age 3 years: The vdaart randomized clinical trial. *JAMA* **2016**, *315*, 362–370. [CrossRef]
21. Wolsk, H.M.; Chawes, B.L.; Litonjua, A.A.; Hollis, B.W.; Waage, J.; Stokholm, J.; Bønnelykke, K.; Bisgaard, H.; Weiss, S.T. Prenatal vitamin D supplementation reduces risk of asthma/recurrent wheeze in early childhood: A combined analysis of two randomized controlled trials. *PLoS ONE* **2017**, *12*, e0186657. [CrossRef]
22. Nordic Council of Ministers. The fortification of foods with vitamins and minerals. In *Tilsætning af Vitaminer og Mineraler til Levnedsmidler*; Nordic Council of Ministers: Copenhagen, Denmark, 1989.
23. Jacobsen, R.; Abrahamsen, B.; Bauerek, M.; Holst, C.; Jensen, C.B.; Knop, J.; Raymond, K.; Rasmussen, L.B.; Stougaard, M.; Sørensen, T.I.A.; et al. The influence of early exposure to vitamin D for development of diseases later in life. *Bmc Public Health* **2013**, *13*, 515. [CrossRef]
24. Pedersen, C.B. The Danish Civil Registration System. *Scand. J. Public Health* **2011**, *39* (Suppl. 7), 22–25. [CrossRef] [PubMed]
25. Lynge, E.; Sandegaard, J.L.; Rebolj, M. The Danish National Patient Register. *Scand. J. Public Health* **2011**, *39* (Suppl. 7), 30–33. [CrossRef] [PubMed]
26. Juul, A.; Teilmann, G.; Scheike, T.; Hertel, N.T.; Holm, K.; Laursen, E.M.; Main, K.M.; Skakkebæk, N.E. Pubertal development in Danish children: Comparison of recent European and US data. *Int. J. Androl.* **2006**, *29*, 247–255. [CrossRef] [PubMed]
27. Moth, G.; Vedsted, P.; Schiøtz, P.O. National registry diagnoses agree with medical records on hospitalized asthmatic children. *Acta Pædiatr.* **2007**, *96*, 1470–1473. [CrossRef] [PubMed]
28. Therneau, T.M.; Grambsch, P.M. *Modeling Survival Data: Extending the Cox Model*; Statistics for Biology and Health; Springer: New York, NY, USA, 2000; Volume XIV, p. 350.
29. Just, J.; Saint Pierre, P.; Amat, F.; Gouvis-Echraghi, R.; Lambert-Guillemot, N.; Guiddir, T.; Annesi Maesano, I. What lessons can be learned about asthma phenotypes in children from cohort studies? *Pediatric Allergy Immunol.* **2015**, *26*, 300–305. [CrossRef] [PubMed]
30. Erkkola, M.; Kaila, M.; Nwaru, B.I.; Kronberg-Kippilä, C.; Ahonen, S.; Nevalainen, J.; Veijola, R.; Pekkanen, J.; Ilonen, J.; Simell, O.; et al. Maternal vitamin D intake during pregnancy is inversely associated with asthma and allergic rhinitis in 5-year-old children. *Clin. Exp. Allergy* **2009**, *39*, 875–882. [CrossRef] [PubMed]
31. Camargo, C.A.; Rifas-Shiman, S.L.; Litonjua, A.A.; Rich-Edwards, J.W.; Weiss, S.T.; Gold, D.R.; Kleinman, K.; Gillman, M.W. Maternal intake of vitamin D during pregnancy and risk of recurrent wheeze in children at 3 y of age. *Am. J. Clin. Nutr.* **2007**, *85*, 788–795. [CrossRef] [PubMed]
32. Devereux, G.; Litonjua, A.A.; Turner, S.W.; Craig, L.C.; McNeill, G.; Martindale, S.; Helms, P.J.; Seaton, A.; Weiss, S.T. Maternal vitamin D intake during pregnancy and early childhood wheezing. *Am. J. Clin. Nutr.* **2007**, *85*, 853–859. [CrossRef] [PubMed]
33. Vuillermin, P.J.; Macia, L.; Nanan, R.; Tang, M.L.; Collier, F.; Brix, S. The maternal microbiome during pregnancy and allergic disease in the offspring. *Semin Immunopathol.* **2017**, *39*, 669–675. [CrossRef]
34. Camargo, C.A.; Ingham, T.; Wickens, K.; Thadhani, R.; Silvers, K.M.; Epton, M.J.; Town, G.I.; Pattemore, P.K.; Espinola, J.A.; Crane, J. Cord-blood 25-hydroxyvitamin D levels and risk of respiratory infection, wheezing, and asthma. *Pediatrics* **2011**, *127*, e180–e187. [CrossRef] [PubMed]
35. Chawes, B.L.; Bonnelykke, K.; Jensen, P.F.; Schoos, A.M.; Heickendorff, L.; Bisgaard, H. Cord blood 25(OH)-vitamin D deficiency and childhood asthma, allergy and eczema: The COPSAC2000 birth cohort study. *PLoS ONE* **2014**, *9*, e99856. [CrossRef]
36. Gazibara, T.; den Dekker, H.T.; de Jongste, J.C.; McGrath, J.J.; Eyles, D.W.; Burne, T.H.; Reiss, I.K.; Franco, O.H.; Tiemeier, H.; Jaddoe, V.W.; et al. Associations of maternal and fetal 25-hydroxyvitamin D levels with childhood lung function and asthma: The Generation R Study. *Clin. Exp. Allergy* **2016**, *46*, 337–346. [CrossRef] [PubMed]

37. Gopal-Kothandapani, J.S.; Evans, L.F.; Walsh, J.S.; Gossiel, F.; Rigby, A.S.; Eastell, R.; Bishop, N.J. Effect of vitamin D supplementation on free and total vitamin D: A comparison of Asians and Caucasians. *Clin. Endocrinol.* **2019**, *90*, 222–231. [CrossRef]
38. Bikle, D.D.; Malmstroem, S.; Schwartz, J. Current Controversies: Are Free Vitamin Metabolite Levels a More Accurate Assessment of Vitamin D Status than Total Levels? *Endocrinol. Metab. Clin. North Am.* **2017**, *46*, 901–918. [CrossRef]
39. Jacobsen, R.; Hypponen, E.; Sorensen, T.I.; Vaag, A.A.; Heitmann, B.L. Gestational and Early Infancy Exposure to Margarine Fortified with Vitamin D through a National Danish Programme and the Risk of Type 1 Diabetes: The D-Tect Study. *PloS ONE* **2015**, *10*, e0128631. [CrossRef]
40. *Nordic Nutrition Recommendations 2012*; Nordic Council of Ministers: Copenhagen, Denmark, 2004; Volume 5.
41. Stevenson, D.K.; Verter, J.; Fanaroff, A.A.; Oh, W.; Ehrenkranz, R.A.; Shankaran, S.; Donovan, E.F.; Wright, L.L.; Lemons, J.A.; Tyson, J.E. Sex differences in outcomes of very low birthweight infants: The newborn male disadvantage. *Arch. Dis. Child. Fetal Neonatal Ed.* **2000**, *83*, F182–F185. [CrossRef]
42. Just, J.; Bourgoin-Heck, M.; Amat, F. Clinical phenotypes in asthma during childhood. *Clin. Exp. Allergy* **2017**, *47*, 848–855. [CrossRef]
43. Guilbert, T.W.; Mauger, D.T.; Lemanske, R.F. Childhood asthma-predictive phenotype. *J. Allergy Clin. Immunol. Pract.* **2014**, *2*, 664–670. [CrossRef]
44. Martinez, F.D.; Wright, A.L.; Taussig, L.M.; Holberg, C.J.; Halonen, M.; Morgan, W.J. Asthma and wheezing in the first six years of life. The Group Health Medical Associates. *N. Engl. J. Med.* **1995**, *332*, 133–138. [CrossRef]
45. Torday, J.S.; Nielsen, H.C.; Fencl Mde, M.; Avery, M.E. Sex differences in fetal lung maturation. *Am. Rev. Respir. Dis.* **1981**, *123*, 205–208.
46. Zosky, G.R.; Hart, P.H.; Whitehouse, A.J.; Kusel, M.M.; Ang, W.; Foong, R.E.; Chen, L.; Holt, P.G.; Sly, P.D.; Hall, G.L. Vitamin D deficiency at 16 to 20 weeks' gestation is associated with impaired lung function and asthma at 6 years of age. *Ann. Am. Thorac. Soc.* **2014**, *11*, 571–577. [CrossRef]
47. Pedersen, C.B.; Gotzsche, H.; Moller, J.O.; Mortensen, P.B. The Danish Civil Registration System. A cohort of eight million persons. *Dan Med. Bull.* **2006**, *53*, 441–449.
48. Schmidt, M.; Schmidt, S.A.; Sandegaard, J.L.; Ehrenstein, V.; Pedersen, L.; Sorensen, H.T. The Danish National Patient Registry: A review of content, data quality, and research potential. *Clin. Epidemiol.* **2015**, *7*, 449–490. [CrossRef] [PubMed]
49. Olsen, J.; Frische, G.; Poulsen, A.O.; Kirchheiner, H. Changing smoking, drinking, and eating behaviour among pregnant women in Denmark. Evaluation of a health campaign in a local region. *Scand. J. Soc. Med.* **1989**, *17*, 277–280. [CrossRef] [PubMed]
50. Bendixen, H.; Holst, C.; Sorensen, T.I.; Raben, A.; Bartels, E.M.; Astrup, A. Major increase in prevalence of overweight and obesity between 1987 and 2001 among Danish adults. *Obes. Res.* **2004**, *12*, 1464–1472. [CrossRef] [PubMed]
51. Ministry of Treasury. *Tre Reformer af Personskatterne 1987–2002*; Ministry of Treasury: Copenhagen, Denmark, 2001.
52. Jensen, A. Kuren der rystede Danmark. Available online: https://www.berlingske.dk/samfund/kuren-der-rystede-danmark (accessed on 23 April 2019).

6

Effectiveness of an Intervention of Dietary Counseling for Overweight and Obese Pregnant Women in the Consumption of Sugars and Energy

Elisa Anleu [1], Marcela Reyes [1], Marcela Araya B [2], Marcela Flores [3], Ricardo Uauy [1,4] and María Luisa Garmendia [1,*]

1 Institute of Nutrition and Food Technology (INTA), University of Chile, 7830490 Santiago, Chile; anleuelisa@gmail.com (E.A.); mreyes@inta.uchile.cl (M.R.); druauy@gmail.com (R.U.)
2 Department of Women and Newborn Health Promotion, Faculty of Medicine, University of Chile, 8380453 Santiago, Chile; marbannout@uchile.cl
3 Corporación de Salud Municipal de Puente Alto, 8210269 Santiago, Chile; marcela.flores@cmpuentealto.cl
4 Department of Pediatrics, School of Medicine, Pontificia Universidad Católica de Chile, 8330023 Santiago, Chile
* Correspondence: mgarmendia@inta.uchile.cl

Abstract: Objective: Evaluate if an intervention based on nutritional counseling decreases total sugars and energy consumption in overweight and obese pregnant women, compared to their previous consumption and compared to women who only received routine counseling. Methods: Randomized study of two groups: dietary counseling (Intervention Group: IG) and routine counseling (Control Group: CG). The intervention consisted of three educational sessions focused on decreasing intake of foods that most contribute to sugars consumption. Changes in sugars and energy consumption were evaluated by a food frequency questionnaire before and after the intervention. Results: We evaluated 433 pregnant women, 272 in IG and 161 in CG, who before intervention had a mean consumption of 140 g total sugars and 2134 kcal energy per day. At the end of the intervention, the IG showed 15 g/day lower consumption of total sugars (95% CI: −25 and −5 g/day), 2% less total energy from sugars (95% CI: −3% and −1% g/day), and 125 kcal/day less energy than the CG (95% CI: −239 and −10 kcal/day). Table sugar, sweets, and soft drinks had the greatest reduction in consumption. Conclusions: The intervention focused on counseling on the decrease in consumption of the foods that most contribute to sugars consumption in overweight and obese pregnant women was effective in decreasing total sugars and energy consumption, mainly in the food groups high in sugars. Future studies should examine if this intervention has an effect on maternal and fetal outcomes.

Keywords: nutritional intervention; pregnant women; overweight; obesity; total sugars; energy

1. Introduction

In recent years, Chile has had one of the highest prevalence rates of overweight and obesity in Latin America [1]. Overweight has 39% prevalence and obesity has 29%; 51% of women in reproductive age have a state of malnutrition due to excess [2]. This situation is of concern for the country, given the consequences it represents for maternal and infant health. Excessive weight during pregnancy and maternal obesity are associated with complications such as fetal trauma, congenital malformations, recurrent abortion, gestational hypertension, preeclampsia, macrosomia (birth weight >4 kg at birth), Caesarean births, and gestational diabetes, among others [3,4]. Long-term complications include the appearance of obesity and noncommunicable diseases in both mother and child.

The appearance of pregnancy complications depends on the pre-gestation nutritional status, but also on gestational weight gain (GWG). One of the most important contributors to GWG are eating habits. Elevated sugars consumption of foods with high energy value and high added sugars predisposes these women to excessive GWG [5,6]. The study by Renault et al. [6] revealed that large GWG is more related to intake of added sugars than to saturated fats. It is of interest to consider the nutritional state of pregnant women, emphasizing the habitual consumption of these foods.

Interventions focused on diet and physical exercise during pregnancy have shown to be efficacious in preventing excessive GWG and in other maternal–fetal outcomes, such as lower incidence of gestational diabetes and Caesarean births [7–9]. The dietary component of the interventions has usually been based on acquiring healthier eating habits (reduction of the glycemic index of foods, restricting the consumption of saturated fats, and increased consumption of fruits and vegetables [10–12]. Others have used recommendations based on food guides, considering preferences and alimentary beliefs [8]. However, there are no studies that show the effect of a nutritional intervention focused on the reduction in consumption of those foods that most contribute to total sugars consumption.

We developed a home intervention strategy in Chile based on diet counseling and omega-3 supplementation in order to decrease the incidence of gestational diabetes mellitus in women who began their pregnancy overweight or obese. The study protocol has been published elsewhere [13] (Trial registration: NCT02574767). Briefly, the intervention attempts to achieve adequate metabolic control for pregnant women and their children resulted in lower incidence of gestational diabetes mellitus and lower incidence of macrosomia in the newborn. The present study evaluates whether the dietary counseling decreased the consumption of total sugars and energy, compared to their consumption before the intervention and compared to women who only received routine counseling.

2. Materials and Methods

2.1. Study Design

The prospective experimental study evaluated the frequency of consumption before and after nutritional counseling of overweight and obese pregnant women, comparing the intervention group (IG) to a control group (CG). The IG received dietary counseling, while the CG received the routine control recommendations provided in the primary health centers of the Chilean Health-Care System.

2.2. Study Population

The study population consisted of pregnant women recruited from March 2016 to May 2018 in health centers of the Puente Alto county of Santiago, Chile: 272 participants in IG and 161 in CG. The inclusion criteria were: gestation of 15 weeks or less in the first prenatal control, 18 years of age or older, single pregnancy, and overweight or obese in the first control. The exclusion criteria were: previous diagnosis of diabetes or treatment with metformin or insulin, eating disorders (bulimia or anorexia), or a risk pregnancy defined in the health center using the definition in the Chilean Health Ministry guide [14].

The original group included 1002 women, 500 randomly assigned to IG and 502 to CG. In the present study we included the subsample of participants who answered the food frequency questionnaire (FFQ) at the beginning and end of the intervention between September 2016 and October 2018. Before the intervention, 408 and 264 participants answered the FFQ, respectively. At 35–37 weeks of pregnancy, 272 participants in the IG and 161 in the CG answered a second FFQ. The main reasons the second FFQs were not obtained are given in the flowchart in Figure 1. No significant differences were found in age, education, or nutritional status between the women who answered two questionnaires with those who answered only one, nor with the women who did not answer the FFQ ($p > 0.05$).

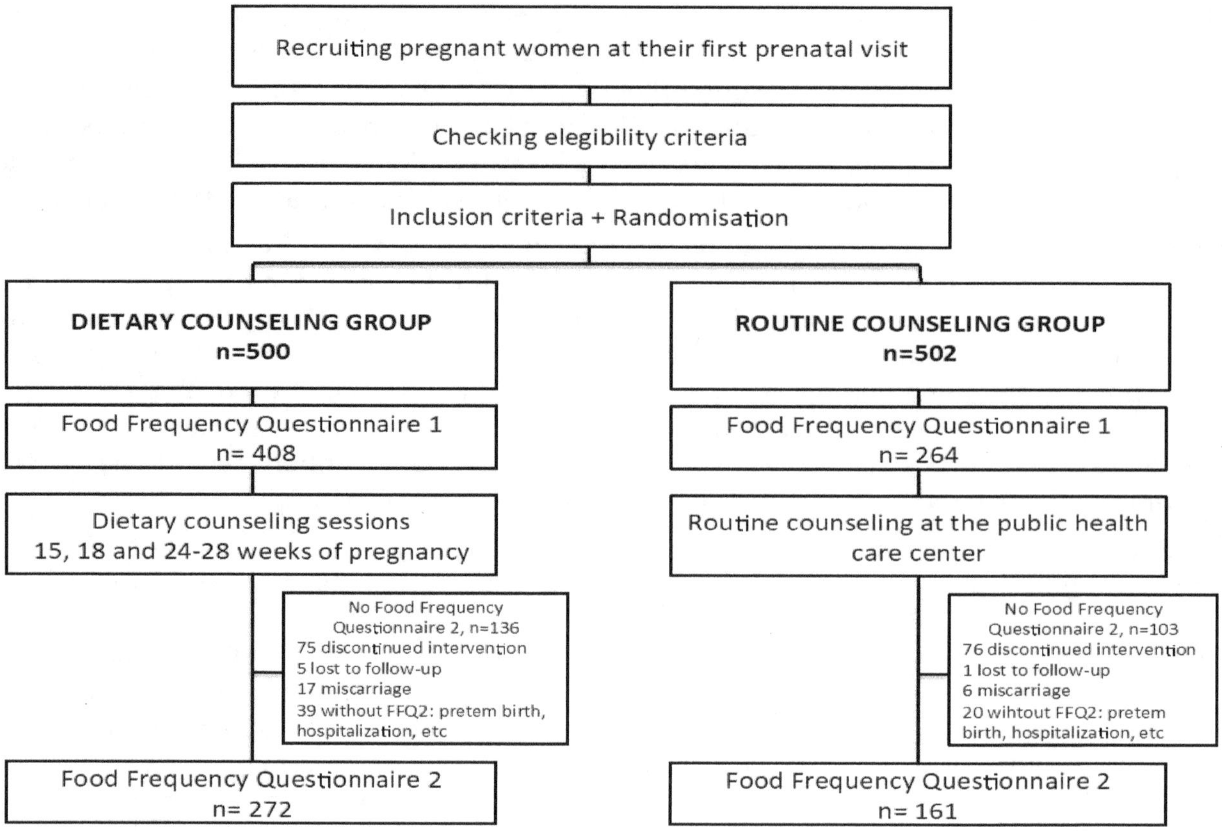

Figure 1. Flow diagram of the recruitment, randomization, and dietary measurements of trial participants.

2.3. Dietary Counseling

The general objective of the dietary intervention is to reduce the consumption of the main sources of total sugars through a culturally tailored intervention culturally with recommendations simple and easy to follow by pregnant women. Nutritional intervention consisted of three teaching sessions focused on decreasing consumption of foods that are a relevant dietary source of sugars as well as the use of behavioral techniques to allow participants to achieve eating behavioral changes. There are no interventions similar to ours in the literature, but several clinical trials have also focused on decreasing the consumption of foods with high glycemic index [15–18]. The consumption of high carbohydrate foods influences maternal glucose levels, which results excessive gestational weight gain and fetoplacental growth [17]. Some interventions focused on reducing foods with high glycemic index have shown beneficial effects on maternal outcomes (gestational weight gain, fasting, and postprandial glucose levels) and offspring birth weight [19].

We previously used a multiple pass 24-h dietary recall (R24h) applied to 114 pregnant women who attended in the same health centers to identify the seven foods that most contributed to their sugars consumption (43.4% of total sugars consumption). The "Top 7" were sweetened soft drinks, juice with added sugar, powdered juices with sugar, cookies, table sugar, sweetened milk products, and bread. The first session took place when the participants had less than 15 weeks gestation, the second session at week 18, and the third between 24–28 weeks.

Session 1: "Introduction to gestational diabetes: sugars consumption during pregnancy and consequences for the baby".

This consisted of showing an animated video with relevant information on gestational diabetes mellitus, illustrating the possible consequences of high sugars consumption on maternal–infant health and recommending general care in this phase of life, including healthy eating and physical activity. Participants were then given 6 photos with the Top 7 foods and a set of sugar cubes equivalent to

5 g each (one teaspoon). Participants were asked to place the sugar cubes that they thought were contained by each food on top of the corresponding photo. Then they were told the real amounts of sugar and given recommendations according to what each participant observed and commented.

Session 2: "Learning to substitute intelligently".

This consisted of presenting information on options of healthy food substitutes for those with high sugars content. Each participant received a magnetic board with images of the Top 7, as well as a number of photos of healthy and unhealthy foods. The participants were asked to choose two alternatives that best substituted for the high-sugars foods in the same meal in which they eat those foods, and to place the two photos of each pair together. Afterwards, the selected choices for each food were analyzed, and recommendations to reinforce the consumption of healthy foods were given.

Session 3: "Identifying my eating habits".

There were two activities in this session. The first activity used a board in the form of a traffic light; the participant was shown five photographs of eating habits of a pregnant woman, and a brief description of exactly what each photograph represented was read to her. The objective was for the participant to place the photograph on the color to which she considered it belonged, where green = healthy, yellow = caution, and red = risky.

The second activity was a roulette game with four colors: red, green, blue, and yellow. Each color represented one of the topics treated in the previous two sessions. The participant spun the wheel five times. According to the color that resulted for each time, she took a card from the stack with that color that had a question on the corresponding topic. There were direct questions and multiple-choice questions with three options, but only one correct.

According to the responses of the participant in the two activities her knowledge was reinforced, emphasizing her weak points, and a general feedback of all the educational sessions was given.

2.4. Routine Counseling

The CG only received the routine counseling given in primary health centers in prenatal controls.

2.5. Data Collection

When participants were enrolled, sociodemographic (age, marital status, occupation, income, composition of the home), obstetric (previous pregnancies and abortions, etc.), and morbidity (personal and family history of depression, type 2 diabetes, hypertension) information was collected, and blood pressure, height, and weight were measured. We also recorded information about the group of omega-3 fatty acids in which women were randomly allocated to receive (200 mg/day or 800 mg/day). By far, this information is not known to the participants or the researchers; thus, we classified this variable for the analyses as group 1 and group 2. GWG was calculated as the difference between the weight at the last visit during pregnancy (35–37 weeks) and pre-pregnancy weight; it was analyzed both as continuous (kg) and as categorical below, within and above the Institute of Medicine (IOM) 2009 guidelines (7–11.5 kg for overweight and 5–9 kg for obesity) [20].

Food consumption was measured using an FFQ applied twice by trained nutritionists. The first was applied when the participant was enrolled in the study (before 15 weeks of gestation) and the second was applied after the last visit (weeks 35–37 of gestation); both measured food consumption in the previous month.

The semi-quantitative FFQ was designed to evaluate the habitual intake of foods that were a relevant dietary source of total sugars and energy and, according to data derived from R24h mentioned above, in which all foods and culinary preparations eaten by the participant were compiled. One R24h was collected for each participant by a single trained dietitian using the multi-pass method [21] and a photographic atlas of standard portions of usual foods and culinary preparations [22,23]. Contents of energy and total sugars of foods were computed according to the weight/volume consumed and based on nutrient composition databases. In the case of natural foods, we used the Chilean database [24] and the United States Department of Agriculture [25] (USDA) nutrient database; in the case of packaged foods, we used a database previously built by our research group, based on nutrient fact panels of packaged foods collected from supermarkets during 2015 [26]. No specific software was used for dietary assessments. Food items consumed by participants were identified with numbers from 1 to 489 and then grouped into 171 food items according to their similarity in physical characteristics or the content of energy or sugars in 100 g of the foods. We then calculated the percentage that each food contributed to the total intake of energy and total sugars of the diet. These food items were listed in decreasing order according to their contribution and the accumulated percentage calculated. Food groups that provided 95% of the energy and total sugars were selected to design the FFQ. The R24H results were also used to estimate the portions of each food usually consumed; these were selected as the standard portions.

The final FFQ instrument contained 86 food items grouped in 16 food groups: cereals, tubers, bread and cakes, cookies, snacks, sugars and sweets, ice cream, soft drinks and juices, fruits, vegetables, legumes, meats, sausages, whole milk products, Chilean prepared foods, and oils. There were six fruits that were asked about in all months, and some that were asked about only during part of the year: an autumn–winter group from 21 March to 20 September and a spring–summer group from 21 September to 2 March.

To help visualize portions and aid in asking about consumption, there was a specific photographic atlas for this project with photographs of the standard portion of each food item, in the same order in which they were asked. The participant answered how much and how often she consumed this food in the month previous to the application of the FFQ.

2.6. Statistical Analysis

Energy and total sugars consumption were estimated by multiplying the consumption frequency of a food by the mass of the standard portion of the FFQ, giving the monthly intake in grams per food item. This was transformed to total daily intake in grams per item and then to daily energy and total sugars consumption using the nutritional information collected at the International Network for Food and Obesity/Non-Communicable Diseases Research, Monitoring and Action Support Project (INFORMAS) of the Instituto de Nutrición y Tecnología de los Alimentos (INTA) of the Universidad de Chile, and from the nutritional composition of foods of the USA Department of Agriculture (USDA).

The continuous variables were described by means and standard deviations, and the categories by frequencies and proportions.

Differences in the consumption of total sugars and energy between the IG and CG in the baseline and after the intervention were evaluated through the Student's *t*-test.

The change in energy and total sugars consumption pre-and post-intervention within each group was evaluated using *t*-test for paired samples.

Finally, the effect of dietary counseling intervention (categorical predictor variable: 0 = no, 1 = yes) on total sugars consumption and energy (outcomes) was tested by multiple linear regression models adjusted for the baseline value and by covariates. We repeated the models considering the change between initial and final values in sugars/energy consumption as outcome.

All analyses were performed on an intention-to-treat basis, according to the treatment group allocated at randomization.

Statistical analyses were performed using the Stata program version 13 (StataCorp LP: College Station, TX, USA). The significance level for all tests was $p < 0.05$.

2.7. Ethical Aspects

The ethics committee of INTA of the Universidad de Chile approved the protocol and informed consent procedure of the study. The women studied accepted to participate by signing an informed consent form.

3. Results

3.1. Characterization of the Participants

The characteristics of the 433 women studied at time of recruitment are shown in Table 1. Mean age was 28 years (SD = 5.8); 63% were obese, no difference between groups. A total of 61% of the participants responded to the FFQ during autumn and winter. A percentage of 74% of the participants had finished secondary school and 55% were married; this percentage was higher in the IG than in the CG ($p < 0.05$). The percentage diagnosis of depression was 27% ($n = 77$), and not different between groups.

Table 1. Characterization of the study sample.

Variables	Control Group N = 161		Intervention Group N = 272		p-Value
	Mean (SD) *	N (%) **	Mean (SD) *	N (%) **	
Age (years)	28.2 (6.1)		27.9 (5.3)		0.629
Nutritional status					
Overweight		67 (42)		94 (35)	0.142
Obese		94 (58)		178 (65)	
Marital state					
Single		82 (51)		100 (37)	0.004
Married		79 (49)		172 (63)	
Level of studies					
Primary school		33 (20)		70 (26)	0.465
High school		119 (74)		188 (69)	
University		9 (6)		14 (5)	
Activity					
Work		80 (50)		129 (47)	0.449
Household labors		54 (33)		106 (39)	
Other		27 (17)		37 (14)	
Number of persons in the home	4.4 (1.9)		4.4 (1.7)		0.651
Monthly household income (US dollars)					
≤ US 717		86 (53)		143(52)	0.333
≥ US 717		64 (40)		99 (36)	
Other (no answer, doesn't know)		11(7)		30 (11)	
Relation to head of household					
Head of household		33 (21)		47 (17)	0.229
Spouse, partner		57 (35)		119 (44)	
Other		71 (44)		106 (39)	
Depression before pregnancy					
Yes		48 (30)		65 (24)	0.211
No		111 (69)		206 (76)	
Doesn't know		2 (1)		1 (0)	
DHA supplementation					
Group 1		82 (51)		138 (51)	0.968
Group 2		79 (49)		134 (49)	
Health center					
Low NSE		79 (49)		120 (44)	0.318
Medium NSE		82 (51)		152 (56)	

* Mean (standard deviation). ** N (%), Number (percentage).

Mean GWG at 35–37 weeks was similar in both groups: 8.6 kg (SD = 4.6) in the IG and 8.7 kg (SD = 4.5) in the CG ($p > 0.05$). The proportion of women who exceeded the IOM recommendations for GWG did not differ between groups (36.2% in the IG and 34.0% in the CG, $p > 0.05$.

3.2. Change in Total Sugars and Energy Consumption between Groups

The total dietary changes in mean intake of total sugars and energy before and after the intervention and the differences between IG and CG are given in Table 2. The mean consumption of total sugars in the group intervened with counseling was 143 g/day before the intervention and 111 g/day after the intervention, with a significant reduction of −33 g/day ($p < 0.05$). There was also a significant reduction in total sugars consumption in the CG, from 137 g/day at the beginning to 124 g/day at the end ($p < 0.05$); however, the reduction in the IG was significantly greater (by 20 g) than in the CG ($p < 0.05$).

Table 2. Change in consumption of total sugars and energy.

	Control Group $N = 161$				Intervention Group $N = 272$				Intervention vs. Control					
	<15 Weeks of Pregnancy [1]	35–37 Weeks of Pregnancy [1]	Change [1]	*p*-Value	15 Weeks of Pregnancy [1]	35–37 Weeks of Pregnancy [1]	Change [1]	*p*-Value	Difference between Groups at < 15 Weeks Pregnancy [2]	*p*-Value	Difference between Groups at 35–37 Weeks Pregnancy [2]	*p*-Value	Difference in the Change [2]	*p*-Value
Total sugars, g/day	136.94 (65.10)	123.94 (53.44)	−13.00 (60.11)	0.006	143.36 (70.33)	110.72 (55.01)	−32.64 (69.74)	<0.001	6.42 (6.80)	0.345	−13.22 (5.41)	0.015	−19.64 (6.59)	0.003
Total kilocalories, kcal/day	2064 (627)	1996 (627)	−68 (658)	0.191	2203 (794)	1924 (652)	−279 (761)	<0.001	139 (73)	0.058	−72 (64)	0.264	−211 (72)	0.003
Kilocalories of energy derived from sugars, kcal/day	548 (260)	496 (214)	−52 (240)	0.007	573 (281)	443 (220)	−130 (279)	<0.001	25 (27)	0.345	−53 (22)	0.015	−78 (26)	0.003
Percentage of energy derived from sugars, %	26 (8)	25 (6)	−1 (8)	0.016	26 (7)	23 (6)	−3 (8)	<0.001	0 (0)	0.519	−2 (1)	0.001	−2 (1)	0.060

Statistical differences were evaluated using Student's *t*-test or *t*-test for paired samples. [1] Mean (standard deviation) [2] Mean difference (standard deviation).

There was also a significant decrease in the total energy consumption in the IG, from 2203 to 1924 kcal/day, a decrease of 279 kcal/day. Total energy consumption also decreased in the CG, from 2064 kcal/day to 1996 kcal/day, but the difference was not significant ($p = 0.191$). The difference between the groups after the intervention (72 kcal/day) was not significant ($p = 0.264$). However, the reduction in energy consumption was significantly greater in the CG ($p < 0.05$).

3.3. Changes in the Consumption of Total Sugars and Energy by Food Group

Tables 3 and 4 show the changes in mean consumption of total sugars and energy, respectively, in the food groups of the FFQ. There were significant decreases in total sugars consumption in the group with dietary counseling in soft drinks and juices, table sugar and sweets, fruits, and milk products, with decreases of 12, 9, 7, and 4 g/day, respectively ($p < 0.05$). Small but significant decreases in sugars consumption were also observed in tubers, ice cream, vegetables, prepared foods, and oils. The CG had significant decreases in sugars and sweets (−4 g/day) and soft drinks and juices (−9 g/day), and very slight decreases in vegetables, prepared foods, and oils. The decrease in consumption was significantly greater in the IG in sugars from fruit (−6 g/day), milk products (−3 g/day), and soft drinks and juices, and it showed a tendency to decrease in ice cream (−1 g/day, $p = 0.08$) and sugars and sweets (−4 g/day, $p = 0.08$). There was a significant reduction of total energy in the IG in the food groups in which the dietary consumption was focused; snacks decreased by 16 kcal/day, sugars and sweets by 44 kcal/day, soft drinks and juices by 50 kcal/day, and whole milk products by 52 kcal/day ($p < 0.05$). There were smaller but significant reductions in ice cream, tubers, fruits, vegetables, prepared meats, and oils ($p < 0.05$).

In the CG, there were significant decreases in the consumption of table sugar and sweets (−22 kcal/day), soft drinks and juices (−39 kcal/day) and a smaller decrease in the energy from vegetables (−3 kcal/day) ($p < 0.05$). Snacks, fruits, and whole milk products that showed greater decrease in the IG after counseling than in the CG, with −14 kcal/day, −30 kcal/day, and −42 kcal/day, respectively ($p < 0.05$).

3.4. Effect of the Nutritional Intervention on Consumption of Sugars and Energy

Table 5 shows the results of the linear and multiple regression models. The multiple model showed that the group with dietary counseling had a significant reduction in total sugars consumption of 15.23 g/day (95% CI −25.01 to −5.46 g/day; $p = 0.002$), in energy by 125 kcal/day (95% CI −239 to −10 kcal/day; $p = 0.032$), and in the percentage of energy derived from sugars by 2% (95% CI −3% to −1%; $p = 0.002$), compared to the control group.

Table 3. Consumption of total sugars (g/day) by food groups.

Food Groups	Control Group $N = 161$				Intervention Group $N = 272$				Intervention Group vs. Control Group					
	<15 Weeks of Pregnancy [1]	35–37 Weeks of Pregnancy [1]	Change [1]	*p*-Value	15 Weeks of Pregnancy [1]	35–37 Weeks of Pregnancy [1]	Change [1]	*p*-Value	Difference between Groups at <15 Weeks of Pregnancy [2]	*p*-Value	Difference between Groups at 35–37 Weeks of Pregnancy [2]	*p*-Value	Difference in the Change [2]	*p*-Value
Cereals	3.88 (4.77)	3.52 (3.68)	−0.35 (5.26)	0.393	3.35 (3.15)	2.97 (3.43)	−0.38 (3.79)	0.099	−0.53 (0.38)	0.161	−0.55 (0.35)	0.116	−0.03 (0.44)	0.952
Tubers	0.57 (0.42)	0.53 (0.44)	−0.04 (0.53)	0.349	0.62 (0.57)	0.52 (0.39)	−0.10 (0.57)	0.003	0.05 (0.05)	0.307	−0.01 (0.04)	0.768	−0.06 (0.05)	0.259
Bread	2.16 (1.81)	2.29 (2.14)	0.13 (2.38)	0.474	2.44 (2.03)	2.36 (1.76)	−0.8 (2.43)	0.594	0.28 (0.19)	0.139	0.07 (0.18)	0.742	−0.21 (0.24)	0.375
Pies and cakes	9.33 (8.08)	9.86 (9.12)	0.53 (10.63)	0.526	10.36 (10.73)	8.92 (8.69)	−1.44 (13.00)	0.068	1.12 (0.97)	0.250	−0.94 (0.88)	0.283	−1.97 (1.21)	0.103
Cookies	3.81 (6.83)	3.57 (4.90)	−0.24 (7.20)	0.672	3.70 (6.26)	3.06 (7.36)	−0.64 (8.09)	0.192	−0.05 (0.64)	0.931	−0.51 (0.65)	0.430	−0.40 (0.77)	0.602
Snacks	1.97 (2.73)	2.46 (3.64)	0.49 (4.36)	0.155	1.75 (2.79)	1.84 (3.43)	0.09 (4.19)	0.701	−0.23 (0.27)	0.394	−0.62 (0.35)	0.077	−0.39 (0.42)	0.353
Sugars and sweets	23.49 (18.69)	19.19 (18.50)	−4.30(20.57)	0.008	27.98 (24.68)	19.38 (19.18)	−8.60 (27.37)	<0.001	4.88 (2.23)	0.029	0.19 (1.88)	0.921	−4.30 (2.49)	0.084
Ice cream	2.28 (4.94)	2.65 (7.39)	0.36 (8.65)	0.595	2.71 (5.23)	1.83 (2.66)	−0.88 (5.95)	0.015	0.70 (0.45)	0.125	−0.82 (0.49)	0.096	−1.24 (0.70)	0.077
Soft drinks and juices	29.23 (35.80)	20.50 (23.96)	−8.73 (31.88)	<0.001	27.08 (32.45)	15.05 (20.51)	−12.03 (34.47)	<0.001	−2.15 (3.35)	0.521	−5.45 (2.17)	0.012	−3.30 (3.33)	0.323
Fruits	31.23 (23.16)	30.69 (23.77)	−0.54 (27.23)	0.799	33.03 (25.71)	26.41 (20.97)	−6.61 (25.29)	<0.001	1.89 (2.46)	0.445	−4.28 (2.18)	0.051	−6.07 (2.58)	0.019
Vegetables	1.79 (1.38)	1.49 (1.08)	−0.30 (1.35)	0.005	2.00 (1.73)	1.59 (1.27)	−0.41 (1.75)	<0.001	0.20 (0.16)	0.208	0.10 (0.12)	0.418	−0.11 (0.16)	0.478
Legumes	0.27 (0.30)	0.28 (0.30)	0.01(0.34)	0.691	0.26 (0.31)	0.27 (0.33)	0.01 (0.40)	0.572	−0.01 (0.03)	0.865	−0.01 (0.03)	0.776	0.00 (0.04)	0.934
Meats	0.29 (0.25)	0.28 (0.19)	−0.01 (0.29)	0.570	0.28 (0.25)	0.26 (0.24)	−0.02 (0.29)	0.295	−0.01 (0.02)	0.839	−0.01 (0.02)	0.579	−0.01 (0.03)	0.845
Sausage	0.20 (0.21)	0.18 (0.19)	−0.02 (0.23)	0.296	0.25 (0.24)	0.20 (0.21)	−0.05 (0.26)	0.002	0.05 (0.02)	0.039	0.02 (0.02)	0.408	-0.03 (0.02)	0.219
Whole milk products	11.67 (14.33)	10.67 (14.58)	−1.00 (15.11)	0.404	12.91 (16.02)	8.51 (13.32)	−4.40 (15.09)	<0.001	1.59 (1.51)	0.294	−2.16 (1.37)	0.115	−3.40 (1.49)	0.023
Low-fat milk products	12.23 (12.19)	14.18 (14.66)	1.95 (15.21)	0.103	10.00 (11.87)	14.19 (15.15)	4.19 (15.74)	<0.001	−2.30 (1.19)	0.054	0.01 (1.48)	0.995	2.24 (1.54)	0.148
Preparations	3.73 (3.68)	3.07 (3.04)	−0.66 (3.49)	0.019	4.54 (8.19)	3.27 (3.63)	−1.27 (7.67)	0.007	0.93 (0.68)	0.171	0.20 (0.34)	0.561	−0.62 (0.64)	0.334
Oils	0.06 (0.06)	0.04 (0.04)	−0.02 (0.06)	0.010	0.07 (0.08)	0.04 (0.04)	−0.03 (0.09)	<0.001	0.01 (0.01)	0.112	0.00 (0.00)	0.665	0.01 (0.01)	0.173

Statistical differences were evaluated using Student's *t*-test or *t*-test for paired samples. [1] Mean (standard deviation) [2] Mean difference (standard deviation).

Table 4. Energy consumption (kcal/day) by food group.

	Control Group N = 161				Intervention Group N = 272				Intervention Group vs. Control Group					
Food Groups	<15 Weeks of Pregnancy [1]	35–37 Weeks of Pregnancy [1]	Change [1]	p-Value	15 Weeks of Pregnancy [1]	35–37 Weeks of Pregnancy [1]	Change [1]	p-Value	Difference between Groups at < 15 Weeks of Pregnancy [2]	p-Value	Difference between Groups at 35–37 Weeks of Pregnancy [2]	p-Value	Difference in the Change [2]	p-Value
Cereals	228 (119)	243 (125)	15 (139)	0.182	238 (132)	231 (143)	−7 (160)	0.527	10 (12)	0.452	-12 (13)	0.391	−21 (15)	0.170
Tubers	48 (35)	43 (34)	−5 (37)	0.070	54 (50)	44 (34)	−10 (50)	<0.001	6 (4)	0.193	1 (3)	0.845	−5 (4)	0.268
Bread	213 (179)	226 (210)	13 (234)	0.472	240 (200)	232 (174)	−8 (240)	0.595	28 (19)	0.139	6 (18)	0.741	−21 (23)	0.375
Pies and cakes	241 (207)	245 (215)	4 (236)	0.813	271 (226)	237 (229)	−34 (286)	0.053	30 (22)	0.172	−8 (22)	0.706	−38 (27)	0.154
Cookies	73 (102)	63 (73)	−10(110)	0.263	70 (102)	60 (114)	−10 (128)	0.208	−3 (10)	0.898	−2 (10)	0.813	0 (12)	0.999
Snacks	46 (51)	44 (49)	−2 (67)	0.785	51 (77)	35 (47)	−16 (79)	<0.001	5 (7)	0.428	−9 (5)	0.047	−14 (7)	0.047
Sugars and sweets	136 (114)	114 (100)	−22(121)	0.019	154 (126)	110 (98)	−44(144)	<0.001	20 (12)	0.087	−3 (9)	0.731	−21 (13)	0.117
Ice cream	22 (47)	25 (72)	3 (84)	0.621	26 (49)	17 (26)	−9 (56)	0.015	7 (4)	0.125	−8 (5)	0.115	−12 (7)	0.086
Soft drinks and juices	123 (151)	84 (104)	−39(135)	<0.001	112 (132)	62 (84)	−50 (140)	<0.001	−11 (14)	0.407	−22 (9)	0.014	−10 (14)	0.451
Fruits	169 (120)	165 (121)	−4(136)	0.692	177 (132)	143 (108)	−34 (130)	<0.001	8 (13)	0.516	−22 (11)	0.047	−30 (13)	0.022
Vegetables	16 (12)	13 (9)	−3 (11)	0.001	18 (15)	14 (11)	−4 (15)	<0.001	2 (1)	0.085	1 (1)	0.268	−1 (1)	0.348
Legumes	31 (31)	32 (30)	1 (37)	0.537	30 (32)	30 (33)	0 (39)	0.793	0 (3)	0.975	−2 (3)	0.520	−1 (4)	0.760
Meats	190 (99)	191 (85)	1 (107)	0.923	189 (100)	188 (97)	−1 (112)	0.891	−1 (9)	0.956	−3 (9)	0.763	−2 (11)	0.873
Sausage	42 (35)	39 (35)	−3 (41)	0.459	48 (41)	42 (38)	−6 (47)	0.021	6 (4)	0.089	2 (4)	0.534	−4 (4)	0.345
Whole milk products	143 (172)	133 (165)	−10 (160)	0.403	164 (171)	112 (135)	−52 (164)	<0.001	24 (17)	0.161	−20 (14)	0.162	−41 (16)	0.010
Low-fat milk products	129 (117)	141 (130)	12 (143)	0.287	115 (135)	145 (139)	30 (156)	0.001	−15 (13)	0.246	4 (13)	0.748	18 (15)	0.218
Preparations	152 (83)	143 (96)	−9 (104)	0.288	159 (106)	150 (96)	−9 (120)	0.236	8 (9)	0.379	7 (9)	0.442	0 (11)	0.994
Oils	75 (50)	69 (44)	−6 (55)	0.134	86 (68)	69 (43)	−17 (69)	<0.001	12 (6)	0.060	0 (4)	0.967	−11 (6)	0.094

Statistical differences were evaluated using Student's t-test or t-test for paired samples. [1] Mean (standard deviation) [2] Mean difference (standard deviation).

Table 5. Effect of the nutritional intervention on the consumption of total sugars and energy. Linear regression models.

	MODEL 1	p-Value	MODEL 2	p-Value	MODEL 3	p-Value
Total sugars consumption post intervention, g/day	−13.22 (−23.85, −2.57)	0.015	−15.44 (−25.04, −5.84)	0.002	−15.23 (−25.01, −5.46)	0.002
Total kilocalorie consumption post intervention, kcal/day	−71 (−197, 54)	0.265	127 (−239, −14)	0.028	−125 (−239, −10)	0.032
Total percentage of energy consumption derived from sugars, %	−2 (−3, −1)	0.001	−2 (−3, −1)	0.001	−2 (−3, −1)	0.002

Reference group is the control group. Figures represent β coefficients of the regression models and 95% confidence intervals. MODEL 1: Sugars/kilocalories/% calories from sugars at 35–37 weeks of pregnancy = β0 + β1 (dietary counseling). MODEL 2: Sugars/kilocalories/% calories from sugars at 35–37 weeks of pregnancy = β0 + β1 (dietary counseling) + β2 (sugars/kilocalories/% calories at < 15 weeks of pregnancy). MODEL 3: Sugars/kilocalories/% calories from sugars at 35–37 weeks of pregnancy = β0 + β1 (dietary counseling) + β2 (sugars/kilocalories/% calories at < 15 weeks of pregnancy) + β3 (marital state) + β4 (persons in home) + β5 (age) + β6 (level of studies) + β7 (monthly income) + β8 (relation to head of household) + β9 (activity) + β10 (depression) + β11 (nutritional status) + β12 (gestational weight gain) + β13 (season) + β14 (health center).

In addition to baseline values, significant covariables in the multivariable models were maternal age (β coefficient = −1.1, 95% CI = −2.1, −0.1) and health care center (β coefficient= −14.7, 95% CI = −24.4, −4.9) for the model of sugars consumption, maternal age (β coefficient −16, 95% CI −27, −5), and GWG (β coefficient 18, 95% CI 6, 30) for the model of energy, and health care center (β coefficient −2, 95% CI −3, −1) for the model of percentage of energy derived from sugars.

We repeated the analysis using the change between initial and final consumption as the response variable in a sensitivity analysis. The multiple models had similar results (Table S1).

4. Discussion

The present study showed that an intervention with dietary counseling in overweight or obese pregnant women was effective in decreasing the consumption of foods that most contribute to total sugars, energy, and the percentage of energy from sugars. Compared to participants who only received routine counseling, the IG reduced the mean consumption of total sugars by 15 g/day and energy by 125 kcal/day, and also reduced the percentage of energy from sugars by 2%.

We did not find reported nutritional interventions focused on decreasing sugars comparable to the present study. However, our results are consistent with other interventions of a similar nature. A study in Mexico determined if the nutritional status of overweight and obese pregnant women improved by implementing a personalized diet. These results indicated that the group of sugars had a greater decrease in consumption (15.1%) than the other food groups evaluated [5]. This could be attributed to the fact that the personalized diet emphasized eating foods with low glycemic index. Poston et al. provided diet counseling to obese pregnant women centered on consumption of foods with low glycemic index, including replacement of sugared soft drinks by ones with low glycemic index and reduction of saturated foods; they showed that intervened participants reduced mean intake of saturated fats, carbohydrates, and total energy, and increased intake of protein and fiber [10]. Petrella et al. [16] evaluated a nutritional intervention in overweight and obese pregnant women in which the primary focus of the dietary intervention was decreasing high-glycemic index foods consumption and substituting them with healthier alternatives. They observed that the group who received the intervention decreased the consumption of sugar and increased the consumption of vegetables and fruits [16]. Wolff et al. [27] performed a dietetic intervention restricted to energy consumption, providing a distribution of macronutrients according to Danish recommendations; they found changes in the composition of the diet and a decrease in total energy consumption similar to that found in our study [27]. In contrast, an Australian randomized LIMIT trial performed an intervention in lifestyle focused on maintaining equilibrium of carbohydrates, fats, and proteins to reduce intake of foods rich in refined carbohydrates and saturated fats. They did not find a significant difference in the mean daily energy consumption between the group of pregnant women randomized to the intervention and the control group [28]. Our intervention may have been more effective because it was focused on the foods that contribute most to sugars consumption, thus it may have been easier for the participants to follow the indications. It has been shown that dietary interventions during pregnancy are more effective than a combination of diet and physical activity in terms of weight gained during pregnancy, suggesting that there may be poorer compliance by participants when a large number of indications are given to the participants [29].

As far as we know, ours is the first Chilean study that presents detailed information on the consumption of energy and total sugars in different food groups of the diet of overweight and obese pregnant women. The dietary counseling was effective in differentially reducing some of the foods that most contribute to sugars consumption (the Top 7). Compared to women in the CG, participants from the IG had significant greater reductions of the intake (calories) of snacks and whole fat milk products, which was also the case for total sugars coming from whole fat milk products. Besides this, the intervention also decreased the intake of energy and sugars coming from fruits, even if fruits were not part of the targeted food groups. The intervention also decreased the consumption (calories) of sugars and sweets, and soft drinks and juices, but this was not significantly different from what happened in the CG. The intake of bread and cookies did not decrease. The decrease in more than 15 g of total sugars intake observed in the adjusted models corresponded to a decrease of 2% of energy from total sugars in the studied population. The baseline intake of total sugars was 26% of calories, which is much greater than the recommendations made for the general population (i.e., <20% of daily energy intake from total sugars) [30]. Thus, the reported intervention helped decrease one-third of the excessive intake of total sugars. Total sugars intake decreased mainly from whole fat milk products and fruits, which could be interpreted as an unexpected outcome. In the case of fruits, the intake of total sugars in the follow-up of the IG was 26 g, which corresponds to 2–3 servings of fruits, according to the recommendations (considering that most of them have about 10% of their weight as sugars). The women counseled also showed greater reduction (42 kcal/day) of intake of whole milk foods and increase of 18 kcal/day in low-fat dairy products. These results comply with the nutritional recommendations of the Health ministry for low-fat dairy products for pregnant women, considered essential during pregnancy [31]. Evidence has shown that the absorption of calcium increases during pregnancy, fulfilling the requirements of bone mineralization of the fetus [32]. The study of Osorio et al. [33] suggests that greater intake of low-fat dairy products is significantly associated with lower risk of gestational diabetes mellitus. These findings lend weight to the context of the present research [33].

The decrease in dairy products also implies a decrease in the consumption of both total and added sugars, since the amount of total sugars among all yogurts and most whole fat milks were 2–3 times the natural content of lactose (about 5% among milks and 7% among yogurts). Thus, the intervention also helped in decreasing the gap between the intake and the recommendation of added sugars [34] even when we cannot indicate in which extent given added sugars were not assessed.

As far as we know, it is not possible to anticipate the exact clinical impact of such dietary improvement, but given the current knowledge on the detrimental impact of an excessive intake of sugars [35] and the better understanding of the Developmental Origin of Disease paradigm [36,37], it is plausible that this changes would imply relevant improvements in women and offspring health. Although the evidence of the effect of dietary interventions in mothers with obesity focused on reducing foods with high glycemic index on maternal and offspring cardiometabolic health is not consistent and needs to be further studied, some animal experiments have shown positive results [19,38]. In our study, the intervention was not associated with differences in GWG or in the percentage of women who exceeded the IOM 2009 recommendations for GWG between groups; therefore, any effect of maternal diet on maternal and offspring outcomes could be not mediated by changes in GWG. However, it is possible that sample size of the present study is not large enough to ensure adequate power to detect differences on GWG between groups.

The strengths of this study include its cohort design with close follow-up of the participants and measurement of multiple variables, which helped fit the models. The construction of an FFQ aimed at the consumption of sugars and energy based on an R24H questionnaire in a population with similar characteristics allowed a reliable representation of daily consumption. FFQ is a method of dietary evaluation used in most epidemiological studies [39,40], considered to provide a valid model of long-term habitual consumption as well as being cheap, rapid, and easy to apply [41]. However, since FFQs are self-reported, they may be subject to report bias. The IG may have reported lower intake than the CG, given the fact that our intervention was not blind. However, the results of consumption in the baseline were similar to those reported in the R24h of women who did not participate in the intervention. Both groups showed decreases in the consumption of sugars and total energy, greater in the IG, although evidence shows that pregnant women tend to increase energy consumption during pregnancy [42]. Part of the decrease in the CG group may be due to the routine counseling received in the prenatal attention.

This study showed that focused dietary counseling provided in only three sessions during a 12-week period can be effective in decreasing the consumption of sugars and energy. This is an alternative to the current guidelines of the Chilean National Health Services, which recommend a generally healthy diet [31]. Future studies should evaluate if these changes produce maternal and child results (lower incidence of gestational diabetes and macrosomia, among others). It would also be interesting to know if these maternal dietary changes that may be motivated by the pregnancy are maintained after the women give birth.

5. Conclusions

The implementation of a dietary intervention with nutritional counseling focused on sugars consumption decreased the consumption of energy and total sugars in overweight and obese pregnant women, mainly in the food groups high in free sugars. Future studies should evaluate if these changes produce short- and long-term maternal and child results. Given its focus, this intervention may be replicable in all primary health centers for pregnant women with the highest nutritional risk.

Author Contributions: M.L.G. helped design the study and provided advice on statistical analysis. E.A. performed the research, inscription of participants, home nutritional counseling, compilation and analysis of data. M.L.G. and E.A. wrote the first version of the manuscript. M.R., M.A.B., M.F., and R.U. read and approved the final manuscript.

Acknowledgments: DSM Nutritional Products donated the capsules for the original study, but had no role in the design of the study, in its analysis, interpretation, nor in its dissemination. The South East Health Service and Puente Alto county have provided kind support for the implementation of the study. We thank all the participants in this study for generously helping us in this research.

References

1. Organización de las Naciones Unidas para la Alimentación y la Agricultura. América Latina y el Caribe. Panorama de la Seguridad Alimentaria y Nutricional. 2017. Available online: http://www.fao.org/americas/publicaciones-audio-video/panorama/es/ (accessed on 10 May 2017).
2. Gobierno de Chile Ministerio de Salud. *Encuesta Nacional de Salud ENS Chile 2009–2010*; Ministerio de Salud: Santiago, Chile, 2010.
3. Araya, B.; Padilla, O.; Garmendia, M.L.; Atalah, E.; Uauy, R. Prevalence of obesity among Chilean women in childbearing ages. *Revista Medica de Chile* **2014**, *142*, 1440–1448.
4. Huidobro, A.; Fulford, A.; Carrasco, E. Incidence of gestational diabetes and relationship to obesity in Chilean pregnant women. *Revista Medica de Chile* **2004**, *132*, 931–938. [PubMed]
5. Sandoval, K.V.; Nieves, E.R.; Luna, M.Á. Efecto de una dieta personalizada en mujeres embarazadas con sobrepeso u obesidad. *Revista Chilena de Nutrición* **2016**, *43*, 233–246. [CrossRef]
6. Renault, K.M.; Carlsen, E.M.; Nørgaard, K.; Nilas, L.; Pryds, O.; Secher, N.J.; Olsen, S.F.; Halldorsson, T.I. Intake of sweets, snacks and soft drinks predicts weight gain in obese pregnant women: Detailed analysis of the results of a randomised controlled trial. *PLoS ONE* **2015**, *10*, e0133041. [CrossRef] [PubMed]
7. Aşcı, Ö.; Rathfisch, G. Effect of lifestyle interventions of pregnant women on their dietary habits, lifestyle behaviors, and weight gain: A randomized controlled trial. *J. Health Popul. Nutr.* **2016**, *35*, 7. [CrossRef] [PubMed]
8. Hui, A.L.; Ludwig, S.; Gardiner, P.; Sevenhuysen, G.; Dean, H.J.; Sellers, E.; McGavock, J.; Morris, M.; Shen, G.X.; Jiang, D.; et al. Effects of lifestyle intervention on dietary intake, physical activity level, and gestational weight gain in pregnant women with different pre-pregnancy Body Mass Index in a randomized control trial. *BMC Pregnancy Childbirth* **2014**, *14*, 331. [CrossRef] [PubMed]
9. Shepherd, E.; Gomersall, J.C.; Tieu, J.; Han, S.; Crowther, C.A.; Middleton, P. Combined diet and exercise interventions for preventing gestational diabetes mellitus. *Cochrane Database Syst Rev.* **2017**, *11*, CD01443. [CrossRef] [PubMed]
10. Poston, L.; Bell, R.; Croker, H.; Flynn, A.C.; Godfrey, K.M.; Goff, L.; Hayes, L.; Khazaezadeh, N.; Nelson, S.M.; Oteng-Ntim, E.; et al. Effect of a behavioural intervention in obese pregnant women (the UPBEAT study): A multicentre, randomised controlled trial. *Lancet Diabetes Endocrinol.* **2015**, *3*, 767–777. [CrossRef]

11. Bruno, R.; Petrella, E.; Bertarini, V.; Pedrielli, G.; Neri, I.; Facchinetti, F. Adherence to a lifestyle programme in overweight/obese pregnant women and effect on gestational diabetes mellitus: A randomized controlled trial. *Matern. Child Nutr.* **2017**, *13*, e12333. [CrossRef]
12. Luoto, R.; Kinnunen, T.I.; Aittasalo, M.; Kolu, P.; Raitanen, J.; Ojala, K.; Mansikkamäki, K.; Lamberg, S.; Vasankari, T.; Komulainen, T.; et al. Primary prevention of gestational diabetes mellitus and large-for-gestational-age newborns by lifestyle counseling: A cluster-randomized controlled trial. *PLoS Med.* **2011**, *8*, e1001036. [CrossRef]
13. Garmendia, M.L.; Corvalán, C.; Casanello, P.; Araya, M.; Flores, M.; Bravo, A.; Kusanovic, J.P.; Olmos, P.; Uauy, R. Effectiveness on maternal and offspring metabolic control of a home-based dietary counseling intervention and DHA supplementation in obese/overweight pregnant women (MIGHT study): A randomized controlled trial-Study protocol. *Contemp. Clin. Trials* **2018**, *70*, 35–40. [CrossRef]
14. Governement of Chile, Ministry of Health. *Guía Perinatal*; Ministry of Health: Santiago, Chile, 2015.
15. Poston, L.; Briley, A.L.; Barr, S.; Bell, R.; Croker, H.; Coxon, K.; Essex, H.N.; Hunt, C.; Hayes, L.; Howard, L.M.; et al. Developing a complex intervention for diet and activity behaviour change in obese pregnant women (the UPBEAT trial); assessment of behavioural change and process evaluation in a pilot randomised controlled trial. *BMC Pregnancy Childbirth* **2013**, *13*, 148. [CrossRef]
16. Petrella, E.; Malavolti, M.; Bertarini, V.; Pignatti, L.; Neri, I.; Battistini, N.C.; Facchinetti, F. Gestational weight gain in overweight and obese women enrolled in a healthy lifestyle and eating habits program. *J. Matern. Fetal Neonatal Med.* **2014**, *27*, 1348–1352. [CrossRef] [PubMed]
17. Moses, R.G.; Casey, S.A.; Quinn, E.G.; Cleary, J.M.; Tapsell, L.C.; Milosavljevic, M.; Petocz, P.; Brand-Miller, J.C. Pregnancy and Glycemic Index Outcomes study: Effects of low glycemic index compared with conventional dietary advice on selected pregnancy outcomes. *Am. J. Clin. Nutr.* **2014**, *99*, 517–523. [CrossRef] [PubMed]
18. Walsh, J.M.; McGowan, C.A.; Mahony, R.; Foley, M.E.; McAuliffe, F.M. Low glycaemic index diet in pregnancy to prevent macrosomia (ROLO study): Randomised control trial. *BMJ* **2012**, *345*, e5605. [CrossRef] [PubMed]
19. Zhang, R.; Han, S.; Chen, G.C.; Li, Z.N.; Silva-Zolezzi, I.; Parés, G.V.; Wang, Y.; Qin, L.Q. Effects of low-glycemic-index diets in pregnancy on maternal and newborn outcomes in pregnant women: A meta-analysis of randomized controlled trials. *Eur. J. Nutr.* **2018**, *57*, 167–177. [CrossRef] [PubMed]
20. Institute of Medicine; National Research Council. *Weight Gain During Pregnancy: Reexamining the Guidelines*; National Academies Press: Washington, DC, USA, 2009.
21. Moshfegh, A.J.; Rhodes, D.G.; Baer, D.J.; Murayi, T.; Clemens, J.C.; Rumpler, W.V.; Paul, D.R.; Sebastian, R.S.; Kuczynski, K.J.; Ingwersen, L.A.; et al. The US Department of Agriculture Automated Multiple-Pass Method reduces bias in the collection of energy intakes. *Am. J. Clin. Nutr.* **2008**, *88*, 324–332. [CrossRef]
22. Mendonça, R.D.; Pimenta, A.M.; Gea, A.; de la Fuente-Arrillaga, C.; Martinez-Gonzalez, M.A.; Lopes, A.C.; Bes-Rastrollo, M. Ultraprocessed food consumption and risk of overweight and obesity: The University of Navarra Follow-Up (SUN) cohort study. *Am. J. Clin. Nutr.* **2016**, *104*, 1433–1440. [CrossRef]
23. Gobierno de Chile Ministerio de Salud. Encuesta Nacional de Consumo Alimentario. 2011. Available online: https://www.minsal.cl/enca/ (accessed on 10 November 2016).
24. Schmidt-Hebbel, H.; Pennacchiotti, I.; Masson, L.; Mella, M. *Tabla de Composición Química de Alimentos Chilenos*, 8th ed.; Facultad de Ciencias Químicas y Farmacéuticas, Departamento de Ciencia de los Alimentos y Tecnología Química, Universidad de Chile: Santiago, Chile, 1992.
25. United States Department of Agriculture, Agricultural Research Service, USDA Food Composition Databases. USDA National Nutrient Database for Standard Reference. Available online: https://ndb.nal.usda.gov/ndb/ (accessed on 15 November 2017).
26. Kanter, R.; Reyes, M.; Corvalán, C. Photographic Methods for Measuring Packaged Food and Beverage Products in Supermarkets. *Curr. Dev. Nutr.* **2017**, *1*, e001016. [CrossRef]
27. Wolff, S.; Legarth, J.; Vangsgaard, K.; Toubro, S.; Astrup, A. A randomized trial of the effects of dietary counseling on gestational weight gain and glucose metabolism in obese pregnant women. *Int. J. Obes. (Lond.)* **2008**, *32*, 495–501. [CrossRef]
28. Dodd, J.M.; Cramp, C.; Sui, Z.; Yelland, L.N.; Deussen, A.R.; Grivell, R.M.; Moran, L.J.; Crowther, C.A.; Turnbull, D.; McPhee, A.J. The effects of antenatal dietary and lifestyle advice for women who are overweight or obese on maternal diet and physical activity: The LIMIT randomised trial. *BMC Med.* **2014**, *12*, 161. [CrossRef]

29. Thangaratinam, S.; Rogozinska, E.; Jolly, K.; Glinkowski, S.; Roseboom, T.; Tomlinson, J.W.; Kunz, R.; Mol, B.W.; Coomarasamy, A.; Khan, K.S. Effects of interventions in pregnancy on maternal weight and obstetric outcomes: Meta-analysis of randomised evidence. *BMJ* **2012**, *344*, e2088. [CrossRef]
30. French Agency for Food, Environmental and Occupational Health & Safety. *Opinion of the French Agency for Food, Environmental and Occupational Health & Safety on the Establishment of Recommendations on Sugar Intake*; Request No 2012-SA-0186; ANSES: Maisons-Alfort, France, 2016.
31. Gobierno de Chile, Ministerio de Salud, Subsecretaria de Salud Pública. *Guía Perinatal*; Ministerio de Salud: Santiago, Chile, 2014.
32. Hacker, A.N.; Fung, E.B.; King, J.C. Role of calcium during pregnancy: Maternal and fetal needs. *Nutr. Rev.* **2012**, *70*, 397–409. [CrossRef] [PubMed]
33. Osorio-Yáñez, C.; Qiu, C.; Gelaye, B.; Enquobahrie, D.A.; Williams, M.A. Risk of gestational diabetes mellitus in relation to maternal dietary calcium intake. *Public Health Nutr.* **2017**, *20*, 1082–1089. [CrossRef] [PubMed]
34. U.S. Department of Health and Human Services and U.S. Department of Agriculture. 2015–2020 DietaryGuidelines for Americans. 8th Edition. December 2015. Available online: http://health.gov/dietaryguidelines/2015/guidelines/ (accessed on 15 January 2019).
35. Vos, M.B.; Kaar, J.L.; Welsh, J.A.; Van Horn, L.V.; Feig, D.I.; Anderson, C.A.M.; Patel, M.J.; Cruz Munos, J.; Krebs, N.F.; Xanthakos, S.A.; et al. Added Sugars and Cardiovascular Disease Risk in Children: A Scientific Statement from the American Heart Association. *Circulation* **2017**, *135*, e1017–e1034. [CrossRef] [PubMed]
36. Gluckman, P.D.; Hanson, M.A.; Beedle, A.S. Early life events and their consequences for later disease: A life history and evolutionary perspective. *Am. J. Hum. Biol.* **2007**, *19*, 1–19. [CrossRef] [PubMed]
37. Uauy, R.; Kain, J.; Corvalan, C. How can the Developmental Origins of Health and Disease (DOHaD) hypothesis contribute to improving health in developing countries? *Am. J. Clin. Nutr.* **2011**, *94*, 1759S–1764S. [CrossRef] [PubMed]
38. Menting, M.D.; Mintjens, S.; van de Beek, C.; Frick, C.J.; Ozanne, S.E.; Limpens, J.; Roseboom, T.J.; Hooijmans, C.R.; van Deutekom, A.W.; Painter, R.C. Maternal obesity in pregnancy impacts offspring cardiometabolic health: Systematic review and meta-analysis of animal studies. *Obes. Rev.* **2019**. [CrossRef]
39. Trinidad Rodríguez, I.; Fernández Ballart, J.; Cucó Pastor, G.; Biarnés Jordà, E.; Arija Val, V. Validación de un cuestionario de frecuencia de consumo alimentario corto: Reproducibilidad y validez. *Nutrición Hospitalaria* **2008**, *23*, 242–252.
40. Rauh, K.; Kunath, J.; Rosenfeld, E.; Kick, L.; Ulm, K.; Hauner, H. Healthy living in pregnancy: A cluster-randomized controlled trial to prevent excessive gestational weight gain-rationale and design of the GeliS study. *BMC Pregnancy Childbirth* **2014**, *14*, 119. [CrossRef]
41. Barbieri, P.; Nishimura, R.Y.; Crivellenti, L.C.; Sartorelli, D.S. Relative validation of a quantitative FFQ for use in Brazilian pregnant women. *Public Health Nutr.* **2013**, *16*, 1419–1426. [CrossRef] [PubMed]
42. Hillier, S.E.; Olander, E.K. Women's dietary changes before and during pregnancy: A systematic review. *Midwifery* **2017**, *49*, 19–31. [CrossRef] [PubMed]

7

Association of Full Breastfeeding Duration with Postpartum Weight Retention in a Cohort of Predominantly Breastfeeding Women

Muna J. Tahir [1,*], Jacob L. Haapala [1], Laurie P. Foster [1], Katy M. Duncan [2], April M. Teague [2], Elyse O. Kharbanda [3], Patricia M. McGovern [4], Kara M. Whitaker [5,6], Kathleen M. Rasmussen [7], David A. Fields [2], Lisa J. Harnack [1], David R. Jacobs Jr. [1] and Ellen W. Demerath [1]

1 Division of Epidemiology and Community Health, University of Minnesota, Minneapolis, MN 55454, USA; jacob.l.haapala@healthpartners.com (J.L.H.); fost0112@umn.edu (L.P.F.); harna001@umn.edu (L.J.H.); jacob004@umn.edu (D.R.J.J.); ewd@umn.edu (E.W.D.)

2 Department of Pediatrics, University of Oklahoma Health Sciences Center, Oklahoma City, OK 73104, USA; Katy-Duncan@ouhsc.edu (K.M.D.); April-Teague@ouhsc.edu (A.M.T.); David-Fields@ouhsc.edu (D.A.F.)

3 HealthPartners Institute, Minneapolis, MN 55425, USA; elyse.o.kharbanda@healthpartners.com

4 Division of Environmental Health Sciences, University of Minnesota, Minneapolis, MN 55455, USA; pmcg@umn.edu

5 Department of Health and Human Physiology, University of Iowa, Iowa City, IA 52242, USA; kara-whitaker@uiowa.edu

6 Department of Epidemiology, University of Iowa, Iowa City, IA 52242, USA

7 Division of Nutritional Sciences, Cornell University, Ithaca, NY 14853, USA; kathleen.rasmussen@cornell.edu

* Correspondence: mtahir@umn.edu

Abstract: Full breastfeeding (FBF) is promoted as effective for losing pregnancy weight during the postpartum period. This study evaluated whether longer FBF is associated with lower maternal postpartum weight retention (PPWR) as compared to a shorter FBF duration. The MILK (Mothers and Infants Linked for Healthy Growth) study is an ongoing prospective cohort of 370 mother–infant dyads, all of whom fully breastfed their infants for at least 1 month. Breastfeeding status was subsequently self-reported by mothers at 3 and 6 months postpartum. Maternal PPWR was calculated as maternal weight measured at 1, 3, and 6 months postpartum minus maternal prepregnancy weight. Using linear mixed effects models, by 6 months postpartum, adjusted means ± standard errors for weight retention among mothers who fully breastfed for 1–3 (3.40 ± 1.16 kg), 3–6 (1.41 ± 0.69 kg), and ≥6 months (0.97 ± 0.32 kg) were estimated. Compared to mothers who reported FBF for 1–3 months, those who reported FBF for 3–6 months and ≥6 months both had lower PPWR over the period from 1 to 6 months postpartum ($p = 0.04$ and $p < 0.01$, respectively). However, PPWR from 3 to 6 months was not significantly different among those who reported FBF for 3–6 versus ≥6 months ($p > 0.05$). Interventions to promote FBF past 3 months may increase the likelihood of postpartum return to prepregnancy weight.

Keywords: full breastfeeding; postpartum; weight retention; obesity

---

1. Introduction

Pregnancy is a period of rapid weight gain and change in body composition [1] as maternal metabolism accommodates the demands of a growing fetus [2]. Gestational weight gain within the recommended ranges based on prepregnancy body mass index (BMI) is important for optimal fetal development [1,3] and accretion of fat depots necessary to support the energy cost of lactation [2].

Unfortunately, 47% of women in the United States have excessive gestational weight gain [4] and 13–20% fail to return to their prepregnancy weight after delivery, weighing approximately 5 kg more at 6–18 months postpartum compared to prepregnancy [5,6]. Excessive postpartum weight retention (PPWR) may in turn initiate a vicious cycle of obesity among women during their reproductive years and contribute to future unhealthy pregnancies, diabetes, and cardiovascular disease [1].

Many factors influence variation in PPWR, including maternal prepregnancy BMI, gestational weight gain, parity, age, race/ethnicity, education, diet, physical activity, and breastfeeding duration [7–10]. Breastfeeding is of particular interest due to its established physical and psychological benefits for both mother and infant during the postpartum period and beyond [11–13]. Prolonged breastfeeding may theoretically promote postpartum weight loss owing to the energy expenditure requirements of lactation [14] and mobilization of pregnancy-related accumulated fat stores [2].

To date, studies examining the association between breastfeeding and PPWR or postpartum weight loss have yielded inconclusive findings [15–17]. In a recent systematic review, Neville et al. concluded that, compared to other forms of infant feeding, there was insufficient evidence indicating that breastfeeding is directly associated with postpartum weight change [18]. Of particular concern is the issue of confounding, whereby women who breastfeed longer are more likely to have intended to breastfeed [19], have greater social support [11], and have lower prepregnancy BMI [20] and gestational weight gain [21] than women who breastfeed for short durations, never breastfeed or breastfeed only partially. All these factors are directly associated with PPWR [7–10]. Most studies included in this comprehensive review had relatively few women who were exclusively breastfeeding to 6 months as recommended, and/or did not adjust for important potentially confounding variables. They also often relied on self-reported maternal weight and lacked repeated measurements to assess patterns of weight retention over time, both of which decrease precision. Additional studies that can characterize the relationship between longer versus shorter full breastfeeding (FBF) and PPWR, including in women who are strongly committed to and initiate full breastfeeding, are therefore warranted.

In this exploratory study, we aimed to examine the association between FBF duration and maternal PPWR from 1 to 6 months postpartum using repeated measures of FBF and objectively measured maternal anthropometry within a cohort of healthy, predominantly breastfeeding women. We hypothesized that, compared to mothers who fully breastfed for 1–3 months and 3–6 months, those who fully breastfed for ≥6 months would exhibit lower PPWR from 1 to 6 months, and from 3 to 6 months, respectively.

2. Materials and Methods

2.1. Study Population

The Mothers and Infants Linked for Healthy Growth (MILK) study is an ongoing prospective cohort of mother–infant dyads recruited from Minneapolis, MN and Oklahoma City, OK [22]. Women were included in the study if they: were 21–45 years of age at delivery; had a prepregnancy BMI of 18.5–40.0 kg/m^2; had a healthy singleton pregnancy (i.e., spent <3 days in the hospital post-delivery for vaginal deliveries and <5 days for caesarean section deliveries); delivered an infant at-term with a birthweight of ≥2500 g but ≤4500 g; and reported an intention to breastfeed exclusively for at least 3 months. Women were excluded from the study if they consumed tobacco or >1 alcoholic drink per week during pregnancy/lactation, had a history of Type 1 or Type II diabetes or current diagnosis of gestational diabetes, were unable to speak or understand English, or if the infant had a known congenital illness affecting feeding and/or growth.

Of the 370 mother–infant dyads enrolled into the MILK study (all fully breastfeeding at 1 month postpartum), 32 were excluded due to missing information on breastfeeding status at 3 or 6 months or maternal prepregnancy weight. The final analytic sample size included 338 mother–infant dyads with complete information on FBF duration, maternal prepregnancy weight, and maternal weight on at least one of the follow-up time points (i.e., at 1, 3 or 6 months postpartum).

Written informed consent was obtained at baseline, and participants were compensated for completion of each visit. All study protocols were approved by the institutional review boards at the University of Minnesota, HealthPartners Institute, and the University of Oklahoma Health Sciences Center.

2.2. Breastfeeding Status

Maternal breastfeeding status was ascertained at the 1-, 3-, and 6-month study visits. Mothers were asked to report their breastfeeding habits, which were further classified as FBF, mixed-feeding or fully formula feeding. Given our inability to discern "exclusive" (no other solid foods/liquids) from "almost exclusive" breastfeeding (water, vitamins and minerals occasionally provided), we defined FBF as maintaining breastfeeding with <24 oz of formula during the entire time period, and only breast milk for the 2 weeks prior to the visit. Mixed feeding was defined as providing infants with >24 oz of formula for each time period but also some breast milk. Fully formula feeding was defined as providing infants only formula for each time period. We categorized the duration of FBF in terms of the number of completed months of FBF as follows: 1–3 months, 3–6 months, and ≥6 months. The frequencies of various barriers to lactation were queried at the 1-month study visit.

2.3. Maternal Anthropometry

Maternal prepregnancy weight (kg) was measured within 6 weeks of conception and abstracted from electronic medical records. Maternal weight was then measured at the 1-, 3-, and 6-month study visits using calibrated digital scales. Standard procedures were followed after cross-training of staff [23]. PPWR was calculated and defined as maternal weight at the 1-, 3-, and 6-month visits minus maternal prepregnancy weight.

2.4. Covariates

Maternal educational attainment (high school/GED/Associates degree, Bachelor's degree, graduate degree), race/ethnicity (white, other), household income (<\$60,000, \$60,000–\$90,000, >\$90,000), physical activity at 3 months postpartum (meets/does not meet moderate-to-vigorous physical activity (MVPA) guidelines of 150 min/week) [24], and frequency of feeds at 1, 3, and 6 months postpartum (≤6, >6 times/day) were self-reported by mothers. Dietary intake was self-reported by mothers at 1 month postpartum using a modified version of the Diet History Questionnaire II to reflect intake during the past month [25]. Maternal age (years), parity (0, 1, ≥2), delivery mode (vaginal, caesarean section), infant birthweight (grams), and infant sex (male, female) were abstracted from the mother's electronic medical records. Maternal gestational weight gain (kg) was calculated by subtracting maternal prepregnancy weight from weight at delivery (measured within 2 weeks of birth and abstracted from medical records).

2.5. Statistical Analyses

Characteristics of the mother–infant dyads were described using raw means ± standard deviations (SD) and raw frequencies stratified by FBF duration. Chi-square tests and one-way ANOVAs were used to compare participant characteristics by FBF duration for categorical and continuous variables, respectively. The purpose of these statistical tests was to identify potential confounding variables. One inclusion criterion for the study included an intention to fully breastfeed for at least 3 months and the presence of breastfeeding support; however, $n = 23$ mothers stopped breastfeeding before 3 months. As such, we examined differences in frequencies of barriers to lactation between women who fully breastfed to 1–3 months and those who fully breastfed for ≥3 months using chi-square tests.

Linear mixed effects models (PROC MIXED) were then used to test the association of FBF duration with repeated within-subject measures of maternal PPWR at 1, 3, and 6 months postpartum using an unstructured covariance matrix. These models can accommodate unbalanced intervals of measurement, time-dependent and independent exposures/covariates, and provide greater statistical power with serial measurements [26]. We first examined the crude association of FBF duration with maternal PPWR. The model was then adjusted for maternal education, race/ethnicity, household income, MVPA at 3 months postpartum, frequency of feeds (time-varying), age, parity, delivery mode, gestational weight gain, and infant birthweight and sex. The main exposure (FBF duration) was included as a main effect and as an interaction with time (time-varying). All covariates were included as main effects, but we only retained an interaction with time if the corresponding estimate for the interaction had a p-value < 0.05. Since maternal prepregnancy weight was part of the outcome variable, it was not included as a potential confounder in adjusted analyses. However, in sensitivity analyses, we adjusted for maternal prepregnancy BMI in final models to assess whether any observed associations persisted after accounting for prepregnancy weight status. In another sensitivity analysis, we included maternal Healthy Eating Index-2015 (HEI-2015) total scores and energy intakes at 1 month postpartum as covariates in the final models. Dietary intake was not included in the main analysis owing to the relatively large number of missing data (approximately 13%). Lastly, we tested whether similar findings were observed in main analyses when maternal postpartum weight loss (defined as maternal weight at 1, 3, and 6 months minus maternal weight at delivery) was utilized as an outcome, rather than PPWR.

Because longitudinal mixed effects regression model estimates can be difficult to interpret in the presence of time interactions, we derived and plotted the adjusted means ± SEs for PPWR from the linear mixed model analysis specified above for each FBF group and each time point. Next, a difference-of-differences analysis was conducted, such that the change in adjusted means of weight retention over time (slopes) within each FBF duration category (e.g., PPWR at 1 month minus PPWR at 6 months) were compared across FBF duration categories. Specifically, differences in PPWR from 1 to 6 months were compared for mothers who fully breastfed for 3–6 and ≥6 versus 1–3 months and differences in PPWR from 3 to 6 months were compared for mothers who fully breastfed for 3–6 versus ≥6 months, with corresponding p-values derived from t-tests presented. Statistical analyses were conducted using SAS, version 9.4 (SAS Institute, Inc., Cary, NC, USA).

3. Results

3.1. Participant Characteristics

Mothers included in the analyses were predominantly white, highly educated, and multiparous; most mothers delivered vaginally, met MVPA guidelines at 3 months postpartum, and fully breastfed for ≥6 months (Table 1). By the 6-month visit, less than half of the women who stopped FBF at 1–3 months were partially breastfeeding (48% were mixed feeding), while 73% of the women who continued to fully breastfeed for 3–6 months were still partially breastfeeding (mixed feeding). Maternal age, race, weight retention at 6 months postpartum, frequency of feeds at 3 and 6 months postpartum, and infant birthweight differed significantly by FBF duration, such that mothers who fully breastfed for longer durations were more likely to be older, white, retain less weight, feed more frequently at 3 and 6 months, and give birth to heavier infants ($p < 0.05$). There were no significant differences in delayed lactogenesis, milk flow, milk supply, sore, cracked or bleeding nipples, breast engorgement, breast yeast infection, clogged milk ducts, infected or abscessed breasts or breast milk leakage between mothers who fully breastfed for 1–3 months versus ≥3 months (all $p > 0.20$; Table S1).

Table 1. Demographic, reproductive, and lifestyle characteristics of mother–infant dyads by full breastfeeding duration ($n = 338$).

Participant Characteristics		Full Breastfeeding Duration			
	Total	1–3 months ($n = 23$)	3–6 months ($n = 63$)	≥6-Months ($n = 252$)	
		n (%) or mean ± SD			p-Value
Maternal Age, years	30.8 ± 4.1	28.7 ± 4.9	30.7 ± 4.1	31.0 ± 4.0	0.03 *

Table 1. *Cont.*

Participant Characteristics	Full Breastfeeding Duration				
	Total	1–3 months (n = 23)	3–6 months (n = 63)	≥6-Months (n = 252)	
	n (%) or mean ± SD				p-Value
Maternal Race					
White	288 (87)	14 (64)	51 (82)	223 (90)	
Other	44 (13)	8 (36)	11 (18)	25 (10)	<0.01 *
Maternal Education					
High school /GED/Associates degree	74 (23)	10 (44)	11 (19)	53 (22)	
Bachelor's degree	135 (41)	9 (39)	27 (47)	99 (40)	
Graduate degree	117 (36)	4 (17)	19 (33)	94 (38)	0.09
Household income					
<$60,000	99 (30)	11 (48)	22 (39)	66 (27)	
$60,000–90,000	80 (25)	4 (17)	15 (26)	61 (25)	
>90,000	147 (45)	8 (35)	20 (35)	119 (48)	0.11
Parity					
0	141 (42)	13 (59)	21 (35)	107 (43)	
1	128 (39)	4 (18)	29 (48)	95 (38)	
≥2	63 (19)	5 (23)	10 (17)	48 (19)	0.17
Delivery Mode					
Vaginal	264 (80)	17 (77)	50 (81)	197 (79)	0.94
Caesarean section	68 (20)	5 (23)	12 (19)	51 (21)	
Prepregnancy BMI, kg/m^2	26.5 ± 5.6	28.1 ± 5.3	26.9 ± 6.9	26.2 ± 5.2	0.24
Gestational weight gain (kg)	12.3 ± 6.6	12.2 ± 8.8	11.7 ± 7.0	12.5 ± 6.3	0.69
Postpartum weight retention (kg)					
1-month	3.9 ± 5.4	4.2 ± 7.2	3.2 ± 6.5	4.0 ± 5.0	0.56
3-months	2.8 ± 5.5	4.6 ± 7.9	1.9 ± 6.4	2.8 ± 4.9	0.13
6-months	1.4 ± 5.9	4.3 ± 7.8	0.9 ± 6.4	1.2 ± 5.5	0.05 *
HEI-2015 score at 1-month postpartum	65.6 ± 8.9	64.8 ± 9.6	63.7 ± 6.3	66.4 ± 8.9	0.16
Energy intake at 1-month postpartum (kcal)	1952 ± 761	1666 ± 770	1889 ± 633	1975 ± 666	0.14
Meets MVPA guidelines at 3-months postpartum (yes)	178 (54)	13 (62)	25 (40)	140 (57)	0.06
Frequency of feeds (per day)					
1-month	9.7 ± 2.1	9.4 ± 2.3	9.4 ± 2.0	9.8 ± 2.1	0.44
3-months	7.6 ± 2.1	4.6 ± 2.1	7.8 ± 2.0	7.7 ± 1.9	<0.01 *
6-months	6.8 ± 2.1	3.6 ± 1.8	6.0 ± 2.8	7.1 ± 1.7	<0.01 *
Breastfeeding status at 6 months postpartum					
Fully breastfeeding	252 (74)			252 (100)	<0.01 *
Mixed-feeding	57 (17)	11 (48)	46 (73)		
Fully formula feeding	29 (9)	12 (52)	17 (27)		
Infant birthweight, (g)	3534 ± 445	3329 ± 482	3620 ± 425	3530 ± 442	0.03 *
Infant sex					
Male	172 (51)	10 (43)	38 (60)	124 (49)	0.22
Female	166 (49)	13 (57)	25 (40)	128 (51)	

Abbreviations: BMI = body mass index; HEI-2015 = Healthy Eating Index-2015; meeting MVPA guidelines: Moderate to vigorous physical activity >150 min/week. * $p < 0.05$ for tests of differences in participant characteristics by full breastfeeding duration using chi-square or one-way ANOVA for categorical and continuous variables, respectively.

3.2. *Full Breastfeeding Duration and Postpartum Weight Retention*

A significant interaction between FBF duration and time was observed, suggesting between-group differences in PPWR over time (Table 2). To illustrate the interaction effect of FBF and time on PPWR,

Figure 1 depicts differences in adjusted means ± SE of maternal PPWR from 1 to 6 months postpartum by FBF duration. By 6 months postpartum, mothers who fully breastfed for 1–3, 3–6, and ≥6 months had adjusted means ± SEs for PPWR of 3.40 ± 1.16 kg, 1.41 ± 0.69 kg, and 0.97 ± 0.32 kg. Compared to mothers who fully breastfed for 1–3 months only, those who fully breastfed for 3–6 and ≥6 months retained significantly less weight from 1 to 6 months postpartum ($p = 0.04$ and $p < 0.01$, respectively). Although mothers who fully breastfed for 6 months or longer weighed approximately 0.45 kg less by 6 months postpartum than those who fully breastfed for 3–6 months only, this difference in PPWR at 6 months and slope of change in PPWR from 3 to 6 months was not significant between these two groups ($p = 0.15$). These findings were independent of the statistical effects of numerous potential confounders included in the model. Significant covariate effects were observed for MVPA and maternal age, and time-dependent effects were observed for GWG, maternal education, parity, and mode of delivery (Table S2).

Table 2. Association of full breastfeeding duration with maternal postpartum weight retention measured from 1 to 6 months postpartum.

	Crude Model ($n = 338$)			Covariate-Adjusted Model [a] ($n = 301$)		
	β	95% CI	p-Value	β	95% CI	p-Value
FBF duration						
1–3 months	Ref	Ref		Ref	Ref	
3–6 months	−1.07	−3.67, 1.54		0.33	−1.55, 2.20	
>6 months	−0.24	−2.57, 2.08	0.18	0.49	−1.18, 2.16	0.53
Time [c]						
1–3 months	Ref.	Ref		Ref	Ref	
3 months	0.39	−0.68, 1.46		0.26	−1.34, 1.86	
6 months	0.04	−1.79, 1.86	<0.01	1.97	−0.66, 4.61	0.20
FBF duration x time [b,c]						
FBF 3–6 months at 3 months	−1.60	−2.86, −0.35		−1.60	−2.95, −0.25	
FBF 3–6 months at 6 months	−2.27	−4.41, −0.13		−2.32	−4.54, −0.09	
FBF ≥6 months at 3 months	−1.55	−2.67, −0.43	0.03	−1.66	−2.86, −0.45	0.04
FBF ≥6 months at 6 months	−2.76	−4.67, −0.85		−2.92	−4.90, −0.94	

Abbreviations: CI = confidence interval; FBF = full breastfeeding. [a] Adjusted for maternal education, race/ethnicity, household income, age, parity, delivery mode, prepregnancy weight, gestational weight gain, frequency of feeds at 1, 3 and 6 months (time-varying), physical activity level at 3 months postpartum, and infant birthweight and sex. [b] Reference category = FBF 1 month. [c] Reference category = time 1 month.

In sensitivity analyses, after including maternal prepregnancy BMI as a potential covariate in the final model examining the association between FBF duration and maternal PPWR, comparable findings were observed for adjusted means and differences in slopes of PPWR over time (data not shown). After additional adjustment for maternal total HEI-2015 scores and energy intake at 1 month postpartum, adjusted means were consistent with those found in the main analyses. In this sensitivity analysis, differences in slopes of change in weight retention from 1 to 6 months for women who fully breastfed to ≥6 versus 1–3 months were similar to those reported above for the main analysis. However, slopes of change in weight retention were no longer significantly greater among those who fully breastfed to 3–6 versus 1–3 months ($p < 0.10$) (data not shown). Lastly, after examining postpartum weight loss (versus PPWR) as an outcome, similar adjusted means and between-group differences in weight loss over time were observed (data not shown).

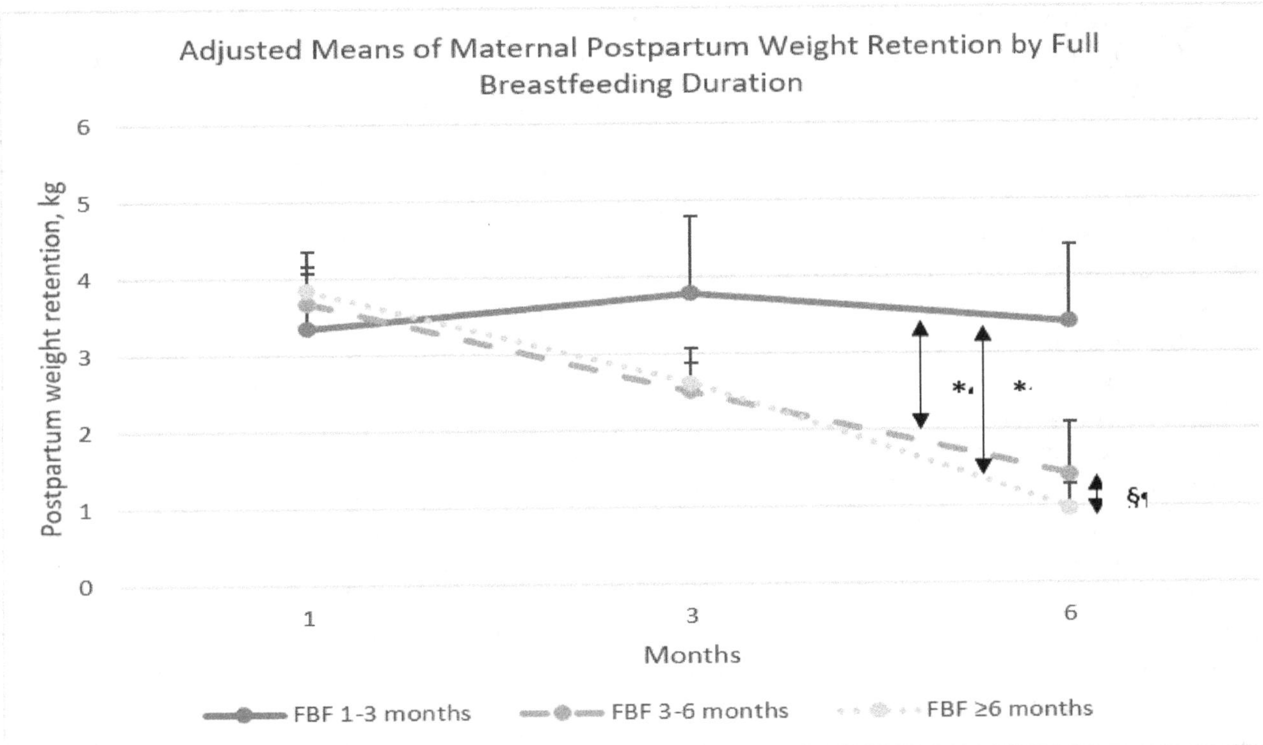

Figure 1. Adjusted means of maternal postpartum weight retention by full breastfeeding duration. Abbreviations: FBF = full breastfeeding; Adjusted for maternal education, race/ethnicity, household income, age, parity, delivery mode, prepregnancy weight, gestational weight gain, frequency of feeds at 1, 3, and 6 months (time-varying), physical activity level at 3 months postpartum, and infant birthweight and sex. * $p < 0.05$ for differences in slopes. § $p > 0.05$ for differences in slopes.

4. Discussion

In this ongoing prospective cohort of mother–infant dyads, we examined the association of FBF duration with maternal weight retention from 1 to 6 months postpartum. We found that, independent of demographic, reproductive, and lifestyle factors, mothers who fully breastfed for longer durations (i.e., greater than 3 months) had significantly greater reductions in PPWR from 1 to 6 months compared to those who fully breastfed to 1–3 months only. Mothers who fully breastfed to 6 months or longer retained approximately 0.45 kg less weight by 6 months postpartum than those who fully breastfed to 3 months only, but differences between these two groups were not statistically significant. The findings from this exploratory analysis suggest that, among healthy women strongly committed and supported to fully breastfeed, encouraging FBF beyond 3 months could reduce PPWR.

The American Academy of Pediatrics recommends exclusive breastfeeding to 6 months, followed by complementary feeding with continued breastfeeding until 1 year and beyond as mutually desired by mothers and their infants [27]. This practice promotes infant health but also has immediate (postpartum) and long-term health benefits for mothers [11–13]. Breastfeeding is hypothesized to mobilize pregnancy-related buildup of visceral and femoral fat stores as a source of energy for milk production [2]. With the concurrent rise in prolactin, lipogenesis is inhibited in peripheral adipose tissue and increases in the mammary glands [28]. Lipoprotein lipase activity in adipocytes (particularly in the femoral region) also surges, resulting in greater weight loss among breastfeeding mothers [29]. Research has demonstrated that maternal total energy expenditure increases by approximately 15–25% during lactation as the production of milk requires an additional 500 kilocalories per day on average [30]. If this excess energy expenditure is not offset by increases in energy intake and decreases in physical activity, the expectation is that mothers will lose weight.

Nonetheless, the 2018 CDC breastfeeding report card suggests that approximately 47% of women in the United States exclusively breastfeed up to 3 months, and only 25% continue to do so up to 6 months with variation between states [31]. A host of social and biological determinants contribute to early cessation of exclusive breastfeeding, including poor family and social support, embarrassment, employment, lactation problems, and perceived lack of sufficient milk supply [32]. Most mothers in the United States do not meet their breastfeeding goals [33], and it is unclear why 23 of the mothers in our highly motivated and supported cohort ceased FBF between 1 and 3 months despite intending to fully breastfeed for at least 3 months. There were no significant differences in early barriers to lactation observed between those with an FBF duration of 1–3 months versus ≥3 months. It is possible that mothers who stopped fully breastfeeding had to return to work, had fewer workplace accommodations for breastfeeding, did not want to pump milk after returning to work or had infants who lost interest in nursing or did not gain enough weight [33]. However, since none of these possible differences are likely to drive postpartum weight loss, they are unlikely to explain the differences we have reported.

Our results on the association between FBF duration and PPWR are in line with those of other studies [15,16,34]. In a cohort of 405 Brazilian women, mean weight retention was approximately 3.6 kg by 9 months postpartum, and longer breastfeeding duration was associated with lower PPWR from 0.5 to 9 months of follow-up [15]. Similarly, Janney et al. reported a mean weight retention of 3.9 kg at 6 months postpartum and lower weight retention from 0.5–18 months postpartum among 110 mothers in the United States who had a longer duration of full and partial breastfeeding [16]. Contrary to our findings, Mullaney et al. reported no association between exclusive breastfeeding and maternal weight change by 4 months postpartum among 470 Irish women enrolled in a prospective cohort study (mean retention at 4 months postpartum was approximately 1.7 kg) [17]. Few studies have had the opportunity to assess the association between prolonged FBF (i.e., up to 6 months) and PPWR due to the limited number of US women who continue to breastfeed beyond 3 months. In one study of over 25,000 mothers in the Danish National Birth Cohort, Baker et al. found that those who breastfed as recommended (i.e., exclusively to 6 months and to any degree for 12 months) had a greater reduction in PPWR at 6 months (regardless of prepregnancy BMI) and at 18 months (among women within the BMI range of 18.5–34.9 kg/m^2) [34].

Discrepancies in findings pertaining to the associations of FBF with PPWR are evident between studies [8,17,35]. Complications in comparisons across research may be attributable to differences in study design, sample sizes (and, accordingly, statistical power), definition and assessment of breastfeeding duration and intensity, time points at which outcomes were assessed and/or periods of collection that were collapsed into one variable, specific outcomes considered and methods used to measure them, quality of exposure and outcome data, duration of follow-up, and confounders included in analyses. It is important to note that our study population is relatively healthy, with 74% of women fully breastfeeding to 6 months (well above the national rates for exclusive breastfeeding) [28] and 55% meeting MVPA guidelines at 3 months postpartum. Among the 63 mothers who breastfed to at least 3 months but not 6 months or more, 73% continued to practice mixed feeding, that is, feeding their infants both breast milk and formula. If only some breastfeeding is required to achieve continued postpartum weight loss, this may explain the similarity in the rate of weight loss from 3 to 6 months in those who breastfed to ≥6 months as compared to only 3–6 months. Further, the mothers in our study are highly educated and had a lower prepregnancy BMI compared to pregnant women in the United States. Our findings of relatively low weight retention by 6 months postpartum even among those with 1–3 months of FBF (3.9 kg) and a nonsignificant difference in PPWR over time between mothers who fully breastfed for 3–6 months versus to 6 months or longer may be attributable to these characteristics.

Our findings can be interpreted within the context of the strengths and limitations of the study. A strength of our study is that the data were drawn from a contemporary, multisite, prospective cohort with serial measurements from 1 to 6 months postpartum, which provides greater statistical power and allows for descriptions of patterns of weight retention over time. Furthermore, we objectively measured weight at 1, 3, and 6 months postpartum, extracted prepregnancy weight from electronic medical records and used rigorous definitions of FBF in real time, which minimizes recall bias. Our study population is well characterized; thus, we were able to adjust for a range of clinical, sociodemographic, and lifestyle potential confounders obtained from detailed questionnaires or medical records, including key elements of energy balance, such as physical activity and dietary intake. A characteristic that distinguishes this cohort from others is that the primary aim of the study was to assess the lactational programming hypothesis. As such, we focused on maternal obesity and breastfeeding as main exposures and were able to adjust for gestational weight gain and frequency of feeds within a day in our primary analyses.

Our study also has important limitations. The MILK study was designed to address the relationship of maternal weight status to breast milk composition in fully breastfeeding women. We were therefore not able to assess the broader questions of whether PPWR differs among women who ever versus never breastfeed, or between women who partially breastfeed for different durations versus those who fully breastfeed. In addition, most of the women were fully breastfeeding for ≥6 months and the samples of women with shorter FBF durations were relatively small. As such, the precision of estimates for the 1–3 and 3–6 months FBF groups were lower than for the ≥6 months FBF group, and we had reduced statistical power to detect PPWR differences between the three groups. Replication of these findings is necessary in larger cohorts of women who initiate FBF but then cease FBF early to characterize the benefit of FBF in reducing PPWR among women who follow breastfeeding guidelines. The mother–infant dyads included in the cohort were primarily non-Hispanic white. Therefore, the generalizability of our results is limited for other race/ethnic groups [35]. We did not collect maternal anthropometry beyond 6 months and consequently could not examine whether the lower weight retention associated with FBF was maintained in the long-term [36]. We also did not have a sufficient sample size to stratify our analysis by maternal obesity [34]. This drawback is important, given the observed differences in initiation and maintenance of FBF [37] and in fat distribution during pregnancy among normal-weight, overweight, and obese women [38]. Maternal prepregnancy weight was measured and abstracted from medical records within 6 weeks of conception, which may lead to variation in assessment of true prepregnancy weight and introduce measurement error. Although we adjusted for numerous theoretical and empirical confounders in our analyses, there may still be residual confounding or confounding by unmeasured variables. Lastly, we only had measures of important energy balance variables (i.e., diet and physical activity) at select time points. These behaviors tend to correlate strongly over time, but this limitation may have resulted in residual confounding that could have biased the estimates somewhat.

5. Conclusions

The perinatal period is one of significant weight and body composition change for women [1]. Consequently, this period is important for preventing excessive gestational weight gain and PPWR, both of which may contribute to future metabolic disease risk. Findings from the present study correspond to some prior research showing that longer FBF duration may be associated with reduced maternal PPWR up to 6 months postpartum [15,16,34]. Coupled with data from other studies, it is evident that, among healthy, predominantly breastfeeding mothers, FBF for prolonged periods (at least 3 months) is associated with significantly less pregnancy weight retention during the postpartum period. FBF for at least 3 months is a potentially modifiable infant feeding choice that not only promotes infant health but also may help to prevent mothers from future development of obesity and cardiometabolic disorders. Studies that identify how to reduce obstacles to prolonged full breastfeeding are critical to advancing the health of both women and their children.

Author Contributions: Conceptualization, D.A.F. and E.W.D.; Data curation, J.L.H.; Formal analysis, M.J.T., D.R.J.J. and E.W.D.; Funding acquisition, D.A.F.; Investigation, L.P.F., K.M.D., and A.M.T.; Supervision, E.W.D.; Writing—original draft, M.J.T.; Writing—review and editing, J.L.H., L.P.F., K.M.D., A.M.T., E.O.K., P.M.M., K.M.W., K.M.R., D.A.F., D.R.J.J., L.J.H., and E.W.D.

Acknowledgments: We would like to thank the mothers and their families for their interest, time, and dedication to the MILK study.

References

1. Rasmussen, K.M.; Yaktine, A.L. *Institute of Medicine (US) and National Research Council (US) Committee to Reexamine IOM Pregnancy Weight Guidelines*; National Academies Press (US): Washington, DC, USA, 2009.
2. Stuebe, A.M.; Rich-Edwards, J.W. The reset hypothesis: Lactation and maternal metabolism. *Am. J. Perinatol.* **2009**, *26*, 81–88. [CrossRef] [PubMed]
3. Rasmussen, K.M.; Catalano, P.M.; Yaktine, A.L. New guidelines for weight gain during pregnancy: What obstetrician/gynecologists should know. *Curr. Opin. Obstet. Gynecol.* **2009**, *21*, 521–526. [CrossRef] [PubMed]
4. Deputy, N.P.; Sharma, A.J.; Kim, S.Y. Gestational Weight Gain—United States, 2012 and 2013. *Morb. Mortal. Wkly. Rep.* **2015**, *64*, 1215–1220. [CrossRef] [PubMed]
5. Gunderson, E.P.; Abrams, B. Epidemiology of gestational weight gain and body weight changes after pregnancy. *Epidemiol. Rev.* **1999**, *21*, 261–275. [CrossRef] [PubMed]
6. Gunderson, E.P. Childbearing and obesity in women: Weight before, during, and after pregnancy. Obstet. Gynecol. *Clin. N. Am.* **2009**, *36*, 317–332.
7. Hollis, J.L.; Crozier, S.R.; Inskip, H.M.; Cooper, C.; Godfrey, K.M.; Harvey, N.C.; Collins, C.E.; Robinson, S.M. Modifiable risk factors of maternal postpartum weight retention: An analysis of their combined impact and potential opportunities for prevention. *Int. J. Obes.* **2017**, *41*, 1091–1098. [CrossRef] [PubMed]
8. Østbye, T.; Peterson, B.L.; Krause, K.M.; Swamy, G.K.; Lovelady, C.A. Predictors of postpartum weight change among overweight and obese women: Results from the Active Mothers Postpartum study. *J. Womens Health (Larchmt)* **2012**, *21*, 215–222. [CrossRef]
9. Endres, L.K.; Straub, H.; McKinney, C.; Plunkett, B.; Minkovitz, C.S.; Schetter, C.D.; Ramey, S.; Wang, C.; Hobel, C.; Raju, T.; et al. Postpartum weight retention risk factors and relationship to obesity at 1 year. *Obstet. Gynecol.* **2015**, *125*, 144–152.
10. Hill, B.; McPhie, S.; Skouteris, H. The Role of Parity in Gestational Weight Gain and Postpartum Weight Retention. *Womens Health Issues* **2016**, *26*, 123–129. [CrossRef]
11. Dieterich, C.M.; Felice, J.P.; O'Sullivan, E.; Rasmussen, K.M. Breastfeeding and health outcomes for the mother-infant dyad. *Pediatr. Clin. N. Am.* **2013**, *60*, 31–48. [CrossRef] [PubMed]
12. Binns, C.; Lee, M.; Low, W.Y. The Long-Term Public Health Benefits of Breastfeeding. *Asia Pac. J. Public Health* **2016**, *28*, 7–14. [CrossRef]
13. Shamir, R. The Benefits of Breast Feeding. In *Nestle Nutrition Institute Workshop Series*; Karger Publishers: Basel, Switzerland, 2016; Volume 86, pp. 67–76.
14. Institute of Medicine (US) Committee on Nutritional Status During Pregnancy and Lactation. *Nutrition During Lactation*; National Academies Press (US): Washington, DC, USA, 1991.
15. Kac, G.; Benício, M.H.; Velásquez-Meléndez, G.; Valente, J.G.; Struchiner, C.J. Breastfeeding and postpartum weight retention in a cohort of Brazilian women. *Am. J. Clin. Nutr.* **2004**, *79*, 487–493. [CrossRef]
16. Janney, C.A.; Zhang, D.; Sowers, M. Lactation and weight retention. *Am. J. Clin. Nutr.* **1997**, *66*, 1116–1124. [CrossRef] [PubMed]
17. Mullaney, L.; O'Higgins, A.C.; Cawley, S.; Kennedy, R.; McCartney, D.; Turner, M.J. Breast-feeding and postpartum maternal weight trajectories. *Public Health Nutr.* **2016**, *19*, 1397–1404. [CrossRef] [PubMed]
18. Neville, C.E.; McKinley, M.C.; Holmes, V.A.; Spence, D.; Woodside, J.V. The relationship between breastfeeding and postpartum weight change—A systematic review and critical evaluation. *Int. J. Obes.* **2014**, *38*, 577–590. [CrossRef] [PubMed]
19. Colaizy, T.T.; Saftlas, A.F.; Morriss, F.H. Maternal intention to breast-feed and breast-feeding outcomes in term and preterm infants: Pregnancy Risk Assessment Monitoring System (PRAMS), 2000–2003. *Public Health Nutr.* **2012**, *15*, 702–710. [CrossRef] [PubMed]
20. Wojcicki, J.M. Maternal prepregnancy body mass index and initiation and duration of breastfeeding: A review of the literature. *J. Womens Health (Larchmt)* **2011**, *20*, 341–347. [CrossRef] [PubMed]
21. Hilson, J.A.; Rasmussen, K.M.; Kjolhede, C.L. Excessive weight gain during pregnancy is associated with earlier termination of breast-feeding among White women. *J. Nutr.* **2006**, *136*, 140–146. [CrossRef] [PubMed]

22. Whitaker, K.M.; Marino, R.C.; Haapala, J.L.; Foster, L.; Smith, K.D.; Teague, A.M.; Jacobs, D.R.; Fontaine, P.L.; McGovern, P.M.; Schoenfuss, T.C.; et al. Associations of Maternal Weight Status Before, During, and After Pregnancy with Inflammatory Markers in Breast Milk. *Obesity* **2017**, *25*, 2092–2099. [CrossRef] [PubMed]
23. Lohman, T.M.R.; Roche, A.F. *Anthropometric Standardization Reference Manual*; Human Kinetics Books: Champaign, IL, USA, 2011.
24. Hayden-Wade, H.A.; Coleman, K.J.; Sallis, J.F.; Armstrong, C. Validation of the telephone and in-person interview versions of the 7-day PAR. *Med. Sci. Sports Exerc.* **2003**, *35*, 801–809. [CrossRef]
25. Subar, A.F.; Thompson, F.E.; Kipnis, V.; Midthune, D.; Hurwitz, P.; McNutt, S.; McIntosh, A.; Rosenfeld, S. Comparative validation of the Block, Willett, and National Cancer Institute food 489 frequency questionnaires: The Eating at America's Table Study. *Am. J. Epidemiol.* **2001**, *154*, 1089–1099. [CrossRef]
26. Gibbons, R.D.; Hedeker, D.; DuToit, S. Advances in analysis of longitudinal data. *Annu. Rev. Clin. Psychol.* **2010**, *6*, 79–107. [CrossRef] [PubMed]
27. Section on Breastfeeding. Breastfeeding and the use of human milk. *Pediatrics* **2012**, *129*, 827–841. [CrossRef] [PubMed]
28. Brandebourg, T.D.; Bown, J.L.; Ben-Jonathan, N. Prolactin upregulates its receptors and inhibits lipolysis and leptin release in male rat adipose tissue. *Biochem. Biophys. Res. Commun.* **2007**, *357*, 408–413. [CrossRef] [PubMed]
29. Rebuffé-Scrive, M.; Enk, L.; Crona, N.; Lönnroth, P.; Abrahamsson, L.; Smith, U.; Björntorp, P. Fat cell metabolism in different regions in women. *Effect of menstrual cycle, pregnancy, and lactation. J. Clin. Investig.* **1985**, *75*, 1973–1976.
30. Gunderson, E.P. Impact of breastfeeding on maternal metabolism: Implications for women with gestational diabetes. *Curr. Diabetes Rep.* **2014**, *14*, 460. [CrossRef] [PubMed]
31. Centers for Disease Control and Prevention. Breastfeeding Report Card-United States. 2018. Available online: https://www.cdc.gov/breastfeeding/pdf/2018breastfeedingreportcard.pdf (accessed on 8 December 2018).
32. U.S. Department of Health and Human Services. *The Surgeon General's Call to Action to Support Breastfeeding*; U.S. Department of Health and Human Services, Office of the Surgeon General: Washington, DC, USA, 2011.
33. Odom, E.C.; Li, R.; Scanlon, K.S.; Perrine, C.G.; Grummer-Strawn, L. Reasons for Earlier Than Desired Cessation of Breastfeeding. *Pediatrics* **2013**, *131*, e726–e732. [CrossRef]
34. Baker, J.L.; Gamborg, M.; Heitmann, B.L.; Lissner, L.; Sørensen, T.I.; Rasmussen, K.M. Breastfeeding reduces postpartum weight retention. *Am. J. Clin. Nutr.* **2008**, *88*, 1543–1551. [CrossRef]
35. Jones, K.M.; Power, M.L.; Queenan, J.T.; Schulkin, J. Racial and ethnic disparities in breastfeeding. *Breastfeed Med.* **2015**, *10*, 186–196. [CrossRef] [PubMed]
36. Jarlenski, M.P.; Bennett, W.L.; Bleich, S.N.; Barry, C.L.; Stuart, E.A. Effects of breastfeeding on postpartum weight loss among U.S. women. *Prev. Med.* **2014**, *69*, 146–150. [CrossRef]
37. Bever Babendure, J.; Reifsnider, E.; Mendias, E.; Moramarco, M.W.; Davila, Y.R. Reduced breastfeeding rates among obese mothers: A review of contributing factors, clinical considerations and future directions. *Int. Breastfeed J.* **2015**, *10*, 21. [CrossRef] [PubMed]
38. Straughen, J.K.; Trudeau, S.; Misra, V.K. Changes in adipose tissue distribution during pregnancy in overweight and obese compared with normal weight women. *Nutr. Diabetes* **2013**, *3*, e84. [CrossRef] [PubMed]

8

Vitamin B_{12} Status in Pregnant Adolescents and their Infants

Julia L. Finkelstein [1,*], Ronnie Guillet [2], Eva K. Pressman [2], Amy Fothergill [1], Heather M. Guetterman [1], Tera R. Kent [1] and Kimberly O. O'Brien [1]

1 Division of Nutritional Sciences, Cornell University, Ithaca, NY 14853, USA; af544@cornell.edu (A.F.); hg384@cornell.edu (H.M.G.); trk8@cornell.edu (T.R.K.); koo4@cornell.edu (K.O.O.)

2 University of Rochester Medical Center, Rochester, NY 14642, USA; ronnie_guillet@urmc.rochester.edu (R.G.); eva_Pressman@urmc.rochester.edu (E.K.P.)

* Correspondence: jfinkelstein@cornell.edu

Abstract: Vitamin B_{12} deficiency has been associated with increased risk of adverse pregnancy outcomes. Few prospective studies have investigated the burden or determinants of vitamin B_{12} deficiency early in life, particularly among pregnant adolescents and their children. The objectives of this study were to determine the prevalence of vitamin B_{12} deficiency and to examine associations between maternal and neonatal vitamin B_{12} status in a cohort study of healthy pregnant adolescents. Serum vitamin B_{12} and folate concentrations were measured in adolescents at mid-gestation (n = 124; 26.4 $\pm$ 3.5 weeks) and delivery (n = 131; 40.0 $\pm$ 1.3 weeks), and in neonates at birth using cord blood. Linear regression was used to examine associations between maternal and neonatal vitamin B_{12} status. Although the prevalence of vitamin B_{12} deficiency (<148.0 pmol/L; 1.6%) in adolescents was low during pregnancy, 22.6% of adolescents were vitamin B_{12} insufficient (<221.0 pmol/L; 22.6%) at mid-gestation. Maternal vitamin B_{12} concentrations significantly decreased from mid-gestation to delivery ($p < 0.0001$), and 53.4% had insufficient vitamin B_{12} status at delivery. Maternal vitamin B_{12} concentrations ($p < 0.001$) and vitamin B_{12} deficiency ($p = 0.002$) at delivery were significantly associated with infant vitamin B_{12} concentrations in multivariate analyses, adjusting for gestational age, maternal age, parity, smoking status, relationship status, prenatal supplement use, pre-pregnancy body mass index, race, and intake of vitamin B_{12} and folate. Maternal vitamin B_{12} concentrations significantly decreased during pregnancy and predicted neonatal vitamin B_{12} status in a cohort of healthy pregnant adolescents.

Keywords: vitamin B_{12}; micronutrients; pregnancy; adolescents; folate

---

1. Introduction

Vitamin B_{12} deficiency (serum vitamin B_{12} <148.0 pmol/L) is a major public health problem globally [1,2]. Although the overall prevalence of vitamin B_{12} deficiency in the United States is estimated to be relatively low (6%), the burden of vitamin B_{12} deficiency is higher in the elderly, pregnant women, and young children (6–25%) [3]. Pregnant adolescents are at increased risk for a variety of micronutrient deficiencies and pregnancy complications, though there is limited data from this high-risk obstetric population.

Vitamin B_{12} deficiency in pregnancy has been associated with increased risk of pregnancy outcomes, including spontaneous abortion, pregnancy loss, intrauterine growth restriction, low birthweight (<2500 g), and neural tube defects (NTDs) [4–15]. Inadequate supply of vitamin B_{12} in pregnancy and early childhood can lead to long-term deficits in growth development in children [16,17].

Maternal vitamin B_{12} concentrations during pregnancy are thought to predict fetal [18–26] and early infant [25,27–29] vitamin B_{12} status. Previous cross-sectional studies in Norway, Turkey, Germany, United Kingdom, Serbia, and Brazil have noted a significant correlation between maternal and infant vitamin B_{12} status at delivery [18,20–22,30–33]; however, in one study in Belgium, maternal and infant vitamin B_{12} concentrations were not significantly correlated [34]. In one study in Germany, maternal serum vitamin B_{12} and holotranscobalamin (holoTC) concentrations at delivery were significantly correlated with cord blood holoTC concentrations ($p < 0.05$) [18]. In contrast, findings from cross-sectional studies examining the associations between maternal and infant vitamin B_{12} concentrations later in the postpartum period have been heterogeneous [35–40]. Maternal vitamin B_{12} and holoTC concentrations were significantly correlated with infant vitamin B_{12} concentrations in the first month (i.e., 2–30 days) postpartum in a study in Turkey [38]. In analyses in mother–infant dyads in the first 6 months postpartum, maternal and infant vitamin B_{12} concentrations were significantly associated in Canada and Cambodia (i.e., 3–27 weeks) [37], but not in India (i.e., 1–6 months) [35].

Prospective studies to date in The Netherlands, Norway, Turkey, India, and Spain have reported significant associations [19,23,24,26,29] between maternal vitamin B_{12} status during pregnancy and infant vitamin B_{12} status in cord blood or serum. In a prospective study in India, maternal vitamin B_{12} status during pregnancy was associated with infant vitamin B_{12} concentrations at 6 weeks of age [28]. In contrast, a study in Norway was conducted to examine the associations between maternal vitamin B_{12} biomarkers during pregnancy and vitamin B_{12} status in infants at birth and 6 months of age; maternal vitamin B_{12} concentrations did not significantly predict cord blood or infant vitamin B_{12} status, although there were significant associations noted for other biomarkers (i.e., maternal holoTC, holohaptocorrin (holoHC), and methylmalonic acid (MMA)) [25]. Although some studies to date have been conducted to examine vitamin B_{12} status in pregnant adolescents [41–43], most studies investigating the associations between maternal and infant vitamin B_{12} status have been conducted among adult pregnant women (i.e., 18 to 40 years). Of these studies, three cross-sectional studies reported participants which included adolescents, with age ranges of 15 to 38 years [32], 16 to 40 years [38], and 17 to 43 years [27]. However, adolescents comprised a small proportion (<15%) of the sample, and data presented were not stratified by age group, which constrained analysis and interpretation of findings for adolescents. There are limited prospective studies on the associations between maternal and infant vitamin B_{12} status conducted in high-risk obstetric groups such as adolescents.

Pregnant adolescents are at increased risk for a variety of micronutrient deficiencies and pregnancy complications [41,44]. The inadequate dietary intake of key nutrients among adolescents in industrialized countries [45], coupled with increased nutritional requirements for growth and development, warrants concern for health outcomes among pregnant adolescents. However, few data exist on the extent of vitamin B_{12} deficiency or its implications for fetal and child health in this high-risk obstetric population, which comprises over 5% of the US population and 11% globally [46,47]. Well-designed prospective studies are needed to elucidate the burden of vitamin B_{12} insufficiency in this key high-risk population and its implications for maternal and child health.

We, therefore, conducted a prospective observational analysis to: (1) determine the prevalence of vitamin B_{12} deficiency and insufficiency in pregnant adolescents and their infants; and (2) examine the associations of maternal and neonatal vitamin B_{12} status in healthy pregnant adolescents.

2. Materials and Methods

2.1. Study Population

Participants included in this study were enrolled in one of two prospective cohort studies funded by the United States Department of Agriculture (USDA). One study examined maternal and fetal bone health among pregnant adolescents ("bone health study") and collected maternal blood samples at mid-gestation and delivery, and cord blood samples at delivery. The other study evaluated iron status and anemia through gestation in pregnant adolescents aged 13 to 18 years and their infants ("anemia study"), and collected maternal and cord blood samples only at delivery. Both studies were observational cohort studies and not clinical trials (and, thus, do not need to be registered, as per protocol for clinical trials). Pregnant adolescents were recruited between 2006 and 2012, from the Rochester Adolescent Maternity Program (RAMP) in Rochester, New York.

Adolescents were eligible to participate if their pregnancies were 12 to 30 weeks in gestation at the time of the adolescents' enrollment in prenatal care at RAMP, and if the adolescents were healthy and carrying a single fetus. Adolescents were excluded if they had any known medical complications, including diabetes, preeclampsia, gestational hypertension, eating disorders, gastrointestinal diseases, HIV infection, or any other diagnosed medical conditions. Data on maternal and neonatal iron status [48,49] and on vitamin B_{12} transporters in placental tissue from this population [50] have been previously reported.

2.2. Ethics

Written informed consent was obtained from all study participants. The research protocol and study procedures were approved by the Institutional Review Boards (IRB) at Cornell University and the University of Rochester. The IRB approval included laboratory analyses of micronutrients in maternal and infant cord blood samples, including vitamin B_{12} and folate concentrations.

2.3. Follow-Up Procedures

Structured interviews were conducted to collect demographic information, including maternal age, educational level, socioeconomic status, and obstetric history at the baseline clinic visit. Detailed clinical, dietary (i.e., 24-h dietary recall), anthropometric, and biochemical data were collected at each visit. The participant recruitment and flow chart are presented in Figure 1. Of 251 participants who delivered at RAMP, a total of 194 participants (n = 138 participants in the bone study, recruited at mid-gestation; n = 56 participants in the anemia study, recruited at delivery) had archived blood samples available for analysis (Figure 1). All adolescents attending the Rochester Adolescent Maternity Program were prescribed a prenatal supplement as standard of care, which contained 27 mg iron, 12 μg vitamin B_{12}, 1000 μg folic acid, and other micronutrients (i.e., 1200 μg vitamin A, 120 mg vitamin C, 10 μg vitamin D_3, 22 mg vitamin E, 1.84 mg thiamin, 3 mg riboflavin, 20 mg niacin, 10 mg vitamin B_6, 200 mg calcium, 25 mg zinc, and 2000 μg copper).

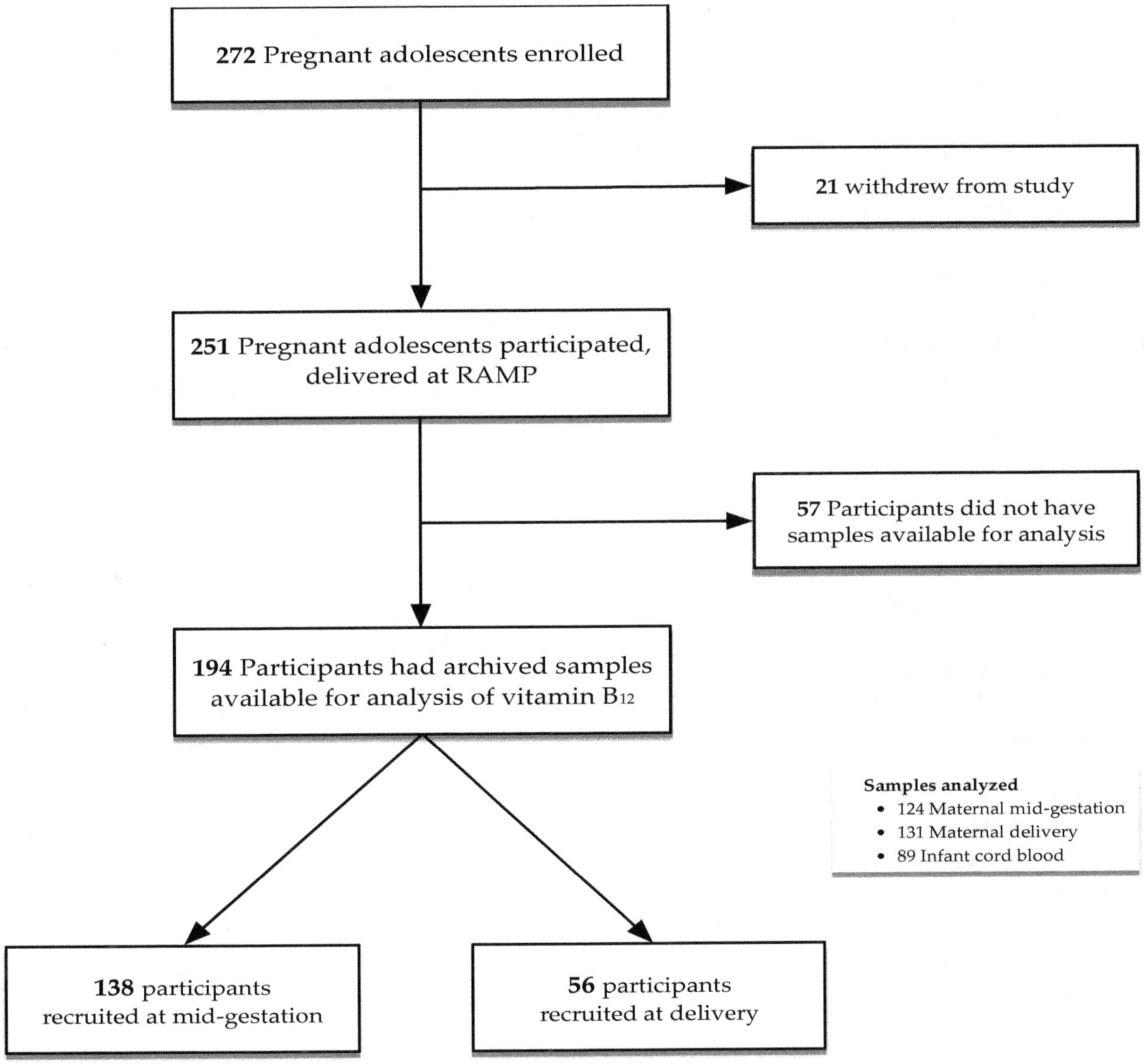

Figure 1. Participant flow diagram.

2.4. Laboratory Analyses

Non-fasting maternal venous blood samples (mid-gestation, delivery) and infant cord blood samples were allowed to clot at room temperature, separated by centrifugation, processed, and stored below −80 °C until analysis. A total of 124 maternal mid-gestation (26.4 ± 3.5 weeks), 131 maternal delivery (40.0 ± 1.3 weeks), and 89 infant cord blood samples were available for analysis.

Vitamin B_{12} concentrations were measured by electrochemiluminescence using the IMMULITE 2000 immunoassay system (Siemens Medical Solutions Diagnostics, Los Angeles, CA, USA). Three levels of controls (Bio-Rad) were used for serum vitamin B_{12}, with inter-assay coefficients of variation (CV) of 4.2% for Level 1 and 4.8% for Level 3. Serum folate concentrations were measured using the IMMULITE 2000 immunoassay system. The Bio-Rad Liquichek Immunoassay Plus Control (High & Low) were used as controls, with intra-assay precision of 6.7% and inter-assay precision of 6.6%.

2.5. Definitions of Outcomes

Conventional cutoffs were used to categorize variables where available; otherwise, medians of variables were defined based on their distributions in the population. Vitamin B_{12} deficiency and insufficiency were defined, following standard Centers for Disease Control and Prevention (CDC) definitions, as less than 148 pmol/L and less than 221.0 pmol/L, respectively [51]. Anemia was defined as hemoglobin <11.0 g/dL during the first and third trimesters, <10.5 g/dL during the second trimester, and <11.0 g/dL at delivery; and anemia status was adjusted for race [52]. Folate deficiency was defined as <6.8 nmol/L [51]. Maternal BMI was defined as the ratio of weight in kg to height in m^2 (kg/m^2), and categorized as <18.5, 18.5 to <25.0, 25.0 to <30.0, and $\geq$30.0 kg/m^2, in accordance with the CDC and World Health Organization (WHO) classifications [53]. Infant low birthweight was defined as <2500 g. Infant ponderal index was calculated as the ratio of weight in g to length in cm^3 ($g/cm^3 \times 100$).

2.6. Statistical Analyses

Binomial and linear regression models were used to examine the associations of maternal vitamin B_{12} status at mid-gestation and delivery with infant vitamin B_{12} status at birth. Binomial regression models were used to obtain risk ratio (RR) estimates for dichotomous variables [54–56]. Non-normally distributed variables were natural logarithmically transformed to ensure normality before further analysis. We also examined the associations between maternal and infant folate status. The values in Table 1 are presented as non-transformed values for interpretation purposes.

We explored potential nonlinearity of the relationships between covariates and outcomes nonparametrically, using stepwise restricted cubic splines [57,58]. If nonlinear associations were not reported, they were not significant. The Rothman and Greenland approach was used to evaluate and adjust for confounding, in which all known or suspected risk factors for the outcome which lead to a >10% change-in-estimate were included in the models [59]. Observations with missing data for covariates were retained in analyses using the missing indicator method [60]. Statistical analyses were conducted using SAS software, version 9.4 (SAS Institute, Inc., Cary, NC, USA).

Table 1. Characteristics of the study population.

Variables [a]	Original Cohort (n = 251)	Current Study (n = 194)	Recruited at Mid-Gestation (n = 138)	Recruited at Delivery (n = 56)
Maternal				
Age at enrollment, years	17.3 (16.5, 18.1)	17.3 (16.5, 18.1)	17.3 (16.4, 18.1)	17.3 (16.6, 18.1)
Age at delivery, years	17.5 (16.7, 18.3)	17.6 (16.8, 18.4)	17.6 (16.7, 18.4)	17.4 (16.9, 18.2)
<16 years, % (n)	12.0 (30)	9.8 (19)	9.4 (13)	10.7 (6)
Gestational age at delivery, weeks	39.9 (38.7, 40.7)	40 (39.0, 40.9)	40.0 (38.9, 40.9)	40.0 (39.2, 41.0)
Pre-term (<37 weeks), % (n)	8.0 (20)	7.8 (15)	8.8 (12)	5.4 (3)
Parity ≥1, % (n)	17.3 (43)	15.1 (29)	8.7 (12)	30.9 (17)
Smoking at enrollment, % (n)				
Never a smoker	77.8 (189)	78.5 (150)	77.5 (107)	81.1 (43)
Past smoker	15.2 (37)	14.4 (27)	12.3 (17)	18.9 (10)
Current smoker	7.0 (17)	7.3 (14)	10.1 (14)	0.0 (0)
Relationship status [b], % (n)	13.5 (33)	10.5 (20)	1.5 (2)	34.0 (18)
WIC [c] program participant	60.9 (148)	63.2 (120)	80.0 (100)	37.7 (20)
Self-reported prenatal supplement use, % (n)				
≥2 pills per week	54.1 (131)	55.5 (106)	56.6 (77)	52.7 (29)
Dietary folate, µg/day	617.2 (397.0, 948.9)	617.2 (400.8, 950.45)	692.7 (464.2, 1020.6)	415.3 (283.9, 624.7)
Dietary vitamin B_{12}, µg/day	4.6 (2.7, 6.5)	4.6 (2.7, 6.6)	5.0 (3.7, 6.9)	2.8 (1.4, 5.2)
Pre-pregnancy BMI, kg/m^2	23.5 (20.8, 28.0)	23.7 (20.8, 28.0)	23.3 (20.8, 28.1)	24.7 (20.8, 27.9)
<18.5 kg/m^2, % (n)	6.9 (17)	7.3 (14)	6.62 (9)	9.1 (5)
≥18.5 to <25 kg/m^2, % (n)	54.3 (133)	52.4 (100)	55.2 (75)	45.5 (25)
≥25.0 to <30 kg/m^2, % (n)	20.8 (51)	21.5 (41)	19.9 (27)	25.5 (14)
≥30 kg/m^2, % (n)	18.0 (44)	18.9 (36)	18.4 (25)	20.0 (11)
Gestational weight gain (GWG), kg	15.9 (11.8, 20.5)	16.4 (11.8, 20.5)	15.5 (11.8, 20.5)	17.3 (12.3, 21.4)
Inadequate [d] GWG, % (n)	15.0 (36)	13.9 (26)	14.3 (19)	13.0 (7)
Within IOM range, % (n)	22.9 (55)	24.0 (45)	26.3 (35)	18.5 (10)
Excessive GWG, % (n)	62.1 (149)	62.0 (116)	59.0 (79)	68.5 (37)
Race, % (n)				
Caucasian	27.9 (70)	29.4 (57)	33.3 (36)	19.6 (11)
African American	71.3 (179)	69.6 (135)	65.2 (90)	80.4 (45)
Native American	0.8 (2)	1.0 (2)	1.5 (2)	0.0 (0)
Ethnicity, % (n)				
Hispanic	24.3 (61)	26.3 (51)	24.6 (34)	30.4 (17)
Infant				
Birthweight, g	3206.0 (2904.0, 3550.0)	3266.0 (2928.0, 3581.0)	3258.0 (2892.0, 3581.0)	3318.5 (3055.5, 3584.0)
Birth length, cm	51.0 (49.0, 52.7)	51.3 (49.5, 52.9)	51.0 (49.5, 52.5)	52.0 (50.0, 53.5)
Weight-for-length z-score < −2, % (n)	27.0 (60)	27.0 (47)	27.3 (35)	26.1 (12)
Ponderal index, g/cm^3 × 100	2.4 (2.2, 2.7)	2.4 (2.3, 2.7)	2.4 (2.2, 2.7)	2.4 (2.3, 2.6)
Male sex, % (n)	52.8 (132)	51.0 (99)	50.7 (70)	51.8 (29)

[a] Values are median interquartile range (IQR) and % (n); [b] Data presented are adolescents that report being in a relationship during pregnancy vs. single; [c] The Special Supplemental Nutrition Program for Women, Infants, and Children (WIC); [d] Gestational Weight Gain: categorized as inadequate or excessive, using Institute of Medicine (IOM) recommendations that vary based on pre-partum body mass index (BMI).

3. Results

3.1. Baseline Characteristics

The characteristics of participants in this study are presented in Table 1. Participants and their infants enrolled in the overall cohort studies and in the current study (i.e., with available serum vitamin B_{12} data) were similar in terms of baseline characteristics, including maternal age, socioeconomic characteristics, and nutritional status. A total of 194 participants had archived samples available for analysis; 138 of these participants were recruited at mid-gestation (bone health study), and 56 participants were recruited at delivery (anemia study) (Figure 1). We also examined potential differences in demographic, socioeconomic, and nutritional factors between participants in the two cohort studies. These variables were identified *a priori* as potential confounders and were considered and adjusted for in all of the multivariate analyses. Vitamin B_{12} and folate concentrations were analyzed in maternal samples that were collected at mid-gestation ($n = 124$) and delivery ($n = 131$); and in infant cord blood samples ($n = 89$).

3.2. Maternal and Neonatal Vitamin B_{12} Status

Maternal and neonatal vitamin B_{12} status are presented in Table 2. At the mid-gestation visit ($n = 124$; 26.4 $\pm$ 3.5 weeks gestation), 1.6% of women were vitamin B_{12} deficient ($n = 2/124$; <148.0 pmol/L), and 22.6% were vitamin B_{12} insufficient ($n = 28/124$; <221.0 pmol/L). Maternal serum vitamin B_{12} concentrations significantly decreased from mid-gestation to delivery ($n = 61$; 39.9 $\pm$ 1.0 weeks; mid-gestation: median = 358.9, interquartile range (IQR) = 233.9, 400.7 vs. delivery: median = 226.2, IQR = 185.2, 311.8; $p < 0.0001$).

The prevalence of maternal vitamin B_{12} insufficiency at delivery ($n = 70/131$; 53.4%) was significantly higher than at mid-gestation ($n = 28/124$; 22.6%, $p < 0.05$). The prevalence of vitamin B_{12} insufficiency was low in infants at birth: 0.0% were vitamin B_{12} deficient (<148.0 pmol/L), and 2.3% were vitamin B_{12} insufficient (<221.0 pmol/L). No mothers or infants were folate deficient (<6.8 nmol/L) or insufficient (<10.0 nmol/L) during this study.

The associations between maternal and infant serum vitamin B_{12} concentrations are presented in Table 3. Maternal vitamin B_{12} status at mid-gestation was not significantly associated with infant serum vitamin B_{12} concentrations ($p > 0.05$).

At delivery, maternal serum vitamin B_{12} concentrations ($p < 0.001$) and vitamin B_{12} deficiency ($p < 0.0001$) were significantly associated with infant serum vitamin B_{12} concentrations in multivariate analyses, adjusting for gestational age at sample collection, maternal age, parity, smoking status, relationship status, reported prenatal supplement use, pre-pregnancy BMI, race, and intake of vitamin B_{12} and folate. Similarly, maternal vitamin B_{12} insufficiency at delivery was significantly associated with infant serum vitamin B_{12} concentrations ($p < 0.01$) in multivariate analyses, adjusting for gestational age at sample collection, maternal age, parity, smoking status, relationship status, reported prenatal supplement use, pre-pregnancy BMI, race, and intake of vitamin B_{12} and folate. Maternal serum folate concentrations were not significantly associated with infant serum vitamin B_{12} concentrations ($p > 0.05$).

The associations between maternal vitamin B_{12} and folate statuses and infant serum folate concentrations are presented in Table 4. Maternal serum folate concentrations at mid-gestation were not significantly associated with infant serum folate concentrations ($p > 0.05$).

Table 2. Maternal and infant vitamin B_{12} and folate status.

	Maternal					Infant	
	Mid-Gestation	Delivery				Cord Blood	
Variables [a]	Total	Total	Recruited at Mid-Gestation	Recruited at Delivery	Total	Mothers Recruited at Mid-Gestation	Mothers Recruited at Delivery
n	124	131	75	56	89	58	31
Serum vitamin B_{12}, pmol/L	343.7 (237.8, 400.7)	216.2 (161.6, 297.8)	216.2 (173.4, 311.8)	211.2 (158.7, 267.0)	597.0 (471.6, 796.3)	569.4 (478.6, 844.3)	602.9 (406.6, 722.1)
<148.0 pmol/L	1.6 (2)	15.3 (20)	14.7 (11)	16.1 (9)	0.0 (0)	0.0 (0)	0.0 (0)
≥148 to <221.0 pmol/L	21.0 (26)	38.2 (50)	37.3 (28)	39.3 (22)	2.3 (2)	0.0 (0)	6.5 (2)
≥221 pmol/L	77.4 (96)	46.6 (61)	48.0 (36)	44.6 (25)	99.8 (87)	100.0 (58)	93.5 (29)
n	122	130	74	56	86	55	31
Serum folate, nmol/L	39.3 (31.7, 50.5)	39.7 (31.8, 50.4)	42.8 (32.2, 51.4)	37.7 (28.8, 48.4)	66.7 (53.1, 85.5)	66.3 (52.1, 84.4)	67.7 (55.5, 98.4)
≤29.45 [b] nmol/L	19.7 (24)	20.0 (26)	13.5 (10)	28.6 (16)	2.3 (2)	3.6 (2)	0.0 (0)
>29.45, ≤35.79 nmol/L	20.5 (25)	16.9 (22)	18.9 (14)	14.3 (8)	2.3 (2)	3.6 (2)	0.0 (0)
>35.79, ≤43.94 nmol/L	19.7 (24)	20.0 (26)	17.6 (13)	23.2 (13)	4.7 (4)	5.5 (3)	3.2 (1)
>43.94, ≤52.66 nmol/L	19.7 (24)	22.3 (29)	29.7 (22)	12.5 (7)	14.0 (12)	12.7 (7)	16.1 (5)
>52.66 nmol/L	20.5 (25)	20.8 (27)	20.3 (15)	21.4 (12)	76.7 (66)	74.6 (41)	80.7 (25)

[a] Values are median and interquartile range (IQR) and (%) *n*. [b] Note: No values of serum folate were <6.8 nmol/L; the cut-offs presented for serum folate are quintiles based on the distribution of serum folate concentrations at mid-gestation.

Table 3. Associations between maternal vitamin B_{12} and folate status with infant serum vitamin B_{12} concentrations.

			Univariate [b]		Multivariate [c]		Multivariate [d]	
Maternal Variables	**Time-Point**	*n*	**β (SE)**	***p*-Value**	**β (SE)**	***p*-Value**	**β (SE)**	***p*-Value**
Serum vitamin B_{12}, [a] pmol/L	Mid-gestation	54	0.29 (0.17)	0.09	0.28 (0.16)	0.08	0.31 (0.16)	0.06
	Delivery (All)	64	0.85 (0.12)	<0.0001	0.74 (0.12)	<0.0001	0.77 (0.12)	<0.001
	Delivery (Recruited at mid-gestation)	33	0.57 (0.20)	0.004	0.53 (0.18)	0.003	0.53 (0.16)	0.001
	Delivery (Recruited at delivery)	31	1.09 (0.13)	<0.0001	0.97 (0.14)	<0.0001	1.02 (0.12)	<0.001
<148.0 pmol/L	Mid-gestation	54	n/a	n/a	n/a	n/a	n/a	n/a
	Delivery (All)	64	−0.65 (0.16)	<0.0001	−0.54 (0.14)	0.0002	−0.62 (0.15)	<0.0001
	Delivery (Recruited at mid-gestation)	33	−0.63 (0.22)	0.004	−0.60 (0.19)	0.002	−0.56 (0.18)	0.002
	Delivery (Recruited at delivery)	31	−0.72 (0.22)	0.001	−0.59 (0.22)	0.008	−0.67 (0.21)	0.002
<221.0 pmol/L	Mid-gestation	54	−0.16 (0.15)	0.28	−0.18 (0.14)	0.20	−0.18 (0.14)	0.21
	Delivery (All)	64	−0.42 (0.12)	0.0007	−0.30 (0.12)	0.01	−0.33 (0.12)	0.008
	Delivery (Recruited at mid-gestation)	33	−0.23 (0.17)	0.17	−0.19 (0.16)	0.22	−0.26 (0.15)	0.07
	Delivery (Recruited at delivery)	31	−0.61 (0.17)	0.0004	−0.44 (0.17)	0.01	−0.41 (0.19)	0.03
Serum folate [a], nmol/L	Mid-gestation	53	−0.24 (0.14)	0.09	−0.24 (0.14)	0.09	−0.28 (0.15)	0.06
	Delivery (All)	64	0.12 (0.16)	0.47	0.07 (0.16)	0.68	0.09 (0.17)	0.61
	Delivery (Recruited at mid-gestation)	33	0.09 (0.22)	0.69	0.12 (0.23)	0.60	0.16 (0.26)	0.54
	Delivery (Recruited at delivery)	31	0.12 (0.25)	0.63	0.06 (0.23)	0.81	0.11 (0.22)	0.62
<40.0 nmol/L	Mid-gestation	53	0.10 (0.12)	0.40	0.11 (0.12)	0.37	0.14 (0.13)	0.28
	Delivery (All)	64	−0.06 (0.13)	0.65	0.02 (0.13)	0.87	0.02 (0.13)	0.88
	Delivery (Recruited at mid-gestation)	33	−0.05 (0.17)	0.76	−0.08 (0.17)	0.64	0.04 (0.20)	0.86
	Delivery (Recruited at delivery)	31	−0.08 (0.21)	0.69	0.11 (0.18)	0.56	0.15 (0.17)	0.39

[a] Statistical analyses: Linear regression models were used to examine associations between maternal vitamin B_{12} and folate status and infant serum vitamin B_{12} concentrations; vitamin B_{12} and folate concentrations were natural logarithmically transformed prior to analyses; [b] Adjusted for gestational age of sample collection; [c] Adjusted for gestational age of sample collection, maternal age at delivery, parity (≥1 vs. 0), ever smoked (yes vs. no), relationship status (single vs. married/in a relationship), self-reported prenatal supplement use (≥2 vs. <2 pills/week), pre-pregnancy BMI, and race (African American vs. other); [d] Adjusted for gestational age of sample collection, maternal age at delivery, parity (≥1 vs. 0), ever smoked (yes vs. no), relationship status (single vs. married/in a relationship), self-reported prenatal supplement use (≥2 vs. <2 pills/week), pre-pregnancy BMI, race (African American vs. other), intake of vitamin B_{12}, and intake of folate.

Table 4. Associations between maternal Vitamin B_{12} and folate status with infant serum folate concentrations.

Maternal Variables	Time-Point	*n*	Univariate [b] β (SE)	Univariate [b] *p*-Value	Multivariate [c] β (SE)	Multivariate [c] *p*-Value	Multivariate [d] β (SE)	Multivariate [d] *p*-Value
Serum vitamin B_{12},[a] pmol/L	Mid-gestation	51	−0.04 (0.16)	0.79	−0.19 (0.14)	0.17	−0.16 (0.13)	0.22
	Delivery (All)	61	−0.02 (0.11)	0.88	−0.08 (0.11)	0.48	−0.08 (0.11)	0.45
	Delivery (Recruited at mid-gestation)	30	−0.20 (0.15)	0.18	−0.20 (0.13)	0.13	−0.22 (0.12)	0.07
	Delivery (Recruited at delivery)	31	0.14 (0.16)	0.37	0.04 (0.15)	0.78	0.06 (0.15)	0.67
<148.0 pmol/L	Mid-gestation	51	n/a	n/a	n/a	n/a	n/a	n/a
	Delivery (All)	61	0.07 (0.13)	0.60	0.16 (0.12)	0.16	0.18 (0.12)	0.14
	Delivery (Recruited at mid-gestation)	30	0.26 (0.17)	0.13	0.26 (0.14)	0.07	0.38 (0.13)	0.005
	Delivery (Recruited at delivery)	31	−0.10 (0.18)	0.57	0.07 (0.17)	0.65	0.03 (0.17)	0.88
<221.0 pmol/L	Mid-gestation	51	−0.05 (0.14)	0.71	0.01 (0.13)	0.91	0.07 (0.12)	0.54
	Delivery (All)	61	−0.01 (0.09)	0.90	0.05 (0.09)	0.58	0.07 (0.09)	0.47
	Delivery (Recruited at mid-gestation)	30	0.18 (0.12)	0.12	0.22 (0.11)	0.04	0.27 (0.10)	0.006
	Delivery (Recruited at delivery)	31	−0.19 (0.13)	0.15	−0.09 (0.12)	0.45	−0.12 (0.13)	0.37
Serum folate [a], nmol/L	Mid-gestation	50	0.27 (0.14)	0.06	0.05 (0.13)	0.69	0.003 (0.13)	0.98
	Delivery (All)	61	0.54 (0.09)	<0.0001	0.47 (0.10)	<0.0001	0.50 (0.10)	<0.0001
	Delivery (Recruited at mid-gestation)	30	0.54 (0.11)	<0.0001	0.55 (0.13)	<0.001	0.53 (0.15)	0.0003
	Delivery (Recruited at delivery)	31	0.57 (0.13)	<0.0001	0.45 (0.13)	0.0005	0.44 (0.12)	0.0003
<40.0 nmol/L	Mid-gestation	50	−0.25 (0.12)	0.03	−0.13 (0.10)	0.21	−0.09 (0.10)	0.39
	Delivery (All)	61	−0.42 (0.08)	<0.0001	−0.40 (0.08)	<0.0001	−0.42 (0.08)	<0.0001
	Delivery (Recruited at mid-gestation)	30	−0.44 (0.09)	<0.0001	−0.43 (0.10)	<0.0001	−0.51 (0.12)	<0.0001
	Delivery (Recruited at delivery)	31	−0.41 (0.12)	0.0006	−0.32 (0.12)	0.01	−0.33 (0.12)	0.006

[a] Statistical analyses: linear regression models were used to examine associations between maternal vitamin B_{12} and folate status and infant serum vitamin B_{12} concentrations; vitamin B_{12} and folate concentrations were natural logarithmically transformed prior to analyses; [b] Adjusted for gestational age of sample collection; [c] Adjusted for gestational age of sample collection, maternal age at delivery, parity (≥1 vs. 0), ever smoked (yes vs. no), relationship status (single vs. married/in a relationship), self-reported prenatal supplement use (≥2 vs. <2 pills/week), pre-pregnancy BMI, and race (African American vs. other); [d] Adjusted for gestational age of sample collection, maternal age at delivery, parity (≥1 vs. 0), ever smoked (yes vs. no), relationship status (single vs. married/in a relationship), self-reported prenatal supplement use (≥2 vs. <2 pills/week), pre-pregnancy BMI, race (African American vs. other), intake of vitamin B_{12}, and intake of folate

Maternal serum folate concentrations at delivery were significantly associated with infant serum folate concentrations ($p < 0.0001$) in multivariate analyses, adjusting for gestational age at sample collection, maternal age, parity, smoking status, relationship status, prenatal supplement use, pre-pregnancy BMI, race, and intake of vitamin B_{12} and folate. Similarly, lower maternal serum folate concentrations (<40.0 nmol/L) at delivery were associated with lower infant serum folate concentrations ($p < 0.0001$) in multivariate analyses, adjusting for gestational age at sample collection, maternal age, parity, smoking status, relationship status, prenatal supplement use, pre-pregnancy BMI, race, and intake of vitamin B_{12} and folate.

4. Discussion

In this prospective analysis among pregnant adolescents, maternal vitamin B_{12} concentrations significantly decreased during pregnancy and predicted neonatal vitamin B_{12} status. Although the prevalence of vitamin B_{12} deficiency (<148.0 pmol/L; 1.6%) was low in adolescents during pregnancy, 22.6% of adolescents were vitamin B_{12} insufficient (<221.0 pmol/L; 22.6%) at mid-gestation. Maternal serum vitamin B_{12} concentrations decreased significantly during pregnancy, and at delivery, 15.3% of mothers were vitamin B_{12} deficient and 53.4% were vitamin B_{12} insufficient (Table 2).

This is among the first studies conducted to date to examine the burden of vitamin B_{12} deficiency in pregnant adolescents and its association with neonatal vitamin B_{12} status in this high-risk obstetric population. The prevalence of vitamin B_{12} deficiency in this study was low (1.6% mid-gestation, 15.3% delivery) and similar to a previous study conducted in Spain among pregnant adolescents (vitamin B_{12} deficiency, T1: 8.3%) [42]. However, the prevalence of vitamin B_{12} deficiency noted in this study was lower than previous studies conducted in pregnant adolescents in Canada (median, T3: 158 pmol/L, IQR: 114, 207 pmol/L; vitamin B_{12} <148.0 pmol/L: 43%) [43] and in Venezuela (vitamin B_{12} <200.0 pg/mL (<148.0 pmol/L), T1: 50.0%, T2: 58.8%, T3: 72.5%) [61]. Maternal vitamin B_{12} concentrations in our study were also higher than in a previous study in pregnant adolescents in the United Kingdom (geometric mean, Trimester 3 (T3): 177 pmol/L, 95% CI: 169, 185 pmol/L) [41].

The prevalence of vitamin B_{12} insufficiency (<221.0 pmol/L), however, was high in this study at both mid-gestation (22.6%) and delivery (53.4%). Although all participants were prescribed prenatal vitamins containing vitamin B_{12} and folic acid, self-reported adherence to prenatal supplements was low. Additionally, while most participants reported dietary intake of vitamin B_{12} at or above the RDA for this group (i.e., median (IQR): 4.5 (2.6, 6.6) μg/day vs. RDA: 2.6 μg/day), approximately 25% of participants reported dietary intake below the RDA. In addition to low dietary intake of vitamin B_{12}, vitamin B_{12} absorption could also be impaired by inadequate bioavailability, losses from processing and cooking animal-source foods, high dose folic acid, metabolic changes during pregnancy (e.g., hemodilution, fetal transfer), gastrointestinal symptoms, infections, and medications [4,62]. For example, since vitamin B_{12} is bound to protein carriers in the food matrix, vitamin B_{12} bioavailability may vary by food source [62,63].

The decline in maternal vitamin B_{12} concentrations during gestation in this study is also consistent with previous studies in adult pregnant women in Canada [64], Spain [26], Norway [25,29], and India [28,65], and in 12 of 13 longitudinal studies included in a systematic review of vitamin B_{12} status and birthweight in adult pregnant women [66]. The observed decrease in vitamin B_{12} concentrations throughout pregnancy could be due to hemodilution, increased protein synthesis, increased requirements for methyl donors during gestation, or a low intake or adherence to prenatal supplements to meet increased requirements [67]. However, there are limited data from pregnant adolescents, who have higher nutritional requirements for their own growth.

The prevalence of vitamin B_{12} deficiency and insufficiency in infants was low in this study (0–3%). Infant vitamin B_{12} concentrations were 2.5-fold higher than maternal vitamin B_{12} concentrations at delivery. These findings are consistent with previous studies in adult pregnant women, which have reported neonatal vitamin B_{12} concentrations 27% to 100% higher than maternal concentrations at delivery [18,19,21,26,30,31,33] and mid-gestation [23], although this has not been reported in all studies [22,25,28,29]. Higher vitamin B_{12} concentrations in offspring indicate active transfer to the fetus, which may occur due to upregulation of placental B_{12} transporter proteins or other active transport mechanisms that have yet to be established.

In this study, maternal vitamin B_{12} status at delivery, but not at mid-gestation, was significantly associated with infant vitamin B_{12} status. Maternal vitamin B_{12} status at delivery has been associated with vitamin B_{12} status in offspring at birth in previous cross-sectional studies [18,20–22,30–33]. There are, however, limited prospective data on maternal vitamin B_{12} status during pregnancy and its association with infant vitamin B_{12} status—particularly among adolescents—to compare findings. Evidence from studies in adult pregnant women have reported significant correlations between maternal vitamin B_{12} status during pregnancy and their infants [19,23,24,26,29]. Few prospective analyses to date have considered potential confounders of these associations in multivariate analyses [25,28]. In a recent study in adult pregnant women (median age = 22, IQR = 20–24 years) in Southern India, maternal vitamin B_{12} status during each trimester was associated with infant vitamin B_{12} status at 6 weeks of age [28], even after adjusting for maternal vitamin B_{12} supplementation. Similarly, a study conducted among pregnant women (mean age = 29.9, SD = 4.4 years) in Norway found that maternal vitamin B_{12} levels did not significantly predict cord blood or infant vitamin B_{12} status, although other vitamin B_{12} biomarkers (i.e., maternal holoTC, holoHC, MMA) were associated [25].

This study has several limitations. Neonatal micronutrient status was assessed at a single time point from cord blood, precluding our ability to evaluate longer-term impacts on infant vitamin B_{12} status or functional outcomes. Longitudinal data on maternal vitamin B_{12} concentrations were available only from a subset of participants in the parent cohort studies, limiting our ability to examine changes in vitamin B_{12} concentrations during pregnancy. Although participants in both cohort studies had similar sociodemographic characteristics (e.g., maternal age, gestational age at initiation of prenatal care, adherence to prenatal vitamins, gestational age at delivery), participants enrolled at mid-gestation (bone study) were more likely to be participants in the Special Supplemental Nutrition Program for Women, Infants, and Children (WIC) program, current smokers, Caucasian, primiparous, and had higher self-reported dietary intake of vitamin B_{12} and folate, compared to participants who were recruited at delivery (anemia). All of these variables were identified *a priori* as potential confounders and were considered and adjusted for in multivariate analyses; however, there may be residual confounding due to additional factors that were not evaluated or adjusted for in these studies. Vitamin B_{12} concentrations assessed at mid-gestation may not reflect vitamin B_{12} status during the relevant etiologic period periconceptionally or for maternal–fetal transfer of cobalamin and subsequent infant status and perinatal outcomes [68]. Additionally, serum folate is a biomarker of short-term dietary intake and does not reflect longer-term or usual intake. Vitamin B_{12} and folate assessments were also based on a single biomarker (i.e., total serum vitamin B_{12} and serum folate concentrations). Inclusion of additional circulating (i.e., holo-transcobalamin) and functional (i.e., methylmalonic acid) biomarkers of vitamin B_{12} metabolism and erythrocyte folate concentrations would improve assessment and interpretation of findings in mother–infant dyads [4]. Additionally, while the low prevalence of vitamin B_{12} deficiency in this study is similar to previous research in pregnant adolescents in Canada and the United Kingdom, a study population of generally adequate vitamin B_{12} status limits the generalizability of results to other populations that may be at greater risk for vitamin B_{12} deficiency, particularly in resource-limited settings [41,43]. Findings should also be interpreted in the context of a folate-replete population (i.e., among participants prescribed high-dose prenatal folic acid (1000 μg) and in a population exposed to folic acid fortification); this also limits the generalizability of findings to other settings. Finally, although findings from this study demonstrated an association of maternal and infant vitamin B_{12} status at delivery, the interpretation of these findings is not causal. Future prospective studies are needed to examine mechanisms of vitamin B_{12} transfer to the fetus and to determine the impact of vitamin B_{12} status on maternal and child health outcomes.

5. Conclusions

In summary, in this cohort of healthy pregnant adolescents, maternal vitamin B_{12} concentrations significantly decreased during pregnancy and predicted infant vitamin B_{12} status. This is one of the first prospective studies to date to evaluate the burden of vitamin B_{12} insufficiency in pregnant adolescents and their infants, a population that is at high risk for both micronutrient deficiencies and pregnancy complications. Findings suggest that vitamin B_{12} deficiency is an important public health problem in this high-risk obstetric population. Future research is needed to increase vitamin B_{12} status and improve the health of adolescent mothers and their children.

Author Contributions: Conceptualization—parent cohort studies, K.O.O., R.G., and E.K.P.; conceptualization—vitamin B_{12} sub-study, J.L.F. and K.O.O.; analysis, J.L.F. and A.F.; writing—original draft manuscript, J.L.F.; writing—review and editing, J.L.F., K.O.O., H.M.G., and A.F.; supervision, R.G., E.K.P., and K.O.O.; project administration, E.K.P.; laboratory analyses, T.R.K.; funding acquisition, K.O.O. and J.L.F. All authors contributed to the development of this manuscript and read and approved the final version.

Acknowledgments: The authors are grateful to the mothers and children, and the midwives of the Strong Midwifery Group, who made this research possible.

References

1. Allen, L.H. How common is vitamin B-12 deficiency? *Am. J. Clin. Nutr.* **2009**, *89*, 693S–696S. [CrossRef] [PubMed]
2. McLean, E.; de Benoist, B.; Allen, L.H. Review of the magnitude of folate and vitamin B_{12} deficiencies worldwide. *Food Nutr. Bull.* **2008**, *29*, S38–S51. [CrossRef] [PubMed]
3. Allen, L.H.; Rosenberg, I.H.; Oakley, G.P.; Omenn, G.S. Considering the case for vitamin B_{12} fortification of flour. *Food Nutr. Bull.* **2010**, *31*, S36–S46. [CrossRef] [PubMed]
4. Finkelstein, J.L.; Layden, A.J.; Stover, P.J. Vitamin B-12 and Perinatal Health. *Adv. Nutr.* **2015**, *6*, 552–563. [CrossRef] [PubMed]
5. Ratan, S.K.; Rattan, K.N.; Pandey, R.M.; Singhal, S.; Kharab, S.; Bala, M.; Singh, V.; Jhanwar, A. Evaluation of the levels of folate, vitamin B_{12}, homocysteine and fluoride in the parents and the affected neonates with neural tube defect and their matched controls. *Pediatr. Surg. Int.* **2008**, *24*, 803–808. [CrossRef]
6. Adams, M.J., Jr.; Khoury, M.J.; Scanlon, K.S.; Stevenson, R.E.; Knight, G.J.; Haddow, J.E.; Sylvester, G.C.; Cheek, J.E.; Henry, J.P.; Stabler, S.P.; et al. Elevated midtrimester serum methylmalonic acid levels as a risk factor for neural tube defects. *Teratology* **1995**, *51*, 311–317. [CrossRef] [PubMed]
7. Wilson, A.; Platt, R.; Wu, Q.; Leclerc, D.; Christensen, B.; Yang, H.; Gravel, R.A.; Rozen, R. A common variant in methionine synthase reductase combined with low cobalamin (vitamin B_{12}) increases risk for spina bifida. *Mol. Genet. Metab.* **1999**, *67*, 317–323. [CrossRef]
8. Gu, Q.; Li, Y.; Cui, Z.L.; Luo, X.P. Homocysteine, folate, vitamin B_{12} and B6 in mothers of children with neural tube defects in Xinjiang, China. *Acta Paediatr.* **2012**, *101*, e486–e490. [CrossRef]
9. Ray, J.G.; Wyatt, P.R.; Thompson, M.D.; Vermeulen, M.J.; Meier, C.; Wong, P.Y.; Farrell, S.A.; Cole, D.E. vitamin B_{12} and the risk of neural tube defects in a folic-acid-fortified population. *Epidemiology* **2007**, *18*, 362–366. [CrossRef]
10. Molloy, A.M.; Kirke, P.N.; Troendle, J.F.; Burke, H.; Sutton, M.; Brody, L.C.; Scott, J.M.; Mills, J.L. Maternal vitamin B_{12} status and risk of neural tube defects in a population with high neural tube defect prevalence and no folic Acid fortification. *Pediatrics* **2009**, *123*, 917–923. [CrossRef]
11. Rowland, A.S.; Baird, D.D.; Shore, D.L.; Weinberg, C.R.; Savitz, D.A.; Wilcox, A.J. Nitrous oxide and spontaneous abortion in female dental assistants. *Am. J. Epidemiol.* **1995**, *141*, 531–538. [CrossRef] [PubMed]
12. Hubner, U.; Alwan, A.; Jouma, M.; Tabbaa, M.; Schorr, H.; Herrmann, W. Low serum vitamin B_{12} is associated with recurrent pregnancy loss in Syrian women. *Clin. Chem. Lab. Med.* **2008**, *46*, 1265–1269. [CrossRef] [PubMed]
13. Reznikoff-Etievant, M.F.; Zittoun, J.; Vaylet, C.; Pernet, P.; Milliez, J. Low Vitamin B(12) level as a risk factor for very early recurrent abortion. *Eur. J. Obs. Gynecol. Reprod. Biol.* **2002**, *104*, 156–159. [CrossRef]

14. Hogeveen, M.; Blom, H.J.; den Heijer, M. Maternal homocysteine and small-for-gestational-age offspring: Systematic review and meta-analysis. *Am. J. Clin. Nutr.* **2012**, *95*, 130–136. [CrossRef] [PubMed]
15. Muthayya, S.; Kurpad, A.V.; Duggan, C.P.; Bosch, R.J.; Dwarkanath, P.; Mhaskar, A.; Mhaskar, R.; Thomas, A.; Vaz, M.; Bhat, S.; et al. Low maternal vitamin B_{12} status is associated with intrauterine growth retardation in urban South Indians. *Eur. J. Clin. Nutr.* **2006**, *60*, 791–801. [CrossRef] [PubMed]
16. Black, M.M. Effects of vitamin B_{12} and folate deficiency on brain development in children. *Food Nutr. Bull.* **2008**, *29*, S126–S131. [CrossRef]
17. Pepper, M.R.; Black, M.M. B12 in fetal development. *Semin. Cell Dev. Biol.* **2011**, *22*, 619–623. [CrossRef]
18. Obeid, R.; Morkbak, A.L.; Munz, W.; Nexo, E.; Herrmann, W. The cobalamin-binding proteins transcobalamin and haptocorrin in maternal and cord blood sera at birth. *Clin. Chem.* **2006**, *52*, 263–269. [CrossRef]
19. Muthayya, S.; Dwarkanath, P.; Mhaskar, M.; Mhaskar, R.; Thomas, A.; Duggan, C.; Fawzi, W.W.; Bhat, S.; Vaz, M.; Kurpad, A. The relationship of neonatal serum vitamin B_{12} status with birth weight. *Asia Pac. J. Clin. Nutr.* **2006**, *15*, 538–543.
20. Balci, Y.I.; Ergin, A.; Karabulut, A.; Polat, A.; Dogan, M.; Kucuktasci, K. Serum vitamin B_{12} and folate concentrations and the effect of the Mediterranean diet on vulnerable populations. *Pediatr. Hematol. Oncol.* **2014**, *31*, 62–67. [CrossRef]
21. Adaikalakoteswari, A.; Vatish, M.; Lawson, A.; Wood, C.; Sivakumar, K.; McTernan, P.G.; Webster, C.; Anderson, N.; Yajnik, C.S.; Tripathi, G.; et al. Low maternal vitamin B_{12} status is associated with lower cord blood HDL cholesterol in white Caucasians living in the UK. *Nutrients* **2015**, *7*, 2401–2414. [CrossRef] [PubMed]
22. Radunovic, N.; Lockwood, C.J.; Stanojlovic, O.; Steric, M.; Kontic-Vucinic, O.; Sulovic, N.; Hrncic, D.; Ackerman Iv, W.E. Fetal and maternal plasma homocysteine levels during the second half of uncomplicated pregnancy. *J. Matern.-Fetal Neonatal Med.* **2014**. [CrossRef] [PubMed]
23. Bergen, N.E.; Schalekamp-Timmermans, S.; Jaddoe, V.W.; Hofman, A.; Lindemans, J.; Russcher, H.; Tiemeier, H.; Steegers-Theunissen, R.P.; Steegers, E.A. Maternal and neonatal markers of the homocysteine pathway and fetal growth: The Generation R Study. *Paediatr. Perinat. Epidemiol.* **2016**, *30*, 386–396. [CrossRef] [PubMed]
24. Kalay, Z.; Islek, A.; Parlak, M.; Kirecci, A.; Guney, O.; Koklu, E.; Kalay, S. Reliable and powerful laboratory markers of cobalamin deficiency in the newborn: Plasma and urinary methylmalonic acid. *J. Matern.-Fetal Neonatal Med.* **2016**, *29*, 60–63. [CrossRef]
25. Hay, G.; Clausen, T.; Whitelaw, A.; Trygg, K.; Johnston, C.; Henriksen, T.; Refsum, H. Maternal folate and cobalamin status predicts vitamin status in newborns and 6-month-old infants. *J. Nutr.* **2010**, *140*, 557–564. [CrossRef]
26. Murphy, M.M.; Molloy, A.M.; Ueland, P.M.; Fernandez-Ballart, J.D.; Schneede, J.; Arija, V.; Scott, J.M. Longitudinal study of the effect of pregnancy on maternal and fetal cobalamin status in healthy women and their offspring. *J. Nutr.* **2007**, *137*, 1863–1867. [CrossRef] [PubMed]
27. Deegan, K.L.; Jones, K.M.; Zuleta, C.; Ramirez-Zea, M.; Lildballe, D.L.; Nexo, E.; Allen, L.H. Breast milk vitamin B-12 concentrations in Guatemalan women are correlated with maternal but not infant vitamin B-12 status at 12 months postpartum. *J. Nutr.* **2012**, *142*, 112–116. [CrossRef] [PubMed]
28. Finkelstein, J.L.; Kurpad, A.V.; Thomas, T.; Srinivasan, K.; Duggan, C. vitamin B_{12} status in pregnant women and their infants in South India. *Eur. J. Clin. Nutr.* **2017**, *71*, 1046–1053. [CrossRef]
29. Varsi, K.; Ueland, P.M.; Torsvik, I.K.; Bjorke-Monsen, A.L. Maternal serum cobalamin at 18 weeks of pregnancy predicts infant cobalamin status at 6 months—A prospective, observational study. *J. Nutr.* **2018**, *148*, 738–745. [CrossRef]
30. Lindblad, B.; Zaman, S.; Malik, A.; Martin, H.; Ekstrom, A.; Amu, S.; Holmgren, A.; Norman, M. Folate, vitamin B_{12}, and homocysteine levels in South Asian women with growth-retarded fetuses. *Acta Obstet. Gynecol. Scand.* **2005**, *84*, 1055–1061. [CrossRef]
31. Bjorke Monsen, A.L.; Ueland, P.M.; Vollset, S.E.; Guttormsen, A.B.; Markestad, T.; Solheim, E.; Refsum, H. Determinants of cobalamin status in newborns. *Pediatrics* **2001**, *108*, 624–630. [CrossRef]
32. Guerra-Shinohara, E.M.; Paiva, A.A.; Rondo, P.H.; Yamasaki, K.; Terzi, C.A.; D'Almeida, V. Relationship between total homocysteine and folate levels in pregnant women and their newborn babies according to maternal serum levels of vitamin B_{12}. *BJOG* **2002**, *109*, 784–791. [CrossRef] [PubMed]

33. Koc, A.; Kocyigit, A.; Soran, M.; Demir, N.; Sevinc, E.; Erel, O.; Mil, Z. High frequency of maternal vitamin B_{12} deficiency as an important cause of infantile vitamin B_{12} deficiency in Sanliurfa province of Turkey. *Eur. J. Nutr.* **2006**, *45*, 291–297. [CrossRef]
34. Jacquemyn, Y.; Ajaji, M.; Karepouan, N.; Jacquemyn, N.; Van Sande, H. vitamin B_{12} and folic acid status of term pregnant women and newborns in the Antwerp region, Belgium. *Clin. Exp. Obstet. Gynecol.* **2014**, *41*, 141–143. [PubMed]
35. Mittal, M.; Bansal, V.; Jain, R.; Dabla, P.K. Perturbing Status of vitamin B_{12} in Indian Infants and Their Mothers. *Food Nutr. Bull.* **2017**, *38*, 209–215. [CrossRef]
36. Dilli, D.; Dogan, N.N.; Orun, U.A.; Koc, M.; Zenciroglu, A.; Karademir, S.; Akduman, H. Maternal and neonatal micronutrient levels in newborns with CHD. *Cardiol. Young* **2018**, *28*, 523–529. [CrossRef] [PubMed]
37. Chebaya, P.; Karakochuk, C.D.; March, K.M.; Chen, N.N.; Stamm, R.A.; Kroeun, H.; Sophonneary, P.; Borath, M.; Shahab-Ferdows, S.; Hampel, D.; et al. Correlations between maternal, breast milk, and infant vitamin B_{12} concentrations among mother-infant dyads in Vancouver, Canada and Prey Veng, Cambodia: An exploratory analysis. *Nutrients* **2017**, *9*, 270. [CrossRef] [PubMed]
38. Coban, S.; Yilmaz Keskin, E.; Igde, M. Association between maternal and infantile markers of cobalamin status during the first month post-delivery. *Indian J. Pediatr.* **2018**, *85*, 517–522. [CrossRef]
39. Williams, A.M.; Stewart, C.P.; Shahab-Ferdows, S.; Hampel, D.; Kiprotich, M.; Achando, B.; Lin, A.; Null, C.A.; Allen, L.H.; Chantry, C.J. Infant serum and maternal milk vitamin b-12 are positively correlated in Kenyan infant-mother dyads at 1–6 months postpartum, irrespective of infant feeding practice. *J. Nutr.* **2018**, *148*, 86–93. [CrossRef]
40. Bellows, A.L.; Smith, E.R.; Muhihi, A.; Briegleb, C.; Noor, R.A.; Mshamu, S.; Sudfeld, C.; Masanja, H.; Fawzi, W.W. Micronutrient deficiencies among breastfeeding infants in Tanzania. *Nutrients* **2017**, *9*, 1258. [CrossRef]
41. Baker, P.N.; Wheeler, S.J.; Sanders, T.A.; Thomas, J.E.; Hutchinson, C.J.; Clarke, K.; Berry, J.L.; Jones, R.L.; Seed, P.T.; Poston, L. A prospective study of micronutrient status in adolescent pregnancy. *Am. J. Clin. Nutr.* **2009**, *89*, 1114–1124. [CrossRef] [PubMed]
42. Baron, M.A.; Solano, L.; Pena, E.; Moron, A. (Nutritional status of folate, vitamin B_{12} and iron in pregnant adolescents). *Arch. Latinoam. Nutr.* **2003**, *53*, 150–156. [PubMed]
43. Gadowsky, S.; Gale, K.; Wolfe, S.A.; Jory, J.; Gibson, R.; O'Connor, D. Biochemical folate, B12, and iron status of a group of pregnant adolescents accessed through the public health system in southern Ontario. *J. Adolsc. Health* **1995**, *16*, 465–474. [CrossRef]
44. Davis, L.M.; Chang, S.C.; Mancini, J.; Nathanson, M.S.; Witter, F.R.; O'Brien, K.O. Vitamin D insufficiency is prevalent among pregnant African American adolescents. *J. Pediatr. Adolesc. Gynecol.* **2010**, *23*, 45–52. [CrossRef] [PubMed]
45. Moran, V. A systematic review of dietary assessments of pregnant adolescents in industrialised countries. *Br. J. Nutr.* **2007**, *97*, 411–425. [CrossRef] [PubMed]
46. Klein, J.D. American Academy of Pediatrics Committee on, A. Adolescent pregnancy: Current trends and issues. *Pediatrics* **2005**, *116*, 281–286. [CrossRef] [PubMed]
47. Sedgh, G.; Finer, L.B.; Bankole, A.; Eilers, M.A.; Singh, S. Adolescent Pregnancy, Birth, and abortion rates across countries: Levels and recent trends. *J. Adolesc. Health* **2015**, *56*, 223–230. [CrossRef]
48. Lee, S.; Guillet, R.; Cooper, E.M.; Westerman, M.; Orlando, M.; Kent, T.; Pressman, E.; O'Brien, K.O. Prevalence of anemia and associations between neonatal iron status, hepcidin, and maternal iron status among neonates born to pregnant adolescents. *Pediatr. Res.* **2016**, *79*, 42–48. [CrossRef]
49. Lee, S.; Guillet, R.; Cooper, E.M.; Westerman, M.; Orlando, M.; Pressman, E.; O'Brien, K.O. Maternal inflammation at delivery affects assessment of maternal iron status. *J. Nutr.* **2014**, *144*, 1524–1532. [CrossRef]
50. Layden, A.J.; O'Brien, K.O.; Pressman, E.K.; Cooper, E.M.; Kent, T.R.; Finkelstein, J.L. vitamin B_{12} and placental expression of transcobalamin in pregnant adolescents. *Placenta* **2016**, *45*, 1–7. [CrossRef]
51. Yetley, E.A.; Pfeiffer, C.M.; Phinney, K.W.; Bailey, R.L.; Blackmore, S.; Bock, J.L.; Brody, L.C.; Carmel, R.; Curtin, L.R.; Durazo-Arvizu, R.A.; et al. Biomarkers of vitamin B-12 status in NHANES: A roundtable summary. *Am. J. Clin. Nutr.* **2011**, *94*, 313S–321S. [CrossRef] [PubMed]
52. Sullivan, K.M.; Mei, Z.; Grummer-Strawn, L.; Parvanta, I. Haemoglobin adjustments to define anaemia. *Trop. Med. Int. Health* **2008**, *13*, 1267–1271. [CrossRef] [PubMed]

53. WHO. *Physical Status: The Use and Interpretation of Anthropometry*; Report of a WHO Expert Committee; World Health Organization: Geneva, Switzerland, 1995; p. 329.
54. Spiegelman, D.; Hertzmark, E. Easy SAS calculations for risk or prevalence ratios and differences. *Am. J. Epidemiol.* **2005**, *162*, 199–200. [CrossRef] [PubMed]
55. Wacholder, S. Binomial regression in GLIM: Estimating risk ratios and risk differences. *Am. J. Epidemiol.* **1986**, *123*, 174–184. [CrossRef] [PubMed]
56. Zou, G. A modified poisson regression approach to prospective studies with binary data. *Am. J. Epidemiol.* **2004**, *159*, 702–706. [CrossRef] [PubMed]
57. Durrleman, S.; Simon, R. Flexible regression models with cubic splines. *Stat. Med.* **1989**, *8*, 551–561. [CrossRef] [PubMed]
58. Govindarajulu, U.S.; Spiegelman, D.; Thurston, S.W.; Ganguli, B.; Eisen, E.A. Comparing smoothing techniques in Cox models for exposure-response relationships. *Stat. Med.* **2007**, *26*, 3735–3752. [CrossRef]
59. Greenland, S. Modeling and variable selection in epidemiologic analysis. *Am. J. Public Health* **1989**, *79*, 340–349. [CrossRef]
60. Miettinen, O. *Theoretical Epidemiology*; John Wiley & Sons: New York, NY, USA, 1985; Volume 107.
61. Garcia-Casal, M.N.; Osorio, C.; Landaeta, M.; Leets, I.; Matus, P.; Fazzino, F.; Marcos, E. High prevalence of folic acid and vitamin B_{12} deficiencies in infants, children, adolescents and pregnant women in Venezuela. *Eur. J. Clin. Nutr.* **2005**, *59*, 1064–1070. [CrossRef]
62. Green, R.; Allen, L.H.; Bjorke-Monsen, A.L.; Brito, A.; Gueant, J.L.; Miller, J.W.; Molloy, A.M.; Nexo, E.; Stabler, S.; Toh, B.H.; et al. vitamin B_{12} deficiency. *Nat. Rev. Dis. Prim.* **2017**, *3*, 17040. [CrossRef]
63. Tucker, K.L.; Rich, S.; Rosenberg, I.; Jacques, P.; Dallal, G.; Wilson, P.W.; Selhub, J. Plasma vitamin B-12 concentrations relate to intake source in the Framingham Offspring study. *Am. J. Clin. Nutr.* **2000**, *71*, 514–522. [CrossRef] [PubMed]
64. Visentin, C.E.; Masih, S.P.; Plumptre, L.; Schroder, T.H.; Sohn, K.J.; Ly, A.; Lausman, A.Y.; Berger, H.; Croxford, R.; Lamers, Y.; et al. Low serum vitamin b-12 concentrations are prevalent in a cohort of pregnant Canadian women. *J. Nutr.* **2016**, *146*, 1035–1042. [CrossRef]
65. Wadhwani, N.S.; Pisal, H.R.; Mehendale, S.S.; Joshi, S.R. A prospective study of maternal fatty acids, micronutrients and homocysteine and their association with birth outcome. *Matern. Child Nutr.* **2015**, *11*, 559–573. [CrossRef] [PubMed]
66. Sukumar, N.; Rafnsson, S.B.; Kandala, N.B.; Bhopal, R.; Yajnik, C.S.; Saravanan, P. Prevalence of vitamin B-12 insufficiency during pregnancy and its effect on offspring birth weight: A systematic review and meta-analysis. *Am. J. Clin. Nutr.* **2016**, *103*, 1232–1251. [CrossRef] [PubMed]
67. Rush, E.C.; Katre, P.; Yajnik, C.S. vitamin B_{12}: One carbon metabolism, fetal growth and programming for chronic disease. *Eur. J. Clin. Nutr.* **2013**, *68*, 2–7. [CrossRef] [PubMed]
68. De-Regil, L.M.; Harding, K.B.; Roche, M.L. Preconceptional nutrition interventions for adolescent girls and adult women: Global guidelines and gaps in evidence and policy with emphasis on micronutrients. *J. Nutr.* **2016**, *146*, 1461S–1470S. [CrossRef] [PubMed]

9

The Function and Alteration of Immunological Properties in Human Milk of Obese Mothers

Ummu D. Erliana * and Alyce D. Fly

Indiana University Bloomington School of Public Health, Bloomington, IN 47405, USA; afly@indiana.edu
* Correspondence: uerliana@indiana.edu

Abstract: Maternal obesity is associated with metabolic changes in mothers and higher risk of obesity in the offspring. Obesity in breastfeeding mothers appears to influence human milk production as well as the quality of human milk. Maternal obesity is associated with alteration of immunological factors concentrations in the human milk, such as C-reactive protein (CRP), leptin, IL-6, insulin, TNF-Alpha, ghrelin, adiponectin, and obestatin. Human milk is considered a first choice for infant nutrition due to the complete profile of macro nutrients, micro nutrients, and immunological properties. It is essential to understand how maternal obesity influences immunological properties of human milk because alterations could impact the nutrition status and health of the infant. This review summarizes the literature regarding the impact of maternal obesity on the concentration of particular immunological properties in the human milk.

Keywords: maternal obesity; gestational weight gain; immunological properties; human milk; nutrition; health

1. Introduction

In 2014, the number of pregnant women with overweight and obesity were estimated at 38.9 million and 14.6 million, respectively, worldwide [1]. The prevalence of women of childbearing age with obesity in the US from 1976 to 2014 increased four-fold, from 7.4% to 27.5% [2,3]. In addition, the prevalence of pre-pregnancy obesity of mothers in the US was more than 20% [4,5]. According to 38 jurisdictions of the District of Columbia, New York City, and 48 states in the United States, the prevalence of mothers that had a normal body weight before pregnancy decreased from 47.3% to 45.1% from 2011 to 2015 [6]. A review by Fields et al. (2016) brought attention to the association between several bioactive components of human milk and adiposity in infancy [7]. There is great interest in understanding the contributions of maternal obesity to changes in the composition or functional properties of human milk. Obesity in lactating mothers was found to be related to changes in the concentration of several bioactive components of their milk [8]. For example, an increased leptin concentration found in human milk is noteworthy because leptin may contribute to maternal obesity [9–14]. Alterations of immunological constituents may influence the genetic, metabolic, and epigenetic processes in the child [15]. The excessive weight gain of an obese child was found to be related the increase in leptin and adiponectin concentrations in the milk from obese mothers [16,17]. Furthermore, increased insulin-like growth factor 1 (IGF-I) and ghrelin in human milk were also correlated with the increased growth rate of an obese infant [16–19].

Human milk consists of nutrients and active factors. In addition to nutritive functions, some milk constituents also have bioactive properties such as whey proteins (immunoglobulin, lactoferrin, and alpha-lactalbumin) and casein proteins (κ-casein and β-casein) [20]. Other bioactive proteins in human milk include immunological factors such as antibodies, live cells, cytokines or signaling molecules; enzymes such as lactoferrin, lysozyme, and bile salt stimulated lipase; glycoproteins or oligosaccharides (oligosaccharide-enriched fraction along with secretory IgA), glycolipids, and high molecular weight protein), alpha-lactalbumin, gut microflora like prebiotic, haptocorrin (vitamin B12-binding protein), and nutrients for the infants' immune system [20]. The activities of these bioactive proteins need further study.

Moreover, human milk composition, both over a single feeding and over the duration of lactation is unique and dynamic. Colostrum is the first milk produced (30 mL/24 h) from 30 to 40 h until a few days postpartum [21,22]. Transitional milk is the milk that is produced from 5 days to 2 weeks postpartum and mature milk is the milk that is produced after 2 weeks postpartum [22]. Mature milk has two types, foremilk and hindmilk. Foremilk is the initial milk of a feeding, while hindmilk is the last milk of feeding (which contains milk fat up to three-fold more than in foremilk [23]. Some characteristics of human milk depend on a multitude of factors of the mother. The DARLING (Davis Area Research on Lactation, Infant Nutrition and Growth) study showed important determinants of human milk composition to include maternal ideal body weight (%IBW), protein intake, nursing frequency, menstruation, and parity [24]. The composition of protein in human milk is also significantly influenced by weaning because weaning was shown to decrease the volume of milk production [25]. Furthermore, this study also showed that milk volume and protein level were inversely associated; if the milk production volume was decreased from >500 to <300 mL, the protein concentration would be increased from 1.23 to 2.01 g/100 mL [25]. The influence of obesity on the quality and quantity of human milk has been demonstrated in several studies. A significantly different and less diverse microbiome in human milk has been demonstrated over lactation period, maternal body mass index (BMI), and delivery mode [26]. The ratio of omega-6 to omega-3 of obese breastfeeding mother is increased, while the concentration of fatty acids (DHA, EPA, DPA,) and carotenoids (lutein) are decreased [15]. Alterations of bioactive properties in the human milk of obese mothers could increase the incidence of obesity, insulin resistance, type 2 diabetes, and other adverse metabolic outcomes [27].

The primary aim of this review is to describe the immunological functions of specific factors in human milk and the alterations that occur in conditions of overweight and obesity mothers. The secondary aim is to explore the other influential factors that stimulate alterations of specific immunological properties that also could influence their functions in human milk.

2. The Function and Alteration of Immunological Properties in Human Milk

Breast milk contains essential bioactive components that have been demonstrated by numerous studies. Many components studied have been found to provide a function, for example to prevent infections, heal diseases, and improve health status [28]. Many bioactive components still remain that are not well studied. Studies are needed to understand the implications of the alteration in the specific bioactive components to maternal and infant health. One study demonstrated that the alteration of specific bioactive components in human milk would influence infant health outcome in both the short term and long term [29]. The understanding of this dynamic variation of human milk is needed because it may suggest practices needed for breastfeeding management and distribution of milk donations [22]. Modification of dietary intake and immunization can optimize the concentration of bioactive components in human milk [30,31]. Table 1 lists the bioactive components of human milk, and whether studies have reported any alterations in the concentration of milk of obese mothers. The functions of these bioactives and details about the changes are described further in the text.

Table 1. Alteration of immunological properties in human milk of obese mothers.

No	Bioactive Components	Alterations	References
1.	Antimicrobial		
	a. Lactoferrin	Increase	Houghton et al., 1985 [32]
	b. Lactadherin	None reported	-
	c. Lactoperoxidase	None reported	-
	d. Lysozyme	None reported	-
	e. Mucins (MUC1 and MUC4)	None reported	-

Table 1. *Cont.*

No	Bioactive Components	Alterations	References
2.	Cells		
	a. Lymphocytes	None reported	-
	b. Macrophages	None reported	-
	c. Neutrophils	Increase	Islam et al., 2006 [33]
	d. Stem cells	Decrease	Twigger et al., 2015 [34]
3.	Chemokines		
	a. Granulocyte Colony Stimulating Factor	None reported	-
	b. Macrophage migration inhibitory factor (MIF)	None reported	-
	c. Chemokine receptors (CXCR1/CXCR2)	None reported	-
	d. CXCL-9 (MIIP)	None reported	-
4.	Cytokines		
	a. Interleukin-1 beta (IL-1β)	None reported	-
	b. Interleukin-2 (IL-2)	Increase	Collado et al., 2012 [35]
	c. Interleukin-4 (IL-4)	Increase (colostrum) Decrease (1-month milk)	Collado et al., 2012 [35]
	d. Interleukin-6 (IL-6)	No alteration Increase	Whitaker et al., 2017 [8] Collado et al., 2012 [35]
	e. Interleukin-7 (IL-7)	None reported	-
	f. Interleukin-8 (IL-8)	None reported	-
	g. Interleukin-10 (IL-10)	Increase	Collado et al., 2012 [35]
	h. Interferon gamma-induced protein 10 (IP-10)	None reported	-
	i. Monocyte chemoattractant protein-1 (MCP-1)	None reported	-
	j. Interferon Gamma (IFN-γ)	Increase (colostrum) Decrease (1-month milk)	Collado et al., 2012 [35]
	k. Transforming growth factor beta (TGF-β)	Decrease	Collado et al., 2012 [35]
	l. Tumor necrosis factor-alpha (TNF-α)	No alteration Increase (colostrum) Decrease (1-month milk)	Fields et al., 2017 [18] Collado et al., 2012 [35]
5.	Cytokines inhibitors		
	a. Tumor necrosis factor receptor-I (TNFR I)	None reported	-
	b. Tumor necrosis factor receptor-II (TNFR II)	None reported	-
6.	Growth Factors		
	a. Epidermal growth factor (EGF)	Decrease	Khodabakhshi et al., 2015 [19]
	b. Heparin-binding EGF-like growth factor (HB-EGF)	None reported	-
	c. Insulin-like growth factor 1 (IGF-1)	Increase	Khodabakhshi et al., 2015 [19]
	d. Nerve growth factor (NGF)	None reported	-
	e. Vascular endothelial growth factor (VEGF)	None reported	-
7.	Hormones		
	a. Adiponectin	Increase	Martin et al., 2006 [36]
	b. Calcitonin	None reported	-
	c. Erythropoietin (Epo)	None reported	-
	d. Insulin	Increase	Fields et al., 2017 [18]
	e. Ghrelin	Decrease	Khodabakhshi et al., 2015 [19]; Zhang N, et al., 2011 [37]
	f. Leptin	Increase	De Luca et al., 2016 [9]; Lemas et al., 2016 [10]; Uysal et al., 2002 [11]; Andreas et al., 2014 [12]; Quinn et al., 2014 [13]; Eilers et al., 2002 [14];
	g. Obestatin	Decrease	Aydin et al., 2008 [38]
	h. Resistin	No alteration	Andreas et al., 2016 [39]; Savino et al., 2012 [40]
	i. Somatostatin	None reported	-
8.	Immunoglobulins		
	a. IgA	Increase (colostrum and serum)	Miranda et al.,1983 [41]; Islam et al., 2006 [33]; Fujimori et al., 2015 [42]
	b. IgG	Increase Decrease Constant (colostrum) Decrease (serum)	Miranda et al., 1983 [41] Islam et al., 2006 [33] Fujimori et al., 2015 [42]
	c. IgM	Increase Increase (colostrum) Decrease (serum)	Islam et al., 2006 [33] Fujimori et al., 2015 [42]
	d. Insulin-like-growth factor-binding proteins (IGFBP)	Decrease	Khodabakhshi et al., 2015 [19]

Table 1. *Cont.*

No	Bioactive Components	Alterations	References
9	Lipids	Increase (triglyceride and cholesterol)	Fujimori et al., 2015 [42]
		Increase (saturated fatty acids) Decrease (n-3 fatty acidss) Decrease (unsaturated to saturated fatty acid ratio) Increase (ratio of n-6 to n-3)	Makela et al., 2013 [43]
		Increase (ratio of n-6 to n-3) Decrease (lutein, docosahexaenoic acid, eicosapentaenoic acid, and docasapentaenoic acid)	Panagos et al., 2016 [15]
10.	Microbiota	*Bifidobacterium* (decrease) *Staphylococcus* (increase)	Delzenne & Cani, 2011 [44]; Collado et al., 2012 [35]
11.	Nucleic Acids	None reported	-
12.	Oligosaccharide and Glycans		
	a. Human milk oligosaccharides (HMOs)	No alteration	Azad et al. 2018 [45]
	b. Gangliosides	None reported	-
	c. Glycosaminoglycans (GAGs)	Decrease	Cerdo et al., 2018 [46]
	d. Osteoprotegerin	None reported	-
	e. Soluble CD14s (SCD14s)	Decrease	Collado et al., 2012 [35]
13.	Other Proteins		
	a. Alpha-Lactalbumin (LALBA)	Increase (6–15 days postpartum) Decrease (16–30 days postpartum) Decrease (31–60 days postpartum) Increase (>60 days postpartum)	Sanchez-Poso et al., 1987 [47]
	b. Alpha-1 Antitrypsin (AAT)	None reported	-
	c. Alpha-Amylase (α-amylase)	None reported	-
	d. Bile Salt Stimulated Lipase (BSSL)	None reported	-
	e. Casein	Decrease	Jevitt et al., 2007 [48]
	f. C-Reactive Protein (CRP)	Increase	Whitaker, 2017 [8]
	f. Folate-Binding Protein (FBP)	None reported	-
	g. Haptocorrin	None reported	-

2.1. Anti-Microbial

Lactoferrin is one of the major iron-binding glycoproteins in colostrum that is immunomodulatory [49]. Lactoferrin is bound to iron and helps in uptake of iron in the cell by specific receptors in the infant intestinal tract [50]. Lactoferrin also functions at the level of DNA, as a transcription factor that influences for example, cell signaling proteins and immune protein synthesis [20,51]. Lactoferrin acts to constrain bacterial growth by binding iron, limiting iron needed for growth of bacteria and other pathogens [52]. The formation of lactoferrin without iron has also been found in human milk. This form was demonstrated to eradicate *Candida albicans*, *Escherichia coli*, *Pseudomonas aeruginosa*, *Streptococcus mutans*, *Streptococcus pneumoniae*, and *Vibrio cholerae* [53]. Lactoferrin concentration was significantly greater in colostrum of mothers who were greater than the 90% Weight for Height, an older surrogate measure for obesity (that corresponds to a BMI > 30 kg/m^2) [32].

Lactadherin is a glycoprotein associated with milk fat globules of human milk together with mucins, xanthine oxidase, and butyrophylin [20]. The main role of lactadherin may be to protect the newborn infant from rotaviral infection, a common cause of diarrheal disease and gastroenteritis [54]. Lactadherin works against the infection by creating apoptosis in infected cells of the infant and decreases inflammation by inhibition of TLR4 and the NF-κB signaling cascade [55–57]. Lactadherin is not digested in the stomach and passes to the intestine to maintain gut health by ameliorating inflammation [57–59]. A study in Mexico with 200 infants demonstrated that infants who were breastfed by milk that contained a low concentration of lactadherin developed severe diarrhea [54]. Other infants who received high levels lactadherin from human milk were asymptomatic of diarrhea.

The catalytic reactions of lactoperoxidase have bactericidal effects that kill Gram-positive and Gram-negative bacteria [60,61]. This bactericidal effect results from catalytic oxidation of substrate such as thiocyanates with hydrogen peroxide resulting in hypothiocyanite ion ($OSCN^-$). The concentration of lactoperoxidase of human milk at the first 6 months was found to be constant between 1–1.5 units/mL [62]. Lactoperoxidase in human milk was shown to detoxify H_2O_2 both in the infant gut and mammary gland of mothers, with additional anti-microbial functions. Whether lactoperoxidase concentration in the human milk of obese mothers is altered has not yet been determined.

Another antimicrobial constituent of milk, lysozyme, is present at a concentration that is 3000-fold higher in human milk than cow's milk. It is an active enzyme that works together with lactoferrin to effectively kill Gram-negative bacteria [63]. A study of the concentration of lysozyme in human milk of obese mothers was not found.

Mucins, another antimicrobial factor, make up one of three major protein fractions of human milk, along with casein and whey [64]. Mucins are a type of glycoprotein that consist of up to 80% carbohydrate, including mannose, as well as sulfonic acid [65]. MUC1 and MUC4 were identified in human milk for the first time by Liu et al. (2012) [66]. Furthermore, their study demonstrated that MUC1 was better than MUC4 in protecting the human epithelium cells (FHs 74 Int cells, CaCo-2 cells) from invasion by Salmonella [66]. Mucins are part of a passive immunity in human milk that protect the infant small intestine and stomach by inhibiting the binding of pathogens [67,68]. There was no study found that compared mucins concentration in the human milk of obese mothers to mothers with normal BMI.

2.2. Cells

The existence of lymphocytes in human milk was first discovered in colostrum [69]. Another study also showed that GFP+ leukocytes were transferred from mothers to their infants through breast milk [70]. T lymphocyte cells (CD8+, CD4+, and CD19+) are produced by GFP+ leukocytes in the Peyer's patches (PPs) [71]. Moreover, Th-2 lymphocytes were shown to contribute to produce specific cytokines such as IL-4, IL-13, IL-15 [56]. This study also demonstrated that the composition of lymphocytes in human milk and blood were different [72]. There were no studies found that compared lymphocyte concentrations in milk of obese mothers with other mothers.

Macrophages and the mammary endothelium support the production of TNF-Alpha in human milk [73,74]. Macrophages protect the infant from the infection by pathogens by activation of T-cells [75,76]. The cells move into the maternal blood and then are shifted to human milk by the mammary epithelial cells [22]. There were no studies found that reported comparisons of macrophage concentration in milk between women with obesity and normal weight conditions.

Neutrophils are another type of leukocyte that are abundant in the colostrum [77]. The three activities of neutrophils in human milk are bactericidal, phagocytic, and enzymatic [78]. Microbiocidal activity occurs through the production of oxidants and granule enzyme activities. In addition, neutrophils demonstrated significant bactericidal activity against *Staphylococcus aureus* [78]. This study by Grazioso and Buescher (1996) also demonstrated the effective ratio for phagocytosis between neutrophils and staphylococci cells at 2:1. A study by Islam et al. (2006) demonstrated that the percentages of breast milk phagocytes (neutrophil-macrophages) of a cell count in mothers with underweight, normal BMI, and overweight were 46.6% ± 19.35, 60.24% ± 6.93, and 55.55% ± 16.16, respectively [33].

Stem cells have been found in human milk that differentiate into luminal, basal, and myoepithelial layers [79]. These stem cells can regulate an octamer-binding transcription factor 4 expression that repairs human cells. The stem cells in human milk protect the cells of the infant [80]. The stem cells in breast milk were hypothesized to function as a neuroprotective factor in a study that used intra-nasal application of breast milk for rescuing preterm neonates from brain injury and to improve long-term neurocognitive improvement of preterm infants [81]. A review by Kakulas (2015) concluded that the number of lactocytes (mature mammary epithelial cells) in obese mothers was lower than other reports of lactocytes in healthy mature milk likely due to lower milk supply of obese mothers. In addition, a study by Twigger et al. (2015) in a review by Kakulas (2015) explained that the number of lactocytes in mothers with obesity was decreased because of the lower expression CK18 expression. Moreover, the lower expression of CK18 expression (a marker of luminal epithelial cell activity such as lactocytes) would reduce epithelial tissue capability to synthesize milk in mammary glands in obese mothers [34,80].

2.3. *Chemokines*

Chemokines are a type of cytokine that may stimulate cell movement [22]. Chemokine production is influenced by lactoferrin and a derivative of lactoferrin [82]. These factors have not been studied with regard to maternal body weight and lactation.

G-CSF functions as a hematopoietic growth factor, to stimulate the proliferation of clonal and neutrophil progenitor differentiation [83]. A study by Wallace et al. (1997) showed that the concentration of G-CSF in 30 samples of mothers with normal BMI ranged from 14 to >2500 pg/mL [84]. Again, there was no information found as to how high maternal body weight affected this factor.

The production of macrophage migration inhibitory factor (MIF) is equivocal with some reports that MIF is not produced by specific human cells [85]. Another study demonstrated that MIF is produced by a large number of T-cells [86]. The specific interleukins found to induce MIF production are tumor necrosis factor-alpha (TNF-α) and interferon gamma (IFNγ) [85,87]. There was no information found regarding how or whether MIF is affected by maternal body weight.

2.4. *Cytokines*

Cytokines interact with the other cells and cross the intestinal barrier to enhance or defend, and reduce inflammation [22]. The cytokines in human milk have roles as immunomodulatory and anti-inflammatory to reduce infection in the infant [88]. Additionally, mammary glands need cytokines for growth and development. Cytokines regulate proliferation and inflammation of cells [89].

Both regulation and development of mammary gland function are mediated by IL-6 and TNF-Alpha [90]. In addition, fever and systemic inflammation also correlate with IL-6, for example IL-6 was higher when mastitis occurred in the lobes [91,92]. IL-6, IL-10, and TGF-β are maternal cytokines associated with maturation of the intestinal immune system. These cytokines also regulate IgA production, development, and differentiation of cells [93]. A study by Whitaker et al. (2017) found no significant association between the maternal weight and IL-6 level [8]. Another study by Fields et al. (2017) also demonstrated similar results of no association between BMI of maternal mothers and IL-6 concentration in their milk [18]. However, a study by Collado (2012) showed contrasting results. IL-6 concentration was higher in colostrum of overweight and obese mothers (81.85 pg/mL) than in colostrum of healthy BMI mothers (62.86 pg/mL), while IL-6 concentrations in 1-month milk of overweight and obese mothers (13.22 pg/mL) was lower than IL-6 concentration of normal BMI mothers (22.12 pg/mL) [35].

The main functions of IL-7 are to support lymphoid development, produce T-cells in the thymus, and assist in T-cell survival at secondary of peripheral lymphoid tissue [94]. IL-7 from human milk is absorbed by the infant through the intestine.

In a study of mothers with varying BMI, the concentrations of TNFα in colostrum and 1-month milk of mothers with normal BMI were reported at 9.87 and 10.60 pg/mL, respectively [35]. However, these values differ greatly from the study by Meki et al. (2003) [91]. This study concluded that TNFα is a proinflammatory cytokine that increased over the course of lactation; however, the values seem to be similar with no standard deviation indicated. These authors also reported that the TNFα concentration in colostrum and 1-month milk of mothers with BMI ≤25 kg/m^2 and BMI >25 kg/m^2 were 11.41 and 10.23 pg/mL, respectively. However, there was no statistically significant difference in the TNFα content of the milk in these mothers [35]. The values for this cytokine are logarithmically different than those reported by others in the literature [35]. Therefore, while no differences were detected by Meki et al. the inconsistency with the literature makes it hard to conclude with certainty that the concentration of TNFα is not influenced by maternal BMI.

2.5. Growth Factors

Epidermal growth factor (EGF) is a growth modulator that can be found in amniotic fluid [95]. The function of EGF in human milk, as a growth and weight regulator, is related to appetite of the infant [19]. Another role of EGF is to support the maturation of infant gut by development, from a high intestinal permeability to become more selectively permeable [95]. A study by Khodabakhshi (2015) demonstrated that the EGF concentration in milk of obese mothers (0.038 ng/mL) was significantly lower ($p = 0.013$) than that of mothers with normal BMI (0.040 ng/mL). Furthermore, low concentration of EGF in the mother's milk was significantly associated with higher infant body weight [19].

HB-EGF is a growth factor that can be found in both amniotic fluid and human milk [96,97]. HB-EGF appears to protect the infant intestine, specifically the intestinal epithelium from cytokine-induced apoptosis and hypoxic necrosis by decreasing the level of nitrogen and reactive oxygen species produced [98–101].

The Insulin-like Growth Factors (IGF)-I in human blood were found in 1968 by Jacobs et al. [102]. IGF-1 has an important role in infant growth where the high concentration of IGF-1 in the human milk promotes rapid growth to the infants that may be associated with overweight and obesity in later life [103]. IGF-1 in breast milk is thought to protect premature infants from retinopathy of prematurity (ROP) in the first 6 weeks of life; IGF-1 deficiency during the first weeks of neonatal life was associated with ROP [104]. In addition, infants who consumed only breast milk had a lower incidence of ROP than the infants who consume infant formula [104]. The concentration of IGF-1 in the human milk of obese mothers (89.63 ng/mL) and normal mothers (75.09) was not significantly different ($p = 0.787$).

Specific neurons of the peripheral nervous system need nerve growth factor (NGF) to survive [105]. NGF has been shown to stimulate the phosphorylation of tyrosine on the TrkA protein receptor in human mast cells-1 (HMC-1) [106]. There was no literature found that described the effect of overweight or obesity in mothers on milk content or functions of NGF.

Human milk contains vascular endothelial growth factor (VEGF) and epidermal growth factor (EGF) at concentrations that are 100 times higher than blood of lactating mothers [107]. The concentration of VEGF from 33 samples of lactating mothers ranged from 12.6 to 155.0 (median 50.0) ng/mL. The concentration of VEGF was significantly positively correlated with the EGF concentration, but negatively correlated with hepatic growth factor (HGF) concentration [107]. VEGF receptors, such as fetal liver kinase 1, are expressed primarily in endothelial cells [108]. There were no studies found that investigated the effect of maternal overweight or obesity on concentrations of VEGF and HGF.

2.6. Hormones

The role of adiponectin is to regulate metabolism of the body, specifically affecting satiety, tissue sensitivity to insulin, stimulate glucose uptake, and decrease energy expenditure [109–111]. Studies by Martin et al. (2006) showed a positive correlation between maternal BMI and the concentration of adiponectin [36]. Furthermore, higher adiponectin in milk increases the risk of being overweight in childhood [109]. In contrast, another study specifically demonstrated lower weight gain and leaner body of neonates [112].

Calcitonin has functions to inhibit gastric acid production, or regulate fluid balance, food intake, and gastrointestinal motility [113–115]. The calcitonin concentration level in the human milk was found to be 10–40-fold greater than the concentration in the serum [116]. Lactating mothers have elevated serum calcitonin which is released into their milk [117]. The effects of maternal obesity on milk calcitonin have not been reported.

Ghrelin was identified by Kojima et al. (1999), as a 28-amino-acid-peptide. It was found to be predominantly expressed in the stomach [118], but it is also expressed in the pituitary, hypothalamus, and pancreas and functions to regulate food intake, sleep, behavior, gastric acid secretion and motility, glucose metabolism, exocrine and endocrine pancreatic function, cardiac performances and vascular resistance, energy metabolism, cell proliferation and survival, stimulates of ghrelin (GH), Arginine vasopressin (AVP), prolactin (PRL), adrenocorticotropic hormone (ACTH) secretion, and inhibits the gonadotropin secretion [119]. Ghrelin in the human milk functions as a growth factor that stimulates feeding by the infant [120]. A study by Khodabakhsh (2015) showed a negative correlation between obese mothers and the concentration of ghrelin in milk [19]. A similar result also was also demonstrated in a study by Zhang et al. (2011), where the concentration of ghrelin in human milk of normal weight mothers was higher than that in mothers with obesity [37].

Insulin in human milk functions as a hormone, and also influences the microbiome community in the lumen of the gastrointestinal tract [10]. Mothers with obesity accumulate more insulin in their human milk than mothers with normal body weight [109,121]. A study by Ley et al. (2012) specifically showed that the insulin concentrations were higher in the milk from obese mothers than mothers with normal BMI at 3 months post-partum [121]. The impact of higher insulin and glucose in human milk is more rapid growth of the infant which may increase risk for childhood obesity because of the higher energy content of diabetic breast milk than breast milk of healthy mothers [122,123]. In addition, Plagemann et al. (2002) observed a positive correlation between infant overweight and volume of diabetic breast milk (DBM) consumed at 2 years of age compared to infants who consumed banked breast milk from non-diabetic mothers [124]. This study showed early neonatal consumption of breastmilk from diabetic mothers was positively correlated to risk of overweight, and impaired glucose tolerance (IGT) during childhood [124].

Leptin is an adipocyte-derived hormone that was first found in 1994 [125]. Opposing the adiponectin function, leptin functions to increase appetite and suppress energy expenditure. It is considered a regulator of long-term energy balance [126]. The mean concentration of leptin at 1 month postpartum in the human milk of 50 normal weight mothers was 2.5 ± 1.5 ng/mL [9]. The concentration of milk leptin significantly decreased, up to 33.7% after 6 months of lactation, this may be in response to the decrease in fat mass of the mothers [18]. A study by Fields et al. (2017) demonstrated other determinants of leptin concentration in human milk such as BMI category, and gender of infant [18]. This study also showed a significant positive correlation between maternal BMI and leptin concentration in human milk. Furthermore, another study demonstrated higher concentrations of leptin in the milk of obese mothers, up to three times the concentration in milk of normal weight mothers [10]. Uysal et al. (2002) also found a significant correlation between high leptin concentration and maternal obesity [11]. The positive association between maternal obesity and leptin concentration in milk also noted by Andreas et al. (2014) and Quinn et al. (2014) [12,13]. At the 3rd and 28th day after delivery, the leptin concentration in milk of mothers who had BMI over 25 showed a significantly higher concentration than the milk of normal weight mothers [14]. Other data supporting this finding, are that increasing concentrations of leptin were found in milk of obese mothers at 1 month postpartum (4.8 ± 2.7 ng/mL) [9].

Obestatin is a hormone that was found in 2005 in the gastrointestinal tract [127]. Obestatin in human milk may control the appetite and gastrointestinal function of infant as the infant adapts to receiving milk [38,128]. The concentration of obestatin is negatively correlated with the BMI of mothers [38]. Therefore, the concentration of obestatin in the milk of overweight and obese mothers will be lower than the concentration of obestatin in milk of normal weight mothers.

Resistin is a hormone in breast milk that regulates fetal growth, appetite, and metabolic development of the infant [129]. The median concentrations of resistin in 23 samples of breast milk were 0.18 ng/mL (IR = 0.44) [40]. Study by Savino et al. (2012) and Andreas at al. (2016) found that the concentration of resistin was not altered in milk of mothers with obese BMI [39,40]. However, the concentration of resistin was higher in the serum of mothers with obese BMI [39]. The higher concentration of resistin in the serum and milk would increase the concentration of hormones (cortisol, estradiol, leptin, progesterone, prolactin, triiodothyronine, and thyroxine) and inflammatory marker (C-reactive protein) [130].

Somatostatin functions to inhibit gastrin secretion [131]. The highest concentration of somatostatin was found on the first day postpartum, in colostrum [132]. The concentration of milk somatostatin is 7.2 times higher than the concentration in the plasma of mothers, due to an active transport process moving somatostatin from blood to mammary gland. Reports of maternal obesity on somatostatin concentration have not been found.

2.7. Immunoglobulins

The major immunoglobulin found in human milk is Secretory IgA (sIgA, 80%–90%). This antibody is transferred from the milk to the infant, at the rate of 0.3 g/kg/day. About 10% is absorbed from the intestines and enters the infant blood [133]. A deficiency of sIgA in the mucous membranes can be substituted by a high concentration of IgM antibodies, particularly for infants with selective IgA deficiency [134]. Carbonare (1997) showed that sIgA fully protects the intestinal tract from enteropathogenic *E. coli* antigens, and is not destroyed by digestion [135]. A study by Islam et al. (2006) also compared the sIgA concentrations among three BMI groups. The study showed that IgA concentration in the human milk of overweight (5.60 ± 1.47 g/L) and normal mothers (5.67 ± 165 g/L) were higher than IgA concentration in malnourished mothers (5.22 ± 1.68 g/L) [63]. The standard deviation of the IgA concentration in the milk of the mothers with normal BMI may be a typographical error as it seems very high.

Unlike IgA, IgG and IgM are completely digested in the small intestine [20]. Thus, intact IgG is not present in significant quantities at the intestinal mucosal surface of infants. IgG is present at a low concentration (0.1 mg/mL) in human milk though it has a role in activating the complement system and antibody-dependent cytotoxicity [136]. The concentrations of IgG in breast milk of mothers with underweight, normal BMI, and overweight were 0.095 ± 024 g/L, 0.096 ± 024 g/L, and 0.093 ± 020 g/L, respectively [33].

IgM concentration in the colostrum of human milk is the second highest of the immunoglobulins. The mean concentration of IgM is 0.47 ± 0.10 g/L [33]. IgM protects the infant intestinal mucosal surface from viruses and bacteria [136]. Islam et al. (2006) demonstrated the mean concentration of overweight mothers and normal mothers were 0.47 ± 0.01 g/L and 0.47 ± 0.09 g/L, respectively.

Insulin-like growth factor-binding proteins can be found in human milk and include insulin growth factor I (IGF-1) and insulin growth factor 2 (IGF-2). Colostrum contains the highest concentration of IGF compared to the later milks [137]. IGF-1 functions to protect the enterocytes in the intestine from damage by oxidative stress, stimulates erythropoiesis, and is related to increasing hematocrit [137]. IGF-binding protein 2 is higher in preterm milk than term milk [138]. IGF-1 concentration is influenced by BMI of mothers whereby IGF-1 concentration was found to decrease significantly in the obese breastfeeding mothers [19].

2.8. Lipids

Lipids contribute up to 44% of the total energy in human milk [139]. Lipids can have an antimicrobial function in the infant intestine [140]. In addition, the activity and development of antimicrobial function in infant's gut is supported by milk fats through provision of nutrients [141]. Cell membranes of bacteria were shown to be damaged by antimicrobial activity of free fatty acids and monoglycerides [142]. A study by Fujimori et al. (2015) demonstrated that both the triglyceride and cholesterol concentration in the colostrum of overweight and obese mothers were higher than concentrations in colostrum of normal weight mothers [42]. Another study by Makela et al. (2013) showed that the fatty acid composition in human milk of overweight mothers was significantly higher in total saturated fatty acids and lower in n-3 fatty acids than in milk of normal weight mothers [43]. Furthermore, unsaturated to saturated fatty acid ratios in milk and the ratio of n-6 to n-3 was higher in overweight mothers versus normal weight mothers. A complete analysis of the various in fatty acids concentration in obese and normal mothers has been conducted by Panagos et al. (2016) [15]. A meta-analysis and a randomized controlled trial (RCT) showed associations between fatty acid composition in human milk and child growth were not significant [143–146].

2.9. Microbiota

Human milk supports proliferation of the milk microbiota by regulating the balance of specific microbiota such as, *Lactobacillus, Bacteroides,* and *Bifidobacteria*. The proliferation of these microbiota stimulates the activation of T regulatory cells and transform intrauterine TH2 predominant to rebalance TH1/TH2 [147]. About 200 kinds of important bacteria grow to constitute the first gut microbiota in the newborn [148]. *Bifidobacterium* and *Lactobacillus* are the primary probiotic in the gut that provide nutrients to the newborn intestine and protect it by establishing an acidic environment rich in short chain fatty acids (SCFAs) [148,149]. Dendritic cells (DCs) and CD18+ cells function to capture the microorganism from the mother's intestinal bacteria and translocate them to lactating mammary glands, therefore the number of DCs and CD18+ cells will increase late in pregnancy and during lactation [150]. A decreasing number of *Bifidobacterium* and increasing number of *Staphylococcus* have been demonstrated in human milk of obese and overweight mothers [35,44]. Furthermore, the higher concentration of *Lactobacillus* and the lower of concentration of *Bifidobacterium* for 3 months may contribute to increased risk of overweight and obesity to the infant [151]. Another study also demonstrated that obese infant and obese children have significantly different microbial flora because of different colonization through breast milk bacteria [152]. The alteration of the microbiota is not the only influence on nutritional status of the infant, but may be related to increased risk of asthma, allergies, inflammatory bowel disease, and type 1 diabetes. Thus, by Turnbaugh et al. (2012), Dibaise et al. (2009), Karvonen et al. (2014), Kostic et al. (2015), Frank et al. (2007) and Cabrera-Rubio et al. (2012) concluded that the bacteria in human milk of obese mothers may influence the health status of their infants [153–158].

2.10. Nucleic Acids

The degradation of milk nucleic acid polymers (RNA) provides nucleotides, which have been found to improve immune function, enhance the bioavailability of iron, adjust the microflora in the intestine, alter plasma lipids, and support growth and maturation of the gut [159–163]. Production of nucleotides in human milk needs further study because there is no study yet that compares the concentration of nucleotides in the milk of mothers with obese and normal BMI.

2.11. Oligosaccharides and Glycans

Human milk oligosaccharides (HMOs) protect infants from microbial infections, protect gut microbiota, prevent microbial adhesion, and invasion in the intestinal mucosa [164]. HMOs are small carbohydrates that bind pathogen bacteria and also facilitate the establishment of a protective microbiome in the intestinal tract of the infant [165]. HMOs are the main glycan and influential in the human milk because they inhibit the growth of pathogenic bacteria by binding to the pathogen and preventing pathogen binding to the intestinal epithelium [165]. HMOs prevent the attachment of viruses and bacteria surface on intestinal epithelium [166]. HMO is involved in development of the submucosa lymphoid structure and intestinal epithelial cell (IEC) barrier [166]. Colostrum contains two kinds of HMOs, 2′-fucosyllactose and 3′-galacto-syllactose, that reduce cytokine production and the inflammatory reactions [167,168]. A study by Azad et al. (2018) showed no significant correlation between the maternal BMI and the concentration of HMO in human milk [45]. This is of interest because a variation of HMO composition in human milk could influence the gut microbiome of the infant and variation in HMO has been shown to be significantly related to growth and body composition of the infant [169].

Prebiotics such as glycosaminoglycans, oligosaccharides, glycoprotein, and glycolipids are needed to support growth of the microbiota in the intestinal tract [166]. Glycosaminoglycans may be protective to infants, particularly the newborn, because the number of these polysaccharides are highest at the first month of lactation [170]. Furthermore, a study by Coppa et al. (2012) also demonstrated that the number of glycosaminoglycans in preterm human milk was higher than in term milk. A study of the association between BMI mothers and metabolic capacity of glycosaminoglycans was shown by Cardo et al. (2018). They found significant degradation of glycosaminoglycan activity in human milk of obese mothers compared to normal BMI mothers [46].

The concentration of soluble CD14 (sCD14) in the colostrum is 20-fold greater than the concentration in maternal serum [171]. A function of sCD14 in the infant intestine is to modulate the innate and adaptive immune response of bacterial colonization [171]. A study by Collado (2012) found that sCD14 in colostrum (28.22 μg/mL) and 1-month milk (5.54 μg/mL) of normal BMI mothers was higher than that of overweight and obese mothers, which contained 23.21 and 4.35 μg/mL, respectively [35]. These differences were not significant.

Osteoprotegerin is part of the TNF super family components that inhibit the activation of TNF-induction to prevent proliferation process of T cells. The concentration of osteoprotegerin in epithelial cells of the human mammary gland and human milk is 1000 times higher than the concentration in human serum [172]. Osteoprotegerin function in the Th1 cells may re-balance the concentration of Th1 and Th2 of newborn infants [173]. However, there was no study found that investigated maternal obesity and overweight on osteoprotegerin concentration in human milk.

2.12. Other Proteins

Alpha-lactalbumin of human milk is a bioactive protein that can be found in the whey fraction of milk [174]. Alpha-lactalbumin is present in both cow milk and human milk, and contains 123 amino acids [175]. Alpha-lactalbumin makes up 22% of total protein and 36% of whey protein in human milk [176,177]. The alpha-lactalbumin functions in synthesis of lactose and regulation of water circulation to human milk through osmotic systems [176]. The level of alpha-lactalbumin in milk is influenced by genetic, environment, and dietary factors [178]. For these reasons, alpha-lactalbumin plays a vital role as a bioactive protein. A previous study showed that the concentration of alpha-lactalbumin in human milk was influenced by nutritional status of mothers. Standard weight (SW) of mothers significantly influenced the concentration of alpha-lactalbumin in human milk [47]. Specifically, the concentration of alpha-lactalbumin in human milk of mothers who had SW, <10% SW, 10%–25% SW, and >25% SW were significantly different at 16–30 days and 31–60 days after delivery.

α1-Antitrypsin is a protease inhibitor in human milk. It has been shown to be an influential protein together with antichymotrypsin [179]. α1-Antitrypsin in human milk can be detected in the stool of human milk-fed infants [180,181]. The function of α1-antitrypsin and antichymotrypsin may be to permit absorption of certain bioactive proteins by limiting the digestibility of certain proteins in the infant gut [182]. Furthermore, α1-antitrypsin and antichymotrypsin affected the total nitrogen balance of infants who are fed by human milk. The inhibitory activity of α1-antitrypsin was not affected by pH (down to pH 2) or temperature [183]. It may be relatedly a protector of bioactive proteins (such as lactoferrin) at the small intestine, particularly in the upper part [183,184]. There was no study found that explored maternal obesity or overweight and α1-Antitrypsin.

Alpha-amylase is another significant bioactive protein in human milk [185]. The newborn infant has low concentrations of salivary amylase and pancreatic amylase activity. Milk amylase therefore may function to compensate for the low infant alpha-amylase from human milk [186]. Future studies should be conducted to better understand the significance of milk alpha-amylase for utilization of carbohydrate in mixed diet-fed infants [182]. There was no report that explored alpha-amylase concentration in milk of overweight and obese mothers.

Bile Salt Stimulated Lipase (BSSL) has been identified in human milk but not cow milk, where it contributes to 1%–2% of total milk protein. BSSL is influential as an active enzyme to digest lipid in the lumen of the infant gut. It hydrolyzes the esters of vitamin A and cholesterol, lyso-phospholipids, and other milk fats such as monoglycerides, diglycerides, and triglycerides [20]. A study by Andersson et al. (2007) demonstrated that BSSL can be destroyed or deactivated by the pasteurization process. Therefore, preterm infants who consume pasteurized milk from donor mothers show reductions in lipid absorption. Anthropometric measurements of length, weight, heel-to-knee of infants who consumed non-pasteurized milk increased more in these growth markers than infants who consumed pasteurized milk [187].

Human milk proteins are often classified according the nature of how the colloids are distributed in milk, as either two components, whey or casein. Casein proteins are distinguished by their arrangement in micelles. Human milk contains 20%–40% caseins [20]. The concentration of β-casein is the highest among other human caseins. β-casein is a highly phosphorylated protein [188]. MUC2 functions to protect the human small intestine layer by multiple mechanisms [189]. The adhesion of *Helicobacter pylori* is prevented by κ-casein activity at the gastric mucosa. More specifically, κ-casein at the epithelial cell surface has role as a soluble receptor analogue which prevents the binding of mucosal epithelium to bacteria [182]. The ratio of the concentration of casein and whey decreases over time [190]. At the first 2 weeks after delivery, the ratio concentration of casein and whey was found to be 20:80. After 2 weeks postpartum the ratio concentration of casein and whey changed to 35:65 and stayed constant. The beta-casein expression was reduced in milk of overfed rats, which suggests a similar effect might occur on beta-casein concentration in the human milk of overweight and obese mothers [48].

C-reactive protein is an inflammatory protein marker that is primarily produced by the liver [191]. Maternal obesity was found to be associated with an alteration of CRP. A study by Whitaker et al. (2017) showed that the concentrations of CRP in the human milk of 126 obese and or mothers with excessive weight gain were significantly higher than mothers with the normal weight gain or lower weight. High concentrations of CRP level in infant serum can increase the risk of cardiovascular disease in the long term due to CRP level functions to control serum cholesterol level [192].

Folate-binding protein regulates the metabolism of the vitamin folic acid, through distribution, absorption, and retention [193]. The soluble folate-binding protein (FBP) function is a glycosylated compound that binds the vitamin in a way that prevents proteolytic degradation in the low gastric pH. The glycosylation appears to provide protection from digestion [194]. Furthermore, folate bound to FBP is gradually released in the small intestine mucosa [195]. There was no study found that reported effects of maternal obesity or overweight on FBP concentration in milk.

Haptocorrin is an anti-microbial substance that was found to reduce *E. coli* and is stable against proteolytic digestive enzymes [196]. In addition, haptocorrin remains undigested at pH 3.5 by pepsin and pancreatic enzymes [196]. High concentrations of haptocorrin are not needed for pathogenic activity. Another function of haptocorrin in human milk is as a substitute for intrinsic factor, that helps in the absorption of Vitamin B_{12} in the newborn (acting as a vitamin B_{12}-binding protein) [197]. There was no study found that reported effects of maternal obesity or overweight on haptocorrin concentration in milk.

3. The Influence of Other Factors on the Levels of Immunological Properties in Human Milk

The composition of human milk is also influenced by other maternal factors, such as diet, age, ethnicity, metabolic health, type of delivery, smoking, amount of sleep, stress, and physical activity. Additionally, it is influenced by physiological factors such as diurnal variation, stage of lactation and stage of nursing, as well as factors related to the infant, including gender, birthweight, body composition, and behavioral factors, such as ad libitum feeding and time between feedings [7]. The main influential factors on human milk composition are preterm delivery and stage of lactation [198]. Studies that demonstrate an influence of other factors that affect immunological properties of milk are reported in Table 2.

Table 2. Alteration of immunological properties by other influential factors.

Influence Factors	Immunological Properties	Alteration
	Lysozyme	A study by Hennart et al. (1991) demonstrated that malnourished mothers had up to four times higher concentration of lysozyme than well-nourished mothers [199].
Malnourishment	Lactoperoxidase	A study by Chang (1990) showed that the concentration of lactoperoxidase in human milk of malnourished Chinese women decreased up to 50% [200].
	sIgA	The concentration of sIgA in milk of malnourished mothers was lower than the concentration of sIgA in milk of normal weight mothers [41].
	IgG	A study by Miranda et al. (1983), with malnourished Colombian mothers, demonstrated lower IgG concentrations compared to milk of well-nourished mothers [41].
	Alpha-lactalbumin	A study by Lonnerdal et al. (1976) in Ethiopian and Swedish mothers demonstrated that alpha-lactalbumin concentration in well-nourished mothers was higher than in milk of malnourished mothers [178].
	Lymphocyte	The mean quantity of lymphocyte plasma cells in colostrum of mothers with low BMI mothers was higher than that of mothers with normal BMI [33].
Lactation Stages	Macrophages	The composition of colostrum is high in macrophages (30%–50% in leukocytes) [201]. However, macrophage concentration was found to decrease after 1 month of lactation and maturation of human milk [22,202].
	G-CSF	A study by Calhoun et al. (2000) demonstrated that the highest concentration of G-CSF in human milk was 1–2 days postpartum. MIF concentration is highest at the first month of lactation and continues to decrease with time of lactation [203].
	IL-6	The IL-6 levels were at similar levels in milk samples taken at 1 month and 3 months postpartum [8].
	IL-7	A showed that mean concentration of IL-7 was influenced by the age of infants. IL-7 concentration in human milk of 6 months breastfed infants (103.5 ± 37.8 pg/dL) was higher than IL-7 concentration of 2 months of breastfed infants (69.8 ± 40 pg/dL) [204]. In a study of healthy mothers' milk over time, the concentration of TNFα in colostrum was higher than the concentration in transitional and mature milk [205]. Another study showed that the TNFα concentration in colostrum (402.80 ± 29.65 pg/mL) and mature milk (178.30 ± 14.41 pg/mL) were higher than the TNFα concentration in transitional milk (135.50 ± 8.26 pg/mL) [91].
	EGF	In milk of 33 mothers at day 1–7 postpartum, the concentration of EGF was reported to range from 33.3 to 184.3 (median 71.2) ng/mL [107].
	IGF-1	A study by Erikkson et al. (1993) showed that the concentration of IGF-1 in the colostrum to transitional milk (decreased five-fold day 1 to day 3, and then remained relatively constant through day 8 of lactation [206].
	NGF	A study by Ai et al. (2012) measured NGF levels of seven healthy breastfeeding mothers on the first 3 days postpartum. Measurement of NGF levels showed very high variation and NGF levels postpartum milk were, 236 ± 332 ng/L, 173 ± 113 ng/L, and 178 ± 248 ng/L, for 1, 2 and 3 days, respectively, but were not significantly different over time [207].
	VEGF	A study by Kobata et el. (2008) demonstrated decreasing concentrations of VEGF from 1 to 7 days postpartum [107].
	Ghrelin	While the ghrelin concentration was high in breast milk, there were significant increases in infants' weight gain at 4 months of age [208]. The negative correlation between ghrelin concentration in serum and infants BMI occurred at the first month of life [146].
		Another study also showed that low concentration of ghrelin in infants would slow the weight gain during the first 3 months [209].
		Transitional milk and colostrum contain small amounts of Immunoglobulin G (IgG) while the amount of IgG is higher in mature milk [20].
	Lipid	Colostrum, transition milk, and mature milk contains lipid concentrations of 3–4, 7.2, and 56.2 g/L respectively [210].
	Gangliosides	Around 6%–10% of total lipid mass in human infant brain consists of gangliosides. This concentration will be increase up to 3-fold from 10-weeks' gestation to 5 years of age [211]. GM1, GM3, and GD3 are three types of gangliosides in human milk that bind pathogens without causing inflammatory reactions [212]. A study by Thakkar et al. (2013) demonstrated that the concentration of gangliosides in human milk was significantly higher at 120 days postpartum in male infants [213].
	α1-antitrypsin	The concentration of α1-antitrypsin from 190 human milk samples of 94 maternal mothers between 1 and 160 days after delivery was found to decrease over time [179].
	Alpha-amylase	The decrease in alpha-amylase concentration could range up to 35% ($p < 0.001$) during the first 3 months [214].

Table 2. *Cont.*

Influence Factors	Immunological Properties	Alteration
Pregnancy length	Chemokines	A study by Michie et al. (1998) showed that there were no differences in chemokines concentration between human milk of mothers that delivered preterm or full term [215].
	G-CSF	The production of G-CSF (at the first 2 days of colostrum) of premature delivered mothers was lower than that of term mothers [216].
	TNFα	A study demonstrated that the concentration of TNFα in colostrum of mothers with premature babies was lower than the mothers with full term babies [205].
	Alpha-amylase	No differences in alpha-amylase concentration were found in the human milk produced for preterm infants or full-term infants [217].
	BSSL	There was no significant difference of characteristics of BSSL found in the human milk produced from mothers with preterm or full-term infants [218].
	Osteoprotegerin	The concentration of osteoprotegerin in the milk of mothers whose deliver their infant prematurely and full term was not significantly different [172].
Type of Breastfeeding	IL-7	A higher concentration of IL-7 was found in exclusively breastfed infants compared to those that received mixed feeding [204].
Nutritional Status of Infant	IGF-1	A study showed that high BMI of infant was negatively correlated with the concentration of IGF-1 in human milk [19].

4. Conclusions

Based on literature that were collected and reviewed, obesity and overweight of mothers appears have a clear influence on the concentration of 29 immunological properties in human milk. An alteration of any of these immunological properties could influence the function of the human milk. An increase or decrease of immunological properties in human milk are predicted to influence the health status of infants in both the short term and long term. Further research is needed to study the correlation of high BMI with the 31 yet unstudied or unreported immunological properties in human milk and the risk of specific diseases to the infants.

There are some limitations of this review. First, the range of years for publications of studies reviewed was not limited. Some current studies might have different results compared to older studies because of different number of participants, data collection methods, immunoassay methods and detection, and statistical analyses. Second, many studies did not classify the samples collected as to whether they were colostrum, hind milk, and fore milk. Differences in the composition of milk over the duration of lactation should have different concentration of immunological properties. Furthermore, these variations might influence the output of immunological actions related to their function as protectors and supporters for infant growth and development.

5. Practice Points

Maternal overweight and obesity has been found to affect 29 immunological properties of human milk. While a complete understanding of the implications of these changes to the infant are not known, they add to the body of evidence supporting healthy weight management:

1. Medical practitioners, dietitian/nutritionists, and nurses should educate the pregnant mothers with BMI > 30 kg/m^2 about the risk of obesity to mother and infant and suggest restricting excessive caloric intake outside of the recommended amounts needed for healthy infant growth. The health care professionals support the pregnant mother in obesity by providing weight management targets and the information about nutrient dense eating plans or menus.
2. After delivery, exclusive breastfeeding can be promoted as another component of energy expenditure which will help prevent further weight gain by the obese mother. Breastfeeding mothers should not follow a weight loss program until 6–8 weeks after delivery because it may influence the quality and quantity of milk production. The overweight and obese mothers should be encouraged and supported to exclusively breastfeed for at least for 6 months.
3. At 6–8 weeks postpartum, obese mothers should be encouraged to pursue healthy weight loss programs with nutrient dense eating plans after lactation is well established. Health professionals can emphasize that achieving a healthier BMI provides health benefits to both the

infants (by normalizing the immunological properties concentration in milk) and to the mothers (by decreasing the risk of metabolic diseases, such as, heart disease, diabetes mellitus, and cancer).

4. Even though composition of some immunological factors in milk changes in obesity, there is not enough evidence at this time to suggest that the changes in the milk should preclude breastfeeding the infant, as the benefits of breastfeeding are well established. In fact, obese mothers in the US, Europe, Brazil, Latin America, Singapore, India, South Africa, and Australia, that cannot breastfeed, can consult with international board certified lactation consultants (IBCLC) and pediatricians to consider obtaining donor milk from a milk bank in one of these countries.

6. Research Agenda

1. The association of maternal obesity with immunological properties reported as unstudied in this review need investigation.
2. The alteration of specific immunological properties and these effects on infant health condition (when breastfed by obese mothers) should be examined both in the short term and long term. A reduction of protective factors could have a negative impact on infant health.
3. The differences in infant health status after exclusive breastfeeding by obese mothers should also be explored for obese mothers that practice nonexclusive breastfeeding. Exclusive breastfeeding has been widely encouraged due to the benefits for mothers and infants. It is conceivable that alterations in the immunological properties due to obesity may affect the usual advantages associated with exclusive breastfeeding.

Author Contributions: Conceptualization, U.D.E. and A.D.F.; Data collection, U.D.E.; Supervision, A.D.F.; Writing—original draft, U.D.E.; Writing—review, A.D.F.; Writing—editing, U.D.E. and A.D.F.

Acknowledgments: This review was supported by Indonesia Endowment Fund for Education (LPDP) and Indiana University Bloomington.

References

1. Chen, C.; Xu, X.; Yan, Y. Estimated global overweight and obesity burden in pregnant women based on panel data model. *PLoS ONE* **2018**, *13*, 1–14. [CrossRef] [PubMed]
2. Singh, G.K.; Siahpush, M.; Hiatt, R.A.; Timsina, L.R. Dramatic Increases in Obesity and Overweight Prevalence and Body Mass Index Among Ethnic-Immigrant and Social Class Groups in the United States, 1976–2008. *J. Community Health* **2010**, *36*, 94–110. [CrossRef] [PubMed]
3. US Department of Health and Human Services. *The National Health Interview Survey, Questionnaires, Datasets, and Related Documentation: 1976–2014 Public Use Data Files*; National Center for Health Statistics: Hyattsville, MD, USA, 2015.
4. Hamilton, B.E.; Martin, J.A.; Michelle, J.L.; Osterman, M.H.S.; Curtin, M.A.; Matthews, M.S. Births: Final data for 2014. *Natl. Vital Stat. Rep.* **2015**, *64*, 1–64. [PubMed]
5. Fisher, S.C.; Kim, S.Y.; Sharma, A.J.; Rochat, R.; Morrow, B. Is obesity still increasing among pregnant women? Prepregnancy obesity trends in 20 states, 2003–2009. *Prev. Med.* **2013**, *56*, 372–378. [CrossRef] [PubMed]
6. Deputy, N.P.; Dub, B.; Sharma, A.J. Prevalence and Trends in Prepregnancy Normal Weight—48 States, New York City, and District of Columbia, 2011–2015. *MMWR Morb. Mortal. Wkly. Rep.* **2018**, *66*, 1402–1407. [CrossRef] [PubMed]
7. Fields, D.A.; Schneider, C.R.; Pavela, G. A narrative review of the associations between six bioactive components in breast milk and infant adiposity. *Obesity (Silver Spring)* **2016**, *24*, 1213–1221. [CrossRef] [PubMed]
8. Whitaker, K.M.; Marino, R.C.; Haapala, J.L.; Foster, L.; Smith, K.D.; Teague, A.M.; Jacobs, D.; Fontaine, P.L.; McGovern, P.M.; Schoenfuss, T.C.; et al. Associations of Maternal Weight Status Before, During, and After Pregnancy with Inflammatory Markers in Breast Milk. *Obesity (Silver Spring)* **2017**, *25*, 2092–2099. [CrossRef]

9. De Luca, A.; Frasquet-Darrieux, M.; Gaud, M.A.; Christin, P.; Boquien, C.Y.; Millet, C.; Herviou, M.; Darmaun, D.; Robins, R.J.; Ingrand, P.; et al. Higher Leptin but Not Human Milk Macronutrient Concentration Distinguishes Normal-Weight from Obese Mothers at 1-Month Postpartum. *PLoS ONE* **2016**, *11*, e0168568. [CrossRef]
10. Lemas, D.J.; Young, B.E.; Baker, P.R.; Tomczik, A.C.; Soderborg, T.K.; Hernandez, T.L.; A de la Houssaye, B.; Robertson, C.E.; Rudolph, M.C.; Patinkin, D.I.Z.W.; et al. Alterations in human milk leptin and insulin are associated with early changes in the infant intestinal microbiome. *Am. J. Clin. Nutr.* **2016**, *103*, 1291–1300. [CrossRef]
11. Uysal, F.K.; Onal, E.E.; Aral, Y.Z.; Adam, B.; Dilmen, U.; Ardicolu, Y. Breast milk leptin: Its relationship to maternal and infant adiposity. *Clin. Nutr.* **2002**, *21*, 157–160. [CrossRef]
12. Andreas, N.J.; Hyde, M.J.; Gale, C.; Parkinson, J.R.; Jeffries, S.; Holmes, E.; Modi, N. Effect of maternal body mass index on hormones in breast milk: A systematic review. *PLoS ONE* **2014**, *9*, 1–25. [CrossRef] [PubMed]
13. Quinn, E.A.; Largado, F.; Borja, J.B.; Kuzawa, C.W. Maternal Characteristics Associated with Milk Leptin Content in a Sample of Filipino Women and Associations with Infant Weight for Age. *J. Hum. Lact.* **2014**, *31*, 273–281. [CrossRef] [PubMed]
14. Eilers, E.; Ziska, T.; Harder, T.; Plagemann, A.; Obladen, M.; Loui, A. Leptin determination in colostrum and early human milk from mothers of preterm and term infants. *Early Hum. Dev.* **2011**, *87*, 415–419. [CrossRef] [PubMed]
15. Panagos, P.G.; Vishwanathan, R.; Penfield-Cyr, A.; Matthan, N.R.; Shivappa, N.; Wirth, M.D.; Hebert, J.R.; Sen, S. Breastmilk from obese mothers has pro-inflammatory properties and decreased neuroprotective factors. *J. Perinatol.* **2016**, *36*, 284–290. [CrossRef] [PubMed]
16. Brunner, S.; Schmid, D.; Zang, K.; Much, D.; Knoeferl, B.; Kratzsch, J.; Amann-Gassner, U.; Bader, B.L.; Hauner, H. Breast milk leptin and adiponectin in relation to infant body composition up to 2 years. *Pediatr. Obes.* **2015**, *10*, 67–73. [CrossRef]
17. Grunewald, M.; Hellmuth, C.; Demmelmair, H.; Koletzko, B. Excessive weight gain during full breast-feeding. *Ann. Nutr. Metab.* **2014**, *64*, 271–275. [CrossRef] [PubMed]
18. Fields, D.A.; George, B.; Williams, M.; Whitaker, K.; Allison, D.B.; Teague, A.; Demerath, E.W. Associations between human breast milk hormones and adipocytokines and infant growth and body composition in the first 6 months of life. *Pediatr. Obes.* **2017**, *12* (Suppl. 1), 78–85. [CrossRef]
19. Khodabakhshi, A.; Ghayour-Mobarhan, M.; Rooki, H.; Vakili, R.; Hashemy, S.I.; Mirhafez, S.R.; Shakeri, M.-T.; Kashanifar, R.; Pourbafarani, R.; Mirzaei, H.; et al. Comparative measurement of ghrelin, leptin, adiponectin, EGF and IGF-1 in breast milk of mothers with overweight/obese and normal-weight infants. *Eur. J. Clin. Nutr.* **2015**, *69*, 614–618. [CrossRef] [PubMed]
20. Lonnerdal, B. Bioactive proteins in breast milk. *J. Paediatr. Child Health.* **2013**, *49* (Suppl. 1), 1–7. [CrossRef]
21. Pang, W.W.; Hartmann, P.E. Initiation of human lactation: Secretory differentiation and secretory activation. *J. Mammary Gland Biol. Neoplasia.* **2007**, *12*, 211–221. [CrossRef]
22. Ballard, O.; Morrow, A.L. Human milk composition: Nutrients and bioactive factors. *Pediatr. Clin. N. Am.* **2013**, *60*, 49–74. [CrossRef] [PubMed]
23. Saarela, T.; Kokkonen, J.; Koivisto, M. Macronutrient and energy contents of human milk fractions during the first six months of lactation. *Acta Paediatr.* **2005**, *94*, 1176–1181. [CrossRef] [PubMed]
24. Nommsen, L.A.; Lovelady, C.A.; Heinig, M.J.; Lonnerdal, B.; Dewey, K.G. Determinants of energy, protein, lipid, and lactose concentrations in human milk during the first 12 mo of lactation- the DARLING Study13. *Am. J. Clin. Nutr.* **1991**, *53*, 457–465. [CrossRef] [PubMed]
25. Dewey, K.G.; Finley, D.A.; Lönnerdal, B. Breast milk volume and composition during late lactation (7–20 months). *J. Pediatric Gastroenterol. Nutr.* **1984**, *3*, 713–720. [CrossRef]
26. Cabrera-Rubio, R.; Collado, M.C.; Laitinen, K.; Salminen, S.; Isolauri, E.; Mira, A. The human milk microbiome changes over lactation and is shaped by maternal weight and mode of delivery. *Am. J. Clin. Nutr.* **2012**, *96*, 544–551. [CrossRef] [PubMed]
27. O'Reilly, J.R.; Reynolds, R.M. The risk of maternal obesity to the long-term health of the offspring. *Clin. Endocrinol. (Oxf.)* **2013**, *78*, 9–16. [CrossRef] [PubMed]
28. Dieterich, C.M.; Felice, J.P.; O'Sullivan, E.; Rasmussen, K.M. Breastfeeding and health outcomes for the mother-infant dyad. *Pediatr. Clin. N. Am.* **2013**, *60*, 31–48. [CrossRef] [PubMed]

29. Horta, B.L.; Victora, C.G. *Long-Term Effects of Breastfeeding: A Systematic Review*; World Health Organization: Geneva, Switzerland, 2013.
30. Steinhoff, M.C.; Omer, S.B. A review of fetal and infant protection associated with antenatal influenza immunization. *Am. J. Obstet. Gynecol.* **2012**, *207*, S21–S27. [CrossRef]
31. Valentine, C.J. Optimizing Humn Milk Fortification for the Preterm Infant. *Pnpg. Build. Block Life.* **2011**, *34*, 9–11.
32. Houghton, M.R.; Gracey, M.; Burke, V.; Bottrell, C.; Spargo, R.M. Breast milk lactoferrin levels in relation to maternal nutritional status. *J. Pediatr. Gastroenterolnutr.* **1985**, *4*, 230–233.
33. Islam, S.K.; Ahmed, L.; Khan, M.N.; Huque, S.; Begum, A.; Yunus, A.B. Immune components (IgA, IgM, IgG, immune cells) of colostrum of Bangladeshi mothers. *Pediatr. Int.* **2006**, *48*, 543–548. [CrossRef] [PubMed]
34. Twigger, A.J.; Hepworth, A.R.; Tat Lai, C.; Chetwynd, E.; Stuebe, A.M.; Blancafort, P.; Hartmann, P.E.; Geddes, D.T.; Kakulas, F. Gene expression in breastmilk cells is associated with maternal and infant characteristics. *Scientific Reports.* **2015**, *5*, 1–14. [CrossRef] [PubMed]
35. Collado, M.C.; Laitinen, K.; Salminen, S.; Isolauri, E. Maternal weight and excessive weight gain during pregnancy modify the immunomodulatory potential of breast milk. *Pediatr. Res.* **2012**, *72*, 77–85. [CrossRef] [PubMed]
36. Martin, L.J.; Woo, J.G.; Geraghty, S.R.; Altaye, M.; Davidson, B.S.; Banach, W.; Dolan, L.M.; Ruiz-Palacios, G.M.; Morrow, A.L. Adiponectin is present in human milk and is associated with maternal factors. *Am. J. Clin. Nutr.* **2006**, *83*, 1106–1111. [CrossRef] [PubMed]
37. Zhang, N.; Yuan, C.; Li, Z.; Li, J.; Li, X.; Li, C.; Li, R.; Wang, S.R. Meta-Analysis of the Relationship Between Obestatin and Ghrelin Levels and the Ghrelin: Obestatin Ratio with Respect to Obesity. *Am. J. Med. Sci.* **2011**, *341*, 48–55. [CrossRef] [PubMed]
38. Aydin, S.; Ozkan, Y.; Erman, F.; Gurates, B.; Kilic, N.; Colak, R.; Gundogan, T.; Catak, Z.; Bozkurt, M.; Akin, O.; et al. Presence of obestatin in breast milk: Relationship among obestatin, ghrelin, and leptin in lactating women. *Nutrition* **2008**, *24*, 689–693. [CrossRef] [PubMed]
39. Andreas, N.J.; Hyde, M.J.; Herbert, B.R.; Jeffries, S.; Santhakumaran, S.; Mandalia, S.; Holmes, E.; Modi, N. Impact of maternal BMI and sampling strategy on the concentration of leptin, insulin, ghrelin and resistin in breast milk across a single feed: A longitudinal cohort study. *BMJ Open.* **2016**, *6*, e010778. [CrossRef] [PubMed]
40. Savino, F.; Sorrenti, M.; Benetti, S.; Lupica, M.M.; Liguori, S.A.; Oggero, R. Resistin and leptin in breast milk and infants in early life. *Early Hum. Dev.* **2012**, *88*, 779–782. [CrossRef] [PubMed]
41. Miranda, R.; Saravia, N.G.; Ackerman, H.; Murphy, N.; Berman, S.; McMurray, D.N. Effect of maternal nutritional statuses on immunological substances in human colostrum and milk. *Am. J. Clin. Nutr.* **1983**, *37*, 632–640. [CrossRef]
42. Fujimori, M.; Franca, E.L.; Fiorin, V.; Morais, T.C.; Honorio-Franca, A.C.; de Abreu, L.C. Changes in the biochemical and immunological components of serum and colostrum of overweight and obese mothers. *BMC Pregnancy Childbirth.* **2015**, *15*, 166. [CrossRef]
43. Makela, J.; Linderborg, K.; Niinikoski, H.; Yang, B.; Lagstrom, H. Breast milk fatty acid composition differs between overweight and normal weight women: The STEPS Study. *Eur. J. Nutr.* **2013**, *52*, 727–735. [CrossRef] [PubMed]
44. Delzenne, N.M.; Cani, P.D. Interaction between obesity and the gut microbiota: Relevance in nutrition. *Annu. Rev. Nutr.* **2011**, *31*, 15–31. [CrossRef] [PubMed]
45. Azad, M.B.; Robertson, B.; Atakora, F.; Becker, A.B.; Subbarao, P.; Moraes, T.J.; Mandhane, P.J.; Turvey, S.E.; Lefebvre, D.L.; Sears, M.R.; et al. Human Milk Oligosaccharide Concentrations Are Associated with Multiple Fixed and Modifiable Maternal Characteristics, Environmental Factors, and Feeding Practices. *J. Nutr.* **2018**, *148*, 1733–1742. [CrossRef] [PubMed]
46. Cerdo, T.; Ruiz, A.; Jauregui, R.; Azaryah, H.; Torres-Espinola, F.J.; Garcia-Valdes, L.; Segura, M.T.; Suárez, A.; Campoy, C. Maternal obesity is associated with gut microbial metabolic potential in offspring during infancy. *J. Physiol. Biochem.* **2018**, *74*, 159–169. [CrossRef] [PubMed]
47. Sanchez-Poso, A.; Lopez-Morales, J.; Ixquierdo, A.; Gil, A. Protein composition of human milk in relation to mother's weight and socio-economic status. *Hum. Nutr. Clin. Nutr.* **1987**, *41*, 115–125.
48. Jevitt, C.; Hernandez, I.; Groer, M. Lactation complicated by overweight and obesity: Supporting the mother and newborn. *J. Midwifery Women's Health* **2007**, *52*, 606–613. [CrossRef]

49. Siqueiros-Cendon, T.; Arevalo-Gallegos, S.; Iglesias-Figueroa, B.F.; Garcia-Montoya, I.A.; Salazar-Martinez, J.; Rascon-Cruz, Q. Immunomodulatory effects of lactoferrin. *Acta Pharmacol. Sin.* **2014**, *35*, 557–566. [CrossRef]
50. Suzuki, Y.A.; Shin, K.; Lönnerdal, B. Molecular cloning and functional expression of a human intestinal lactoferrin receptor. *Biochemistry.* **2002**, *40*, 15771–15779. [CrossRef]
51. Liao, Y.; Jiang, R.; Lonnerdal, B. Biochemical and molecular impacts of lactoferrin on small intestinal growth and development during early life. *Biochem. Cell Biol.* **2012**, *90*, 476–484. [CrossRef]
52. Wakabayashi, H.; Yamauchi, K.; Takase, M. Inhibitory effects of bovine lactoferrin and lactoferricin B on Enterobacter sakazakii. *Biocontrol. Sci.* **2008**, *13*, 29–32. [CrossRef]
53. Arnold, R.R.; Brewer, M.; Gauthier, J.J. Bactericidal Activity of Human Lactoferrin: Sensitivity of a Variety of Microorganisms. *Infect. Immun.* **1980**, *28*, 893–898. [PubMed]
54. Newburg, D.S.; Peterson, J.A.; Ruiz-Palacios, G.M.; Matson, D.O.; Morrow, A.L.; Shults, J.; de Lourdes Guerrero, M.; Chaturvedi, P.; Newburg, S.O.; Scallan, C.D.; et al. Role of human-milk lactadherin in protectoin against symptomatic rotavirus infection. *Lancet.* **1998**, *351*, 1160–1164. [CrossRef]
55. Aziz, M.; Jacob, A.; Matsuda, A.; Wang, P. Review: Milk fat globule-EGF factor 8 expression, function and plausible signal transduction in resolving inflammation. *Apoptosis.* **2011**, *16*, 1077–1086. [CrossRef] [PubMed]
56. Shi, J.; Heegaard, C.W.; Rasmussen, J.T.; Gilbert, G.E. Lactadherin binds selectively to membranes containing phosphatidyl-L-serine and increased curvature. *Biochim. Biophys. Acta.* **2004**, *1667*, 82–90. [CrossRef] [PubMed]
57. Kusunoki, R.; Ishihara, S.; Aziz, M.; Oka, A.; Tada, Y.; Kinoshita, Y. Roles of milk fat globule-epidermal growth factor 8 in intestinal inflammation. *Digestion* **2012**, *85*, 103–107. [CrossRef] [PubMed]
58. Chogle, A.; Bu, H.F.; Wang, X.; Brown, J.B.; Chou, P.M.; Tan, X.D. Milk fat globule-EGF factor 8 is a critical protein for healing of dextran sodium sulfate-induced acute colitis in mice. *Mol. Med.* **2011**, *17*, 502–507. [CrossRef]
59. Peterson, J.; Hamosh, M.; Scallan, C.; Ceriani, R.; Henderson, T.; Mehta, N.; Armand, M.; Hamosh, P. Milk fat globule glycoproteins in human milk and in gastric aspirates of mother's milk-fed preterm infants. *Pediatr. Res.* **1998**, *44*, 499–506. [CrossRef] [PubMed]
60. Steele, W.F.; Morrison, M. Antistreptococcal activity of lactoperoxidase. *J. Bacteriol.* **1969**, *97*, 635–639.
61. Björck, L.; Rosén, C.G.; Marshall, V.; Reiter, B. Antibacterial activity of lactoperoxidase system in milk against pseudomonas and other gram negative bacteria. *Appl. Microbiol.* **1975**, *30*, 199–204.
62. Shin, K.; Tomita, M.; Lonnerdal, B. Identification of lactoperoxidase in mature human milk. *J. Nutr. Biochem.* **2000**, *11*, 94–102. [CrossRef]
63. Ellison, R.; Giehl, T.J. Killing of Gram-negative Bacteria by Lactofernn and Lysozyme. *J. Clin. Investig.* **1991**, *88*, 1080–1091. [CrossRef] [PubMed]
64. Mosca, F.; Gianni, M.L. Human milk: Composition and health benefits. *Pediatr. Med. Chir.* **2017**, *39*, 155. [CrossRef] [PubMed]
65. Bansil, R.; Turner, B.S. Mucin structure, aggregation, physiological functions and biomedical applications. *Curr. Opin. Colloid Interface Sci.* **2006**, *11*, 164–170. [CrossRef]
66. Liu, B.; Yu, Z.; Chen, C.; Kling, D.E.; Newburg, D.S. Human milk mucin 1 and mucin 4 inhibit Salmonella enterica serovar Typhimurium invasion of human intestinal epithelial cells in vitro. *J Nutr.* **2012**, *142*, 1504–1509. [CrossRef] [PubMed]
67. Kvistgaard, A.S.; Pallesen, L.T.; Arias, C.F.; López, S.; Petersen, T.E.; Heegaard, C.W.; Rasmussen, J.T. Inhibitory Effects of Human and Bovine Milk Constituents on Rotavirus Infections. *J. Dairy Sci.* **2004**, *87*, 4088–4096. [CrossRef]
68. Schroten, H.; Hanisch, F.G.; Plogmann, R.; Hacker, J.; Uhlenbruck, G.; Nobis-Bosch, R. Inhibition of Adhesion of S-Fimbriated Escherichia coli to Buccal Epithelial Cells by Human Milk Fat Globule Membrane Components- a Novel Aspect of the Protective Function of Mucins in the Nonimmunoglobulin Fraction. *Infect Immun.* **1992**, *60*, 2893–2899. [PubMed]
69. Smith, C.W.; Goldman, A.S. Interactions of lymphocytes and macrophages from human colostrum- Electron microscopic studies of the interacting lymphocyte. *J. Reticuloendothel.* **1970**, *8*, 91–104.
70. Zhou, L.; Yoshimura, Y.; Huang, Y.; Suzuki, R.; Yokoyama, M.; Okabe, M.; Shimamura, M. Two independent pathways of maternal cell transmission to offspring-through placenta during pregnancy and by breast-feeding after birth. *Immunology* **2000**, *101*, 570–580. [CrossRef]

71. Cabinian, A.; Sinsimer, D.; Tang, M.; Zumba, O.; Mehta, H.; Toma, A.; Sant'Angelo, D.; Laouar, Y.; Laouar, A. Transfer of Maternal Immune Cells by Breastfeeding: Maternal Cytotoxic T Lymphocytes Present in Breast Milk Localize in the Peyer's Patches of the Nursed Infant. *PLoS ONE* **2016**, *11*, e0156762. [CrossRef] [PubMed]
72. Minniti, F.; Comberiati, P.; Munblit, D.; Piacentini, G.L.; Antoniazzi, E.; Zanoni, L.; Boner, A.L.; Peroni, D.G. Breast-Milk Characteristics Protecting Against Allergy. *Endocr. Metab. Immune Disord. Drug Targets* **2014**, *14*, 9–15. [CrossRef]
73. Buescher, E.; Malinowska, I. Soluble Receptors and Cytokine Antagonists in Human Milk. *Pediatr. Res.* **1996**, *40*, 839–844. [CrossRef] [PubMed]
74. English, B.K.; Burchett, S.K.; English, J.D.; Ammann, A.J.; Wara, D.W.; Wilson, C.B. Production of lymphotoxin and tumor necrosis factor by human neonatal mononuclear cells. *Pediatr. Res.* **1988**, *24*, 717–722. [CrossRef] [PubMed]
75. Ichikawa, M.; Sugita, M.; Takahashi, M.; Satomi, M.; Takeshita, T.; Araki, T.; Takahashi, H. Breast milk macrophages spontaneously produce granulocyte—Macrophage colony-stimulating factor and differentiate into dendritic cells in the presence of exogenous interleukin-4 alone. *Immunology* **2003**, *108*, 189–195. [CrossRef] [PubMed]
76. Yagi, Y.; Watanabe, E.; Watari, E.; Shinya, E.; Satomi, M.; Takeshita, T.; Takahashi, H. Inhibition of DC-SIGN-mediated transmission of human immunodeficiency virus type 1 by Toll-like receptor 3 signalling in breast milk macrophages. *Immunology* **2010**, *130*, 597–607. [CrossRef]
77. Jackson, K.M.; Nazar, A.M. Breastfeeding, the Immune Response, and Long-term Health. *J. Am. Osteopath Assoc.* **2006**, *106*, 203–207. [PubMed]
78. Grazioso, C.F.; Buescher, E.S. Inhibition of Neutrophil Function by Human Milk. *Cell Immunol.* **1996**, *168*, 125–132. [CrossRef] [PubMed]
79. Hassiotou, F.; Beltran, A.; Chetwynd, E.; Stuebe, A.M.; Twigger, A.J.; Metzger, P.; Trengove, N.; Lai, C.T.; Filgueira, L.; Blancafort, P.; et al. Breastmilk is a novel source of stem cells with multilineage differentiation potential. *Stem Cells* **2012**, *30*, 2164–2174. [CrossRef] [PubMed]
80. Kakulas, F. Breast milk: A source of stem cells and protective cells for the infant. *Infant* **2015**, *11*, 3.
81. Keller, T.; Korber, F.; Oberthuer, A.; Schafmeyer, L.; Mehler, K.; Kuhr, K.; Kribs, A. Intranasal breast milk for premature infants with severe intraventricular hemorrhage-an observation. *Eur. J. Pediatr.* **2019**, *178*, 199–206. [CrossRef] [PubMed]
82. Cacho, N.T.; Lawrence, R.M. Innate Immunity and Breast Milk. *Front. Immunol.* **2017**, *8*, 584. [CrossRef] [PubMed]
83. Avalos, B. Molecular analysis of the granulocyte colony-stimulating factor receptor. *Blood* **1996**, *88*, 761–777. [PubMed]
84. Wallace, J.M.; Ferguson, S.J.; Loane, P.; Kell, M.; Millar, S.; Gillmore, W.S. Cytokines in human breast milk. *Br. J. Biomed. Sci.* **1997**, *54*, 85–87. [PubMed]
85. Calandra, T.; Bernhagen, J.; Mitchell, R.A.; Bucala, R. The Macrophage Is an Important and Previously Unrecognized Source of Macrophage Migration Inhibitory Factor. *J. Exp. Med.* **1994**, *179*, 1895–1902. [CrossRef] [PubMed]
86. Bacher, M.; Metz, C.N.; Calandra, T.; Mayer, K.; Chesney, J.; Lohoff, M.; Gemsa, D.; Donnelly, T.; Bucala, R. An essential regulatory role for macrophage migration inhibitory factor in T-cell activation. *Proc. Natl. Acad. Sci. USA* **1996**, *93*, 7849–7854. [CrossRef] [PubMed]
87. Magi, B.; Bini, L.; Liberatori, S.; Marzocchi, B.; Raggiaschi, R.; Arcuri, F.; Tripodi, S.A.; Cintorino, M.; Tosi, P.; Pallini, V. Charge heterogeneity of macrophage migration inhibitory factor (MIF) in human liver and breast tissue. *Electrophoresis* **1998**, *19*, 2010–2013. [CrossRef]
88. Lonnerdal, B. Nutritional and physiologic significance of human milk proteins. *Am. J. Clin. Nutr.* **2003**, *77*, 1537S–1543S. [CrossRef] [PubMed]
89. Brenmoehl, J.; Ohde, D.; Wirthgen, E.; Hoeflich, A. Cytokines in milk and the role of TGF-beta. *Best Pract. Res. Clin. Endocrinol. Metab.* **2018**, *32*, 47–56. [CrossRef] [PubMed]
90. Basolo, F.; Fiore, L.; Fontanini, G.; Giulio, P.; Simonetta, C.; Falcone, V. Expression of response to interleukin 6 (IL6) in human mammary tumors. *Cancer Res.* **1996**, *56*, 3118–3122. [PubMed]
91. Meki, A.-R.; Saleem, T.H.; Al-Ghazali, M.H.; Sayed, A.A. Interleukins -6, -8 and -10 and tumor necrosis factor-alpha and its soluble receptor I in human milk at different periods of lactation. *Nutr. Res.* **2003**, *23*, 845–855. [CrossRef]

92. Mizuno, K.; Hatsuno, M.; Aikawa, K.; Takeichi, H.; Himi, T.; Kaneko, A.; Kodaira, K.; Takahashi, H.; Itabashi, K. Mastitis Is Associated with IL-6 Levels and Milk Fat Globule Size in Breast Milk. *J. Hum. Lact.* **2012**, *28*, 529–534. [CrossRef]
93. Bottcher, M.F.; Jenmalm, M.C.; Garofalo, R.P.; Bjorksten, B. Cytokines in breast milk from allergic and nonallergic mothers. *Pediatr. Res.* **2000**, *47*, 157–162. [CrossRef] [PubMed]
94. Aspinall, R.; Prentice, A.M.; Ngom, P.T. Interleukin 7 from maternal milk crosses the intestinal barrier and modulates T-cell development in offspring. *PLoS ONE* **2011**, *6*, e20812. [CrossRef] [PubMed]
95. Wagner, C.L.; Taylor, S.N.; Johnson, D. Host factors in amniotic fluid and breast milk that contribute to gut maturation. *Clin. Rev. Allergy Immunol.* **2008**, *34*, 191–204. [CrossRef] [PubMed]
96. Higashiyama, S.; Abraham, J.A.; Miller, J.; Fiddes, J.C.; Klagsbrun, M. A heparin-binding growth factor secreted by macrophage-like cells that is related to EGF. *Science* **1991**, *251*, 936–939. [CrossRef] [PubMed]
97. Michalsky, M.P.; Lara-Marquez, M.; Chun, L.; Besner, G.E. Heparin-binding EGF-like growth factor is present in human amniotic fluid and breast milk. *J. Pediatr. Surg.* **2002**, *37*, 1–6. [CrossRef] [PubMed]
98. Pillai, S.B.; Turman, M.A.; Besner, G.E. Heparin-Binding EGF-Like Growth Factor Is Cytoprotective for Intestinal Epithelial Cells Exposed to Hypoxia. *J. Pediatr. Surg.* **1998**, *33*, 973–978. [CrossRef]
99. Michalsky, M.P.; Kuhn, A.; Mehta, V.; Besner, G.E. Heparin-binding EGF-like growth factor decreases apoptosis in intestinal epithelial cells in vitro. *J. Pediatr. Surg.* **2001**, *36*, 1130–1135. [CrossRef] [PubMed]
100. Xia, G.; Martin, A.E.; Besner, G.E. Heparin-binding EGF-like growth factor downregulates expression of adhesion molecules and infiltration of inflammatory cells after intestinal ischemia/reperfusion injury. *J. Pediatr. Surg.* **2003**, *38*, 434–439. [CrossRef] [PubMed]
101. Kuhn, M.A.; Xia, G.; Mehta, V.B.; Glenn, S.; Michalsky, M.P. Antioxidants & redox signaling.-Heparin-binding EGF-like growth factor (HB-EGF) decreases oxygen free radical production in vitro and in vivo. *Antioxid. Redox Signal.* **2002**, *4*, 639–646. [PubMed]
102. LeBon, T.R.; Jacobs, S.; Cuatrecasas, P.; Kathuria, S.; Fujita-Yamaguchi, Y. Purification of Insulin-like Growth Factor I Receptor from Human Placental Membranes. *J. Biol. Chem.* **1986**, *261*, 7685–7689.
103. Larnkjaer, A.; Ong, K.K.; Carlsen, E.M.; Ejlerskov, K.T.; Molgaard, C.; Michaelsen, K.F. The Influence of Maternal Obesity and Breastfeeding on Infant Appetite- and Growth-Related Hormone Concentrations: The SKOT Cohort Studies. *Horm. Res. Paediatr.* **2018**, *90*, 28–38. [CrossRef] [PubMed]
104. Fonseca, L.T.; Senna, D.C.; Eckert, G.U.; Silveira, R.C.; Procianoy, R.S. Association between human breast milk and retinopathy of prematurity. *Arq. Bras. Oftalmol.* **2018**, *81*, 102–109. [CrossRef] [PubMed]
105. Bradshaw, R.A. Nerve growth factor. *Annu. Rev. Biochem.* **1978**, *47*, 191–216. [CrossRef] [PubMed]
106. Tam, S.Y.; Tsai, M.; Yamaguchi, M.; Yano, K.; Butterfield, J.H.; Galli, S.J. Expression of Functional TrkA Receptor Tyrosine Kinase in the HMC-1 Human Mast Cell Line and in Human Mast Cells. *Blood* **1997**, *90*, 1807–1820. [PubMed]
107. Kobata, R.; Tsukahara, H.; Ohshima, Y.; Ohta, N.; Tokuriki, S.; Tamura, S.; Mayumi, M. High levels of growth factors in human breast milk. *Early Hum. Dev.* **2008**, *84*, 67–69. [CrossRef] [PubMed]
108. Quinn, T.; Peters, K.G.; de Vries, C.; Ferrara, N.; Williams, L.T. Fetal liver kinase 1 is a receptor for vascular endothelial growth factor and is selectively expressed in vascular endothelium. *Proc. Natl. Acad. Sci. USA* **1993**, *90*, 7533–7537. [CrossRef] [PubMed]
109. Weyermann, M.; Brenner, H.; Rothenbacher, D.A. Adipokines in human milk and risk of overweight in early childhood: A Prospective Cohort Study. *Epidemiology* **2007**, *18*, 722–729. [CrossRef] [PubMed]
110. Catli, G.; Dundar, N.O.; Dundar, B.N. Adipokines in breast milk: An update. *J. Clin. Res. Pediatr. Endocrinol.* **2014**, *6*, 192–201. [CrossRef] [PubMed]
111. Savino, F.; Petrucci, E.; Nanni, G. Adiponectin: An intriguing hormone for paediatricians. *Acta Paediatr.* **2008**, *97*, 701–705. [CrossRef] [PubMed]
112. Woo, J.G.; Guerrero, M.L.; Altaye, M.; Ruiz-Palacios, G.M.; Martin, L.J.; Dubert-Ferrandon, A.; Newburg, D.S.; Morrow, A.L. Human milk adiponectin is associated with infant growth in two independent cohorts. *Breastfeed. Med.* **2009**, *4*, 101–109. [CrossRef] [PubMed]
113. Konturek, S.J.; Radecki, T.; Konturek, D.; Dimitreascu, T. Effect of Calcitonin on Gastric and Pancreatic Secretion and Peptic Ulcer Formation in Cats. *Dig. Dis. Sci.* **1974**, *19*, 235–241. [CrossRef]
114. Bueno, L.; Ferre, J.P.; Fioramonti, J.; Honde, C. Effects of intracerebroventricular administration of neurotensin, substance P and calcitonin on gastrointestinal motility in normal and vagotomized rats. *Regul. Pept.* **1983**, *6*, 197–205. [CrossRef]

115. Appelgren, B.H.; Arver, S.; Sagulin, G.B. Effect of intracerebroventricular calcitonin on renal hydromineral excretion in sheep. *Am. J. Physiol. Regul. Integr. Comp. Physiol.* **1986**, *250*, R980–R983. [CrossRef] [PubMed]
116. Arver, S.; Bucht, E.; Sjoberg, E. Calcitonin-like immunoreactivity in human milk, longitudinal alterations andl divalent cations. *Acta Physiol. Scand.* **1984**, *122*, 461–464. [CrossRef] [PubMed]
117. Root, A.W. *Disorders of Calcium and Phosphorus Homeostasis in the Newborn and Infant*, 4th ed.; Elseviers: Amsterdam, The Netherlands, 2014.
118. Kojima, M.; Hosoda, H.; Date, Y.; Nakazato, M.; Matsuo, H.; Kangawa, K. Ghrelin is a growth-hormone-releasing acylated peptide from stomach. *Nature* **1999**, *402*, 652–660. [CrossRef] [PubMed]
119. van der Lely, A.J.; Tschop, M.; Heiman, M.L.; Ghigo, E. Biological, physiological, pathophysiological, and pharmacological aspects of ghrelin. *Endocr. Rev.* **2004**, *25*, 426–457. [CrossRef] [PubMed]
120. Cesur, G.; Ozguner, F.; Yilmaz, N.; Dundar, B. The relationship between ghrelin and adiponectin levels in breast milk and infant serum and growth of infants during early postnatal life. *J. Physiol. Sci.* **2012**, *62*, 185–190. [CrossRef] [PubMed]
121. Ley, S.H.; Hanley, A.J.; Sermer, M.; Zinman, B.; O'Connor, D.L. Associations of prenatal metabolic abnormalities with insulin and adiponectin concentrations in human milk. *Am. J. Clin. Nutr.* **2012**, *95*, 867–874. [CrossRef] [PubMed]
122. Butte, N.F.; Garza, C.; Burr, R.; Goldman, A.S.; Kennedy, K.; Kitzmiller, J.L. Milk composition of insulin-dependent diabetic women. *J. Pediatr. Gastroenterol. Nutr.* **1987**, *6*, 936–941. [CrossRef] [PubMed]
123. Jovanovic-Peterson, L.; Fuhrmann, K.; Hedden, K.; Walker, L.; Peterson, C.M. Maternal milk and plasma glucose and insulin levels: Studies in normal and diabetic subjects. *J. Am. Coll. Nutr.* **1989**, *8*, 125–131. [CrossRef] [PubMed]
124. Plagemann, A.; Harder, T.; Franke, K.; Kohlhoff, R. Long-term impact of neonatal breast feeding on body weight and glucose tolerance in children of diabetic mothers. *Diabetes Care.* **2002**, *25*, 16–22. [CrossRef] [PubMed]
125. Zhang, Y.; Proenca, R.; Maffei, M.; Barone, M.; Leopold, L.; Friedman, J.M. Positional cloning of the mouse obese gene and its human homologue. *Nature (London)* **1994**, *372*, 425–432. [CrossRef] [PubMed]
126. Friedman, J.M. Leptin at 14 y of age: An ongoing story. *Am. J. Clin. Nutr.* **2009**, *89*, 973S–979S. [CrossRef] [PubMed]
127. Lacquaniti, A.; Donato, V.; Chirico, V.; Buemi, A.; Buemi, M. Obestatin: An interesting but controversial gut hormone. *Ann. Nutr. Metab.* **2011**, *59*, 193–199. [CrossRef] [PubMed]
128. Zhang, J.V.; Ren, P.G.; Avsian-Kretchmer, O.; Luo, C.W.; Rauch, R.; Klein, C.; Hsueh, A.J. Obestatin, a peptide encoded by the ghrelin gene, opposes ghrelin's effects on food intake. *Science* **2005**, *310*, 996–999. [CrossRef]
129. Savino, F.; Liguori, S.A.; Fissore, M.F.; Oggero, R. Breast milk hormones and their protective effect on obesity. *Int. J. Pediatr. Endocrinol.* **2009**, *2009*, 327505. [CrossRef] [PubMed]
130. Ilcol, Y.O.; Hizli, Z.B.; Eroz, E. Resistin is present in human breast milk and it correlates with maternal hormonal status and serum level of C-reactive protein. *Clin. Chem. Lab. Med.* **2008**, *46*, 118–124. [CrossRef] [PubMed]
131. Marchini, G.; Winberg, J.; Uvnas-Mobergi, K. Plasma concentrations of gastrin and somatostatin after breast feeding in 4 day old infants. *Arch. Dis. Child.* **1988**, *63*, 1218–1221. [CrossRef]
132. Hoist, N.; Jenssen, T.G.; Burhol, P.G. A characterization of immunoreactive somastostatin in human milk. *J. Pediatr. Gastroenterol. Nutr.* **1990**, *10*, 47–52.
133. Brandtzaeg, P.; Kiyono, H.; Pabst, R.; Russell, M.W. Terminology: Nomenclature of mucosa-associated lymphoid tissue. *Mucosal. Immunol.* **2008**, *1*, 31–37. [CrossRef] [PubMed]
134. Palmeira, P.; Costa-Carvalho, B.T.; Arslanian, C.; Pontes, G.N.; Nagao, A.T.; Carneiro-Sampaio, M.M. Transfer of antibodies across the placenta and in breast milk from mothers on intravenous immunoglobulin. *Pediatr. Allergy Immunol.* **2009**, *20*, 528–535. [CrossRef] [PubMed]
135. Carbonare, S.B.; Silva, M.L.M.; Palmeira, P.; Carneiro-Sampaio, M.M. Human colostrum IgA antibodies reacting to enteropathogenic Escherichia coli antigens and their persistence in the faeces of a breastfed infant. *J. Diarrhoeal. Dis. Res.* **1997**, *15*, 53–58. [PubMed]
136. Hanson, L.A.; Korotkova, M.; Lundin, S.; Håversen, L.; Silfverdal, S.A.; Mattsby-Baltzer, I.; Strandvik, B.; Telemo, E. The transfer of immunity from mother to child. *N. Y. Acad. Sci.* **2003**, *987*, 199–206. [CrossRef]
137. Kling, P.J.; Taing, K.M.; Dvorak, B.; Woodward, S.S.; Philipps, A.F. Insulin-like growth factor-I stimulates erythropoiesis when administered enterally. *Growth Factors* **2006**, *24*, 218–223. [CrossRef] [PubMed]

138. Blum, J.W.; Baumrucker, C.R. Colostral and milk insulin-like growth factors and related substances- Mammary gland and neonatal (intestinal and systemic) targets. *Domest. Anim. Endocrinol.* **2002**, *23*, 101–110. [CrossRef]
139. Grote, V.; Verduci, E.; Scaglioni, S.; Vecchi, F.; Contarini, G.; Giovannini, M.; Koletzko, B.; Agostoni, C. Breast milk composition and infant nutrient intakes during the first 12 months of life. *Eur. J. Clin. Nutr.* **2016**, *70*, 250–256. [CrossRef] [PubMed]
140. Milani, C.; Duranti, S.; Bottacini, F.; Casey, E.; Turroni, F.; Mahony, J.; Belzer, C.; Delgado Palacio, S.; Arboleya Montes, S.; Mancabelli, L.; et al. The first microbial colonizers of the human gut: Composition, activities, and health implications of the infant gut microbiota. *Microbiol. Mol. Biol. Rev.* **2017**, *81*, e00036-17. [CrossRef]
141. German, J.B.; Dillard, C.J. Composition, structure and absorption of milk lipids: A source of energy, fat-soluble nutrients and bioactive molecules. *Crit. Rev. Food Sci. Nutr.* **2006**, *46*, 57–92. [CrossRef]
142. Bergsson, G.; Arnfinnsson, J.; Karlsson, S.M.; Steingrimsson, O.; Thormar, H. In Vitro Inactivation of Chlamydia trachomatis by Fatty Acids and Monoglycerides. *Antimicrob. Agents Chemother.* **1998**, *42*, 2290–2294. [CrossRef]
143. Gibson, R.A.; Chen, W.; Makrides, M. Randomized trials with polyunsaturated fatty acid interventions in preterm and term infants: Functional and clinical outcomes. *Lipids* **2001**, *36*, 873–883. [CrossRef]
144. Lapillonne, A.; Carlson, S.E. Polyunsaturated fatty acids and infant growth. *Lipids* **2001**, *36*, 901–911. [CrossRef] [PubMed]
145. Makrides, M.; Gibson, R.A.; Udell, T.; Ried, K.; International LUPUFA Investigators. Supplementation of infant formula with long-chain polyunsaturated fatty acids does not influence the growth of term infants. *Am. J. Clin. Nutr.* **2005**, *81*, 1094–1101. [PubMed]
146. Savino, F.; Benetti, S.; Lupica, M.M.; Petrucci, E.; Palumeri, E.; Cordero di Montezemolo, L. Ghrelin and obestatin in infants, lactating mothers and breast milk. *Horm. Res. Paediatr.* **2012**, *78*, 297–303. [CrossRef] [PubMed]
147. Walker, W.A.; Iyengar, R.S. Breast milk, microbiota, and intestinal immune homeostasis. *Pediatr. Res.* **2015**, *77*, 220–228. [CrossRef] [PubMed]
148. Toscano, M.; De Grandi, R.; Grossi, E.; Drago, L. Role of the Human Breast Milk-Associated Microbiota on the Newborns' Immune System: A Mini Review. *Front. Microbiol.* **2017**, *8*, 2100. [CrossRef] [PubMed]
149. Bode, L. Human milk oligosaccharides: Every baby needs a sugar mama. *Glycobiology* **2012**, *22*, 1147–1162. [CrossRef] [PubMed]
150. Rodriguez, J.M. The origin of human milk bacteria: Is there a bacterial entero-mammary pathway during late pregnancy and lactation? *Adv. Nutr.* **2014**, *5*, 779–784. [CrossRef] [PubMed]
151. Kozyrskyj, A.L.; Kalu, R.; Koleva, P.T.; Bridgman, S.L. Fetal programming of overweight through the microbiome: Boys are disproportionately affected. *J. Dev. Orig. Health Dis.* **2016**, *7*, 25–34. [CrossRef] [PubMed]
152. Gregora, M. Lactobacillus Species in Breast Milk. In *Probiotics—Current Knowledge and Future Prospects*; IntechOpen: London, UK, 2018.
153. Turnbaugh, P.J.; Hamady, M.; Yatsunenko, T.; Cantarel, B.L.; Duncan, A.; Ley, R.E.; Sogin, M.L.; Jones, W.J.; Roe, B.A.; Affourtit, J.P.; et al. A core gut microbiome in obese and lean twins. *Nature* **2009**, *457*, 480–484. [CrossRef] [PubMed]
154. DiBaise, J.K.; Frank, D.N.; Mathur, R. Impact of the Gut Microbiota on the Development of Obesity: Current Concepts. *Am. J. Gastroenterol. Suppl.* **2012**, *1*, 22–27. [CrossRef]
155. Karvonen, A.M.; Hyvarinen, A.; Rintala, H.; Korppi, M.; Taubel, M.; Doekes, G.; Gehring, U.; Renz, H.; Pfefferle, P.I.; Genuneit, J.; et al. Quantity and diversity of environmental microbial exposure and development of asthma: A birth cohort study. *Allergy* **2014**, *69*, 1092–1101. [CrossRef] [PubMed]
156. Kostic, A.D.; Gevers, D.; Siljander, H.; Vatanen, T.; Hyötyläinen, T.; Hämäläinen, A.-M.; Peet, A.; Tillmann, V.; Pöhö, P.; Mattila, I.; et al. The dynamics of the human infant gut microbiome in development and in progression toward type 1 diabetes. *Cell Host Microbe* **2015**, *17*, 260–273. [CrossRef] [PubMed]
157. Frank, D.N.; Amand, A.L.S.; Feldman, R.A.; Boedeker, E.C.; Harpaz, N.; Pace, N.R. Molecular-phylogenetic characterization of microbial community imbalances in human inflammatory bowel diseases. *Proc. Natl. Acad. Sci. USA* **2007**, *104*, 13780–13785. [CrossRef] [PubMed]
158. Kalliomäki, M.; Carmen Collado, M.; Salminen, S.; Isolauri, E. Early differences in fecal microbiota composition in children may predict overweight. *Am. J. Clin. Nutr.* **2012**, *96*, 544–551. [CrossRef] [PubMed]

159. Thorell, L. Nucleotides in human milk: Sources and metabolism by the newborn infant. *Pediatr. Res.* **1996**, *40*, 845–852. [CrossRef] [PubMed]
160. Uauy, R. *Dietary Nucleotides and Requirements in Early Life: Text-Book of Gastroenterology and Nutrition in Infancy*; Raven Press Ltd.: New York, NY, USA, 1989.
161. Quan, R.; Barness, L.A.; Uauy, R. Do Infants Need Nucleotide Supplemented Formula for Optimal Nutrition? *J. Pediatr. Gastroenterol. Nutr.* **1990**, *11*, 429–433.
162. Carver, J.D.; Walker, W.A. The role of nucleotides in human nutrition. *J. Nutr. Biochem.* **1995**, *6*, 58–72. [CrossRef]
163. Gil, A.; Uauy, A. Nucleotides and related compounds in human and bovine milks. In *Handbook of Milk Composition*; Jensen, R.G., Ed.; Academic Press: San Diego, CA, USA, 1995.
164. Plaza-Diaz, J.; Fontana, L.; Gil, A. Human Milk Oligosaccharides and Immune System Development. *Nutrients* **2018**, *10*, 1038. [CrossRef] [PubMed]
165. Newburg, D.S.; Walker, W.A. Protection of the neonate by the innate immune system of developing gut and of human milk. *Pediatr. Res.* **2007**, *61*, 2–8. [CrossRef]
166. Newburg, D.S.; He, Y. Neonatal gut microbiota and human milk glycans cooperate to attenuate infection and inflammation. *Clin. Obstet. Gynecol.* **2015**, *58*, 814–826. [CrossRef]
167. He, Y.; Liu, S.; Leone, S.; Newburg, D.S. Human colostrum oligosaccharides modulate major immunologic pathways of immature human intestine. *Mucosal. Immunol.* **2014**, *7*, 1326–1339. [CrossRef] [PubMed]
168. Newburg, D.S.; Morelli, L. Human milk and infant intestinal mucosal glycans guide succession of the neonatal intestinal microbiota. *Pediatr. Res.* **2015**, *77*, 115–120. [CrossRef] [PubMed]
169. Alderete, T.L.; Autran, C.; Brekke, B.E.; Knight, R.; Bode, L.; Goran, M.I.; Fields, D.A. Associations between human milk oligosaccharides and infant body composition in the first 6 mo of life. *Am. J. Clin. Nutr.* **2015**, *102*, 1381–1388. [CrossRef]
170. Coppa, G.V.; Gabrielli, O.; Zampini, L.; Galeazzi, T.; Maccari, F.; Buzzega, D.; Galeotti, F.; Bertino, E.; Volpi, N. Glycosaminoglycan content in term and preterm milk during the first month of lactation. *Neonatology* **2012**, *101*, 74–76. [CrossRef] [PubMed]
171. Blewett, H.J.H.; Cicalo, M.C.; Holland, C.D.; Field, C.J. The Immunological Components of Human Milk. In *Advances in Food and Nutrition Research*; Academic Press: Cambridge, MA, USA, 2008; pp. 45–80.
172. Vidal, K.; Van Den Broek, P.; Lorget, F.; Donnet-Hughes, A. Osteoprotegerin in Human Milk: A Potential Role in the Regulation of Bone Metabolism and Immune Development. *Pediatr. Res.* **2004**, *55*, 1001–1008. [CrossRef]
173. Vidal, K.; Serrant, P.; Schlosser, B.; van den Broek, P.; Lorget, F.; Donnet-Hughes, A. Osteoprotegerin production by human intestinal epithelial cells- a potential regulator of mucosal immune responses. *Am. J. Physiol. Gastrointest. Liver Physiol.* **2004**, *287*, G836–G844. [CrossRef]
174. Phillips, N.I.; Jennes, R. Isolation and properties of human alpha-lactalbumin. *Biochim. Biophys. Acta* **1971**, *229*, 407–410. [CrossRef]
175. Permyakov, E.; Berliner, L.J. Alpha-Lactalbumin structure and function. *Fed. Eur. Biochem. Soc.* **2000**, *473*, 269–274. [CrossRef]
176. Heine, W.E.; Klein, P.D.; Reeds, P.J. The importance of alpha-lactalbumin in infant nutrition. *J. Nutr.* **1991**, *121*, 277–283. [CrossRef]
177. Kunz, C.; Lönnerdal, B. Re-evaluation of the whey protein:casein ratio of human milk. *Acta Paediatr.* **1992**, *81*, 107–112. [CrossRef]
178. Lönnerdal, B.; Forsum, E.; Gebre-Medhin, M.; Hambraeus, L. Breast milk composition in Ethiopian and Swedish mothers. II. Lactose, nitrogen, and protein contents. *Am. J. Clin. Nutr.* **1976**, *9*, 1134–1141. [CrossRef] [PubMed]
179. Lindberg, T.; Ohlsson, K.; Weström, B. Protease inhibitors and their relation to proteases in human milk. *Pediatr. Res* **1982**, *16*, 479–483. [CrossRef] [PubMed]
180. Davidson, L.A.; Lönnerdal, B. Persistence of human milk proteins in the breast fed infant. *Acta Paediatr. Scand.* **1987**, *76*, 733–740. [CrossRef] [PubMed]
181. Davidson, L.A.; Lönnerdal, B. Fecal alpha1 antitrypsin in breast fed infants is derived from human milk and is not indicative of enteric protein loss. *Acta Paediatr. Scand.* **1990**, *79*, 137–141. [CrossRef] [PubMed]
182. Lonnerdal, B.; Lien, E.L. Nutritional and Physiologic Significance of Alpha Lactalbumin in Infants. *Nutr. Rev.* **2003**, *61*, 295–305. [CrossRef] [PubMed]

183. Lonnerdal, B. Bioactive proteins in human milk: Mechanisms of action. *J. Pediatr.* **2010**, *156*, S26–S30. [CrossRef] [PubMed]
184. Chowanadisai, W.; Lonnerdal, B. α(1)-antitrypsin and antichymotrypsin in human milk: Origin, concentrations, and stability. *Am. J. Clin. Nutr.* **2002**, *76*, 828–833. [CrossRef] [PubMed]
185. Lindberg, T.; Skude, G. Amylase in human milk. *Pediatrics* **1982**, *70*, 235–238.
186. Heitlinger, L.A.; Lee, P.C.; Dillon, W.P.; Lebenthal, E. Mammary amylase: A possible alternate pathway of carbohydrate digestion in infancy. *Pediatr. Res.* **1979**, *13*, 969–972. [CrossRef]
187. Andersson, Y.; Savman, K.; Blackberg, L.; Hernell, O. Pasteurization of mother's own milk reduces fat absorption and growth in preterm infants. *Acta Paediatr.* **2007**, *96*, 1445–1449. [CrossRef]
188. Greenberg, R.; Groves, M.L.; Dower, H.J. Human beta-casein. Amino acid sequence and identification of phosphorylation sites. *J. Biol. Chem.* **1984**, *259*, 5128–5132.
189. Plaisancie, P.; Claustre, J.; Estienne, M.; Henry, G.; Boutrou, R.; Paquet, A.; Léonil, J. A novel bioactive peptide from yoghurts modulates expression of the gel-forming MUC2 mucin as well as population of goblet cells and Paneth cells along the small intestine. *J. Nutr. Biochem.* **2013**, *24*, 213–221. [CrossRef] [PubMed]
190. Haschke, F.; Haiden, N.; Thakkar, S.K. Nutritive and Bioactive Proteins in Breastmilk. *Ann. Nutr. Metab.* **2016**, *69* (Suppl. 2), 17–26. [CrossRef]
191. Sproston, N.R.; Ashworth, J.J. Role of C-Reactive Protein at Sites of inflammation and infection. *Front. Immunol.* **2018**, *9*, 1–11. [CrossRef] [PubMed]
192. Williams, M.J.; Williams, S.M.; Poulton, R. Breast feeding is related to C reactive protein concentration in adult women. *J. Epidemiol. Community Health* **2006**, *60*, 146–148. [CrossRef] [PubMed]
193. Henderson, G.B. Folate-Binding Proteins. *Annu. Rev. Nutr.* **1990**, *10*, 319–335. [CrossRef]
194. Antony, A.C.; Utley, C.S.; Marcell, P.D.; Kolhouse, J.F. Isolation, characterization, and comparison of the solubilized particulate and soluble folate binding proteins from human milk. *J. Biol. Chem.* **1982**, *257*, 10081–10089. [PubMed]
195. Said, H.M.; Horne, D.W.; Wagner, C. Effect of human milk folate binding protein on folate intestinal transport. *Arch. Biochem. Biophys.* **1986**, *251*, 114–120. [CrossRef]
196. Adkins, Y.; Lönnerdal, B. Potential host-defense role of a human milk vitamin B-12–binding protein, haptocorrin, in the gastrointestinal tract of breastfed infants, as assessed with porcine haptocorrin in vitro. *Am. J. Clin. Nutr.* **2003**, *77*, 1234–1240. [CrossRef] [PubMed]
197. Adkins, Y.; Lönnerdal, B. Mechanisms of vitamin B12 absorption in breast-fed infants. *J. Pediatr. Gastroenterol. Nutr.* **2002**, *35*, 192–198. [CrossRef] [PubMed]
198. Chung, M.Y. Factors affecting human milk composition. *Pediatr. Neonatol.* **2014**, *55*, 421–422. [CrossRef] [PubMed]
199. Hennart, P.F.; Brasseur, D.J.; Delogne-Desnoeck, J.B.; Dramaix, M.M.; Robyn, C.E. Lysozyme, lactoferrin, and secretory immunoglobulin A content in breast milk: Influence of duration of lactation, nutrition status, prolactin status, and parity of mother. *Am. J. Clin. Nutr.* **1991**, *53*, 32–39. [CrossRef] [PubMed]
200. Chang, S.J. Antimicrobial proteins of maternal and cord sera and milk in relation to maternal nutritional status. *Am. J. Clin. Nutr.* **1990**, *51*, 183–187. [CrossRef] [PubMed]
201. Wirt, D.P.; Adkins, L.T.; Palkowetz, K.H.; Schmalstieg, F.C.; Goldman, A.S. Activated and memory T lymphocytes in human milk. *Cytometry* **1992**, *13*, 282–290. [PubMed]
202. Hassiotou, F.; Geddes, D.T. Immune cell-mediated protection of the mammary gland and the infant during breastfeeding. *Adv Nutr.* **2015**, *6*, 267–275. [CrossRef] [PubMed]
203. Vigh, E.; Bodis, J.; Garai, J. Longitudinal changes in macrophage migration inhibitory factor in breast milk during the first three months of lactation. *J. Reprod. Immunol.* **2011**, *89*, 92–94. [CrossRef]
204. Hossny, E.M.; El-Ghoneimy, D.H.; El-Owaidy, R.H.; Mansour, M.G.; Hamza, M.T.; El-Said, A.F. Breast milk interleukin-7 and thymic gland development in infancy. *Eur. J. Nutr.* **2019**. [CrossRef]
205. Ustundag, B.; Yilmaz, E.; Dogan, Y.; Akarsu, S.; Canatan, H.; Halifeoglu, I.; Cikim, G.; Aygun, A.D. Levels of cytokines (IL-1beta, IL-2, IL-6, IL-8, TNF-α) and trace elements (Zn, Cu) in breast milk from mothers of preterm and term infants. *Mediat. Inflamm.* **2005**, *2005*, 331–336. [CrossRef]
206. Eriksson, U.; Duc, G.; Froesch, E.R.; Zapf, J. Insulin-like growth factors (IGF) I and I1 and IGF binding proteins (IGFBPs) in human colostrum:transitory milk during the first week postpartum. *Biochem. Biophys. Res. Commun.* **1993**, *196*, 267–273. [CrossRef]

207. Ai, Z.; Yumei, Z.; Titi, Y.; Qinghai, S.; Xiaohong, K.; Peiyu, W. The concentrations of some hormones and growth factors in bovine and human colostrums: Short communication. *Int. J. Dairy Technol.* **2012**, *65*, 507–510. [CrossRef]
208. Savino, F.; Fissore, M.; Grassino, E.; Nanni, G.; Oggero, R.; Silvestro, L. Ghrelin, leptin and IGF-I levels in breast-fed and formula-fed infants in the first years of life. *Acta Paediatr.* **2005**, *94*, 531–537. [CrossRef] [PubMed]
209. James, R.J.; Drewett, R.F.; Cheetham, T.D. Low cord ghrelin levels in term infants are associated with slow weight gain over the first 3 months of life. *J. Clin. Endocrinol. Metab.* **2004**, *89*, 3847–3850. [CrossRef] [PubMed]
210. Bitman, J.; Freed, L.M.; Neville, M.C.; Wood, D.L.; Hamosh, P.; Hamosh, M. Lipid composition of prepartum human mammary secretion and postpartum milk. *J. Pediatr. Gastroenterol. Nutr.* **1986**, *5*, 608–615. [CrossRef] [PubMed]
211. Svennerholm, L.; Bostrom, K.; Fredman, P.; Mansson, J.E.; Rosengren, B.; Rynmark, B.M. Human brain gangliosides: Developmental changes from early fetal stage to advanced age. *Biochim. Biophys. Acta* **1989**, *1005*, 109–117. [CrossRef]
212. Liu, B.; Newburg, D.S. Human milk glycoproteins protect infants against human pathogens. *Breastfeed. Med.* **2013**, *8*, 354–362. [CrossRef] [PubMed]
213. Thakkar, S.K.; Giuffrida, F.; Cristina, C.H.; De Castro, C.A.; Mukherjee, R.; Tran, L.-A.; Steenhout, P.; Lee, L.Y.; Destaillats, F. Dynamics of human milk nutrient composition of women from Singapore with a special focus on lipids. *Am. J. Hum. Biol.* **2013**, *25*, 770–779. [CrossRef] [PubMed]
214. Dewit, O.; Dibba, B.; Prentice, A. Breast-milk amylase activity in English and Gambian mothers: Effects of prolonged lactation, maternal parity, and individual variations. *Pediatr. Res* **1990**, *28*, 502–506. [CrossRef] [PubMed]
215. Michie, C.A.; Tantscher, E.; Schall, T.; Rot, A. Physiological secretion of chemokines in human breast milk. *Eur. Cytokine Netw.* **1998**, *9*, 123–129. [PubMed]
216. Calhoun, D.A.; Lunoe, M.; Du, Y.; Christensen, R.D. Granulocyte colony stimulating factor is present in human milk and its receptor is present in human fetal intestine. *Pediatrics* **2000**, *105*, 1–6. [CrossRef]
217. Hegardt, P.; Lindberg, T.; Börjesson, J.; Skude, G. Amylase in human milk from mothers of preterm and term infants. *J. Pediatr. Gastroenterol. Nutr.* **1984**, *3*, 563–566. [CrossRef]
218. Freed, L.M.; York, C.M.; Hamosh, P.; Mehta, N.R.; Hamosh, M. Bile Salt-Stimulated Lipase of Human Milk Characteristics of the Enzyme in the Milk of Mothers of Premature and Full-Term Infants. *J. Pediatr. Gastroenterol. Nutr.* **1987**, *6*, 598–604. [CrossRef] [PubMed]

10

Associations between the Prenatal Diet and Neonatal Outcomes—A Secondary Analysis of the Cluster-Randomised GeliS Trial

Julia Günther [1], Julia Hoffmann [1], Monika Spies [1], Dorothy Meyer [1], Julia Kunath [1], Lynne Stecher [1], Eva Rosenfeld [2], Luzia Kick [2], Kathrin Rauh [1,2] and Hans Hauner [1,*]

1 Else Kröner-Fresenius-Centre for Nutritional Medicine, School of Medicine, Klinikum rechts der Isar, Technical University of Munich, Georg-Brauchle-Ring 62, 80992 Munich, Germany
2 Competence Centre for Nutrition (KErn), Am Gereuth 4, 85354 Freising, Germany
* Correspondence: hans.hauner@tum.de

Abstract: The prenatal lifestyle, including maternal dietary behaviour, is an important determinant of offspring health. This secondary cohort analysis of the GeliS ("healthy living in pregnancy") trial investigated associations between antenatal dietary factors and neonatal weight parameters. The cluster-randomised GeliS trial included 2286 pregnant women. Dietary information was collected with food frequency questionnaires before or in the 12th (T0) and after the 29th week of gestation (T1). Consumption of vegetables (41.28 g per portion at T0, $p = 0.001$; 36.67 g per portion at T1, $p = 0.001$), fruit (15.25 g per portion at T1, $p = 0.010$) and dietary quality, measured with a Healthy Eating Index (39.26 g per 10 points at T0, $p = 0.004$; 42.76 g per 10 points at T1, $p = 0.002$) were positively associated with birth weight. In contrast, sugar-sweetened beverages (10.90 g per portion at T0, $p = 0.003$; 8.19 g per portion at T1, $p = 0.047$), higher sugar consumption at T0 (8.27 g per 10 g, $p = 0.032$) and early pregnancy alcohol intake (15.32 g per g, $p = 0.039$) were inversely associated with birth weight. Most other dietary factors were not associated with neonatal weight. Some components reflecting a healthy maternal diet were associated with a modest increase in offspring birth weight, whereas some unhealthy components slightly reduced neonatal weight.

Keywords: lifestyle intervention; pregnancy; dietary behaviour; neonatal outcomes; birth weight; large for gestational age (LGA); small for gestational age (SGA); obesity prevention

---

1. Introduction

In recent decades, concern about childhood obesity has grown worldwide. The intrauterine environment has been found to have a profound impact on body weight and health development during childhood and adulthood. Offspring birth weight and weight-related parameters such as a high birth weight and large for gestational age (LGA) at birth have been suggested to modify the risk of future health consequences, including obesity [1] and metabolic diseases such as diabetes mellitus [2].

Maternal over-nutrition can result in excessive gestational weight gain (GWG) and has been found to increase the risk of a high birth weight by its influence on the intrauterine environment [3]. Ultimately, excessive GWG can increase the risk of childhood overweight and obesity [4,5] and may promote health complications in the offspring, including metabolic and cardiovascular diseases [6,7]. Several studies have investigated the specific role of the maternal diet in offspring growth and development [8,9]. While clear associations between the antenatal diet and offspring birth weight have been shown in malnourished women [10], the findings in well-nourished women were less conclusive.

Although some components of the maternal diet have been suggested to influence the offspring's birth weight including for instance, milk [11], fruit and vegetables [12] and fish [13], evidence in this field is sparse [8]. Comprehensive data on the impact of the overall antenatal maternal diet on neonatal growth parameters are lacking [14].

The importance of a healthy lifestyle during pregnancy, including adequate GWG, a healthy diet, and regular physical activity, has been increasingly recognised. Different approaches aiming to improve the antenatal maternal lifestyle have been developed. While some of these trials have been effective in reducing excessive GWG, data on diet and physical activity have been less often reported [15]. The large-scale cluster-randomised controlled GeliS study ("Gesund leben in der Schwangerschaft"/healthy living in pregnancy), which primarily aimed to reduce excessive GWG using a routine care approach, extensively reported on pregnancy and obstetric outcomes, as well as behavioural parameters after a lifestyle intervention [16]. Data on the effects of the intervention on GWG, as well as on maternal and infant outcomes, have recently been published [17]. The large GeliS cohort, recruited in the setting of routine prenatal care, collated a large and diverse maternal and offspring data set which provides a valuable opportunity to comprehensively analyse associations between maternal antenatal behaviour and infant growth and health parameters. This secondary analysis aims to investigate associations between the maternal diet during early and late pregnancy and neonatal outcomes in the GeliS cohort. The impact of mean daily intake of food groups, energy and macronutrients as well as dietary quality by means of a Healthy Eating Index (HEI) on offspring weight parameters at birth was elucidated herein.

2. Materials and Methods

2.1. Study Design

The cluster-randomised, controlled GeliS trial was conducted within the German routine care setting in medical practices. In five administrative regions of Bavaria, pairs of ten urban and rural areas were randomised into one intervention and one control area per pair. The randomisation process and study procedures have been described in detail in the published study protocol [16].

Study procedures were conducted in accordance with the declaration of Helsinki as well as with local regulatory requirements and laws. The study protocol was approved by the ethics committee of the Technical University of Munich and is registered at the ClinicalTrials.gov Protocol Registration System (NCT01958307).

2.2. Study Participants

Pregnant women were recruited before or in the 12th week of gestation in gynaecological and midwifery practices. Inclusion criteria were fulfilled if women were aged between 18 and 43 years, had a body mass index (BMI) between 18.5 and 40.0 kg/m^2, had a singleton pregnancy, sufficient German language skills and provided written informed consent for participation in the trial. Women were excluded in case of a multiple or complicated pregnancy and if severe illnesses were diagnosed [16].

2.3. The Lifestyle Intervention Program

In the intervention group (IV), women attended a structured lifestyle intervention programme attached to routine prenatal care visits. They participated in three individual antenatal and one postpartum counselling sessions. Counselling included standardised information about an adequate GWG, a balanced diet and regular physical activity during pregnancy, and was conducted according to German recommendations [18]. Lifestyle counselling was performed by specifically trained midwives, gynaecologists and medical assistants in their practices.

Women in the control group (C) received routine prenatal care, complemented by a leaflet with general recommendations on a healthy antenatal lifestyle.

2.4. Study Outcomes

The primary outcome of the trial was the proportion of women showing excessive GWG as defined by the American Institute of Medicine (IOM) [19]. Data on the effect of the intervention on excessive GWG and some secondary outcomes have been published recently [17]. Despite a slight difference in offspring birth weight and length, no considerable between-group differences in maternal and neonatal outcomes were found [17]. Data from IV and C were thus pooled to form one cohort for the investigation of potential associations between the maternal diet and neonatal weight parameters.

2.5. Data Collection and Processing

Baseline characteristics of study participants were recorded by means of a screening questionnaire at study entry (≤12th week of gestation).

Maternal diet was assessed in both groups in early (≤12th week of gestation, T0) and late pregnancy (>29th week of gestation, T1) with food frequency questionnaires (FFQ). The self-administered FFQ was developed and validated by the Robert Koch Institute, Berlin, Germany for the "German Health Examination Survey for Adults" (DEGS) study [20] and was slightly modified for use in the GeliS trial. In the modified version, mean consumption frequency over the last four weeks was ranked by study participants from "never" to "more than five times per day" for 54 food items. Mean portion size was reported in standard measures such as cups, glasses, plates or bowls, and daily intake was calculated by combining frequency and portion size. If more than 20 out of the 54 food item questions were not answered, questionnaires were excluded from dietary analyses. Further, data of women reporting implausibly high daily intakes (either liquids >15 kg, or solid foods >10 kg, or both liquids >4 kg and solid foods >6 kg) were discarded due to over-reporting of food intake (according to personal communication by Dr. Gert Mensink, Robert Koch Institute, Berlin, Germany, 2018).

Recorded food items were summarised in food groups. Estimations of energy and macronutrient intake were made on the basis of information retrieved from the German food composition database ("Bundeslebensmittelschlüssel", version 3.02, Max Rubner Institute (MRI), Karlsruhe, Germany) using OptiDiet PLUS software (version 6.0, GOE mbH, Linden, Germany). Some questions in the FFQ referred to food groups in sum and not to single food items. For these food groups, data of the German National Consumption Survey II (NVS II) assessing typical patterns in the consumption of food items within food groups were considered (personal communication from MRI, Federal Research Institute of Nutrition and Food, "Verzehrsmengen ausgewählter Lebensmittel aus der Nationalen Verzehrsstudie II" (NVS II), Karlsruhe, Germany, July 2018). Data of women were excluded from analyses of energy and macronutrient consumption if their estimated mean energy intake was below 4500 kJ or exceeded 20,000 kJ per day [21].

Dietary quality was rated by means of a Healthy Eating Index (HEI) specifically developed for the applied DEGS-FFQ from the Robert Koch Institute [22]. Intake of 14 food groups assessed with the FFQ was compared with the German Nutrition Society (DGE) recommendations for a healthy diet and scored from 0 (no adherence to recommendations) to 100 (high adherence to recommendations) points. Correspondingly, a HEI-score was calculated as mean from the group scores [22].

Information on birth weight and length was retrieved from birth records collected from medical practices. Neonatal weight below the 10th percentile for gestational age was defined as "small for gestational age" (SGA), weight above the 90th percentile for gestational age as "large for gestational age" (LGA). Offspring were considered to have a low birth weight if they weighed less than 2500 g and to have a high birth weight if they weighed more than 4000 g.

2.6. Statistical Analysis

Women were included in the analyses if dietary data on at least one assessment point as well as neonatal data (body weight and length) were available. Women dropping out of the study due to a miscarriage or pregnancy termination, severe pregnancy complications or maternal death were excluded from the analyses. IV and C were pooled to form one cohort. Baseline characteristics are presented as mean ± standard deviation or proportion if appropriate.

For the analysis of associations between dietary variables (as mean daily portion or percent of energy if appropriate) and continuous offspring outcomes (birth weight, BMI), linear regression models were applied. Portions sizes were defined according to the FFQ for the different food items. For the analysis of dichotomous outcomes (SGA, LGA, low birth weight, high birth weight), binary logistic regression models were applied. Regression models were adjusted for group assignment, maternal pre-pregnancy age, BMI category and parity. Results are presented as effect sizes or odds ratios with 95% confidence intervals. p-values below 0.05 were considered as statistically significant. All analyses were conducted using SPSS software (IBM SPSS Statistics for Windows, version 24.0, IBM Corp, Armonk, NY, USA).

3. Results

3.1. Study Participants and Baseline Characteristics

Altogether, 2286 women were recruited for participation in the GeliS trial. A total of 112 women dropped out during the course of pregnancy (Figure 1). Women were further excluded from cohort analyses if they did not provide the relevant infant parameters (n = 156), resulting in a total of 2018 eligible participants. The maternal and neonatal characteristics of this sample are shown in Table 1. Dietary intake data were provided by 1995 of the 2018 women. After exclusion of invalid questionnaires and over-reporters, dietary data of 1902 (T0) and 1861 (T1) women were analysed in relation to neonatal weight parameters.

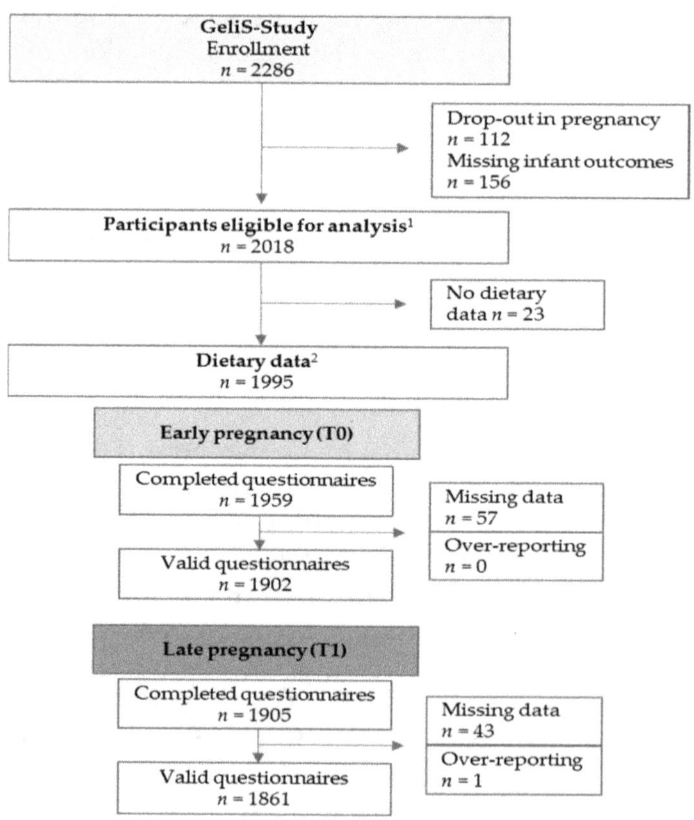

Figure 1. Participant flow. [1] Women without miscarriages, late loss of pregnancy, terminations, pregnancy complications that interfered with the intervention, maternal deaths and/or lack of infant outcomes (birth weight, birth length). [2] Women who provided dietary data at T0 or T1. T0: Dietary assessment before or in the 12th week of gestation; T1: Dietary assessment after the 29th week of gestation.

Table 1. Characteristics of study participants eligible for cohort analyses.

Maternal and Neonatal Characteristics	Total (n = 2018)
Maternal characteristics	
Pre-pregnancy age, years	30.3 ± 4.4 [a]
Pre-pregnancy weight, kg	68.2 ± 13.4 [a]
Pre-pregnancy BMI, kg/m^2	24.4 ± 4.5 [a]
Pre-pregnancy BMI category	
BMI 18.5–24.9 kg/m^2	1311/2018 (65.0%)
BMI 25.0–29.9 kg/m^2	464/2018 (23.0%)
BMI 30.0–40.0 kg/m^2	243/2018 (12.0%)
Educational level	
General secondary school	320/2014 (15.9%)
Intermediate secondary school	856/2014 (42.5%)
(Technical) High school	838/2014 (41.6%)
Country of birth	
Germany	1790/2014 (88.9%)
Others	224/2014 (11.1%)
Further maternal characteristics	
Nulliparous	1162/2018 (57.6%)
Living with a partner	1939/2011 (96.4%)
Full-time employed	1056/1996 (52.9%)
Gestational diabetes mellitus [b]	209/1940 (10.8%)
Pregnancy hypertension [c]	161/2015 (8.0%)
Preterm delivery [d]	131/2016 (6.5%)
Neonatal characteristics	
Birth weight, g	3337.6 ± 517.8 [a]
Birth length, cm	51.3 ± 2.6 [a]
Head circumference, cm	34.7 ± 1.6 [a]
BMI, kg/m^2	12.7 ± 1.3 [a]
SGA	172/2016 (8.5%)
LGA	148/2016 (7.3%)
Low birth weight	101/2018 (5.0%)
High birth weight	169/2018 (8.4%)

[a] mean ± SD. [b] diagnosed with a 2-h oral glucose tolerance test at weeks 24–28 of gestation according to national and international standards [23,24]. [c] Systolic blood pressure > 140 mmHg or diastolic blood pressure > 90 mmHg at at least two time points. [d] < 37 weeks of gestation. BMI: body mass index; SGA: Small for gestational age; LGA: Large for gestational age.

3.2. Associations between the Maternal Diet and Infant Weight and Weight-Related Parameters

Associations between antenatal food intake and neonatal birth weight and BMI are shown in Table 2. Associations with BMI z-scores are shown in Supplementary Table S1. There was evidence for a positive association between maternal fruit and vegetable consumption and infant birth weight (Table 2). An increase in offspring weight at birth by 41.28 g (95% CI 17.87 to 64.70 g, $p = 0.001$) was observed per portion of vegetables (150 g) in early pregnancy, and by 36.67 g/portion in late pregnancy (95% CI 15.95 to 57.39 g, $p = 0.001$). These observations were also reflected in the BMI of the neonates (T0: $p = 0.017$, T1: $p = 0.002$). A significant association between fruit intake and birth weight and BMI was found for the late pregnancy dietary assessment (birth weight: 15.25 g increase per portion of fruit (95% CI 3.67 to 26.83 g, $p = 0.010$), BMI: 0.04 kg/m^2 increase per portion (95% CI 0.01 to 0.07, $p = 0.009$)), but not for early pregnancy (birth weight: $p = 0.322$, BMI: $p = 0.172$). In contrast, maternal consumption of sugar-containing beverages was significantly inversely associated with weight at birth. In early pregnancy, one glass of soft drinks (200 mL) consumed by the mother reduced offspring birth weight by 10.90 g (95% CI −18.17 to −3.64 g, $p = 0.003$). In late pregnancy, there was evidence of a reduction by 8.19 g (95% CI −16.26 to −0.11 g, $p = 0.047$) per consumed glass of soft drinks. The association between soft drink intake and weight was not reflected in the BMI of the neonates (T0: $p = 0.076$, T1: $p = 0.437$). For the other food groups, such as dairy products, fast food and meat, no significant association between the consumed amount and offspring weight and BMI could be shown, either in early or in late pregnancy (Table 2).

Table 2. Associations between maternal food intake and offspring birth weight and body mass index.

Food Groups	Birth Weight (g)		BMI (kg/m^2)	
	Adjusted Effect Size [a] (95% CI)	Adjusted p Value [a]	Adjusted Effect Size [a] (95% CI)	Adjusted p Value [a]
Soft drinks [b] (200 mL/day)				
T0	−10.90 (−18.17, −3.64)	0.003	−0.02 (−0.03,0.00)	0.076
T1	−8.19 (−16.26, −0.11)	0.047	−0.01 (−0.03,0.01)	0.437
Light drinks [c] (200 mL/day)				
T0	−5.70 (−17.59,6.19)	0.347	−0.00 (−0.03,0.03)	0.919
T1	−5.89 (−18.34,6.55)	0.353	0.01 (−0.02,0.04)	0.577
Vegetables (150 g/day)				
T0	41.28 (17.87,64.70	0.001	0.07 (0.01,0.13)	0.017
T1	36.67 (15.95,57.39)	0.001	0.09 (0.03,0.14)	0.002
Fruit (150 g/day)				
T0	5.55 (−5.44,16.55)	0.322	0.02 (−0.01,0.05)	0.172
T1	15.25 (3.67,26.83)	0.010	0.04 (0.01,0.07)	0.009
Dairy products (200 g/day)				
T0	8.41 (−5.60,22.41)	0.239	0.00 (−0.03,0.04)	0.838
T1	3.13 (−9.37,15.62)	0.624	0.02 (−0.01,0.05)	0.233
Meat and meat products (150 g/day)				
T0	6.79 (−54.36,67.94)	0.828	0.00 (−0.15,0.15)	0.993
T1	3.35 (−60.86,67.55)	0.919	0.00 (−0.16,0.17)	0.966
Sweets and snacks (50 g/day)				
T0	11.69 (−8.07,31.44)	0.246	0.00 (−0.05,0.05)	0.895
T1	−4.97 (−21.12,11.18)	0.547	0.00 (−0.04,0.05)	0.855
Fast food (250 g/day)				
T0	9.08 (−153.36,171.52)	0.913	0.08 (−0.32,0.48)	0.702
T1	−95.15 (−273.51,83.22)	0.296	−0.17 (−0.63,0.29)	0.470

Estimated is the regression coefficient describing the association between the intake of a portion of a food item or food group and infant weight and BMI. Portion sizes are defined according to the applied food frequency questionnaire. [a] linear regression models adjusted for pre-pregnancy BMI, age, parity and group assignment. [b] sugar-containing sweetened beverages. [c] low or non-caloric sweetened beverages. BMI: body mass index; T0: assessment before or in the 12th week of gestation; T1: assessment after the 29th week of gestation.

Table 3 shows associations between antenatal food intake and infant weight-related outcomes. Fruit consumption in early pregnancy was significantly associated with increased odds of having a LGA neonate (OR 1.08 per portion, 95% CI 1.02 to 1.15, $p = 0.016$). Moreover, fast food consumption in early pregnancy but not in late pregnancy increased the odds of the offspring weighing > 4000 g at birth (T0: OR 3.14 per 250 g portion, 95% CI 1.26 to 7.84, $p = 0.014$).

Table 3. Associations between maternal food intake and neonatal weight-related parameters.

Food Groups	Low Birth Weight		High Birth Weight		SGA		LGA	
	Adjusted Odds Ratio [a] (95% CI)	Adjusted p Value [a]	Adjusted Odds Ratio [a] (95% CI)	Adjusted p Value [a]	Adjusted Odds Ratio [a] (95% CI)	Adjusted p Value [a]	Adjusted Odds Ratio [a] (95% CI)	Adjusted p Value [a]
Soft drinks [b] (200 mL/day)								
T0	1.04(0.99,1.09)	0.150	0.95(0.88,1.02)	0.149	1.03(0.99,1.08)	0.123	0.94(0.87,1.02)	0.155
T1	1.01(0.94,1.09)	0.766	0.95(0.88,1.03)	0.221	1.00(0.94,1.07)	0.973	0.95(0.87,1.03)	0.212
Light drinks [c] (200 mL/day)								
T0	0.98(0.87,1.11)	0.778	0.99(0.91,1.08)	0.858	1.01(0.93,1.10)	0.783	1.00(0.92,1.09)	0.971
T1	1.01(0.90,1.14)	0.864	1.01(0.94,1.10)	0.763	1.05(0.98,1.12)	0.213	1.02(0.94,1.10)	0.627
Vegetables (150 g/day)								
T0	0.85(0.67,1.08)	0.184	1.09(0.94,1.27)	0.262	0.98(0.84,1.16)	0.841	1.13(0.96,1.32)	0.138
T1	0.81(0.63,1.05)	0.113	1.14(1.00,1.31)	0.058	0.88(0.74,1.05)	0.146	1.14(0.98,1.32)	0.081
Fruit (150 g/day)								
T0	1.05(0.96,1.14)	0.284	1.06(0.99,1.13)	0.094	0.97(0.89,1.05)	0.460	1.08(1.02,1.15)	0.016
T1	1.07(0.96,1.18)	0.224	1.05(0.97,1.14)	0.197	0.90(0.81,1.01)	0.063	1.06(0.97,1.14)	0.187
Dairy products (200 g/day)								
T0	0.95(0.82,1.10)	0.458	1.04(0.95,1.14)	0.387	1.05(0.96,1.14)	0.294	1.06(0.97,1.16)	0.177
T1	0.98(0.85,1.13)	0.772	0.95(0.85,1.06)	0.321	0.95(0.84,1.06)	0.343	0.99(0.90,1.10)	0.903
Meat and meat products (150 g/day)								
T0	1.40(0.87,2.25)	0.172	1.20(0.82,1.76)	0.349	0.85(0.54,1.33)	0.474	1.16(0.77,1.72)	0.481
T1	1.52(0.82,2.82)	0.183	1.25(0.79,1.98)	0.347	1.00(0.61,1.63)	0.998	1.19(0.73,1.94)	0.486
Sweets and snacks (50 g/day)								
T0	1.07(0.91,1.25)	0.423	1.02(0.90,1.17)	0.722	0.97(0.84,1.12)	0.683	1.06(0.93,1.20)	0.424
T1	1.14(0.99,1.30)	0.066	0.96(0.84,1.09)	0.496	1.00(0.88,1.13)	0.963	0.93(0.81,1.07)	0.308
Fast food (250 g/day)								
T0	1.35(0.36,5.09)	0.655	3.14(1.26,7.84)	0.014	1.10(0.37,3.25)	0.862	2.31(0.85,6.33)	0.103
T1	1.87(0.34,10.36)	0.473	2.21(0.64,7.61)	0.210	1.68(0.47,5.97)	0.427	1.04(0.26,4.16)	0.955

Estimated is the regression coefficient describing the association between the intake of a portion of a food item or food group and infant weight-related parameters. Portion sizes are defined according to the applied food frequency questionnaire. [a] linear regression models adjusted for pre-pregnancy BMI, age, parity and group assignment; [b] sugar-containing sweetened beverages; [c] low or non-caloric sweetened beverages. BMI: body mass index; LGA: large for gestational age; SGA: small for gestational age; T0: assessment before or in the 12th week of gestation; T1: assessment after the 29th week of gestation.

There was no evidence for an association between energy or macronutrient intake as percent of energy and offspring birth weight and BMI (Table 4). With increasing saccharose intake (per 10 g of sugar) in early pregnancy, a slight reduction in birth weight by 8.27 g (95% CI −15.83 to −0.70 g, $p = 0.032$) was observed. There was no statistical evidence for such an association in late pregnancy ($p = 0.074$). Similarly, alcohol consumption in early but not late pregnancy was related to a reduction in offspring weight at birth by 15.32 g per g (95% CI −29.83 to −0.80 g, $p = 0.039$).

Table 4. Associations between maternal energy, macronutrient intake and dietary quality and offspring birth weight and body mass index.

Energy and Macronutrient Intake	Birth Weight (g)		BMI (kg/m^2)	
	Adjusted Effect Size [a] (95% CI)	Adjusted p Value [a]	Adjusted Effect Size [a] (95% CI)	Adjusted p Value [a]
Energy [100 kcal/day]				
T0	−0.04 (−3.89,3.80)	0.984	−0.01 (−0.02,0.00)	0.224
T1	3.15 (−0.45,6.76)	0.087	0.01 (−0.00,0.02)	0.218
Carbohydrates [10 E%]				
T0	−8.69 (−39.35,21.97)	0.579	0.01 (−0.06,0.09)	0.769
T1	9.16 (−22.26,40.58)	0.568	0.01 (−0.07,0.09)	0.764
Saccharose [10 g/day]				
T0	−8.27 (−15.83,−0.70)	0.032	−0.02 (−0.04,0.00)	0.074
T1	3.72 (−3.90,11.34)	0.339	0.01 (−0.01,0.03)	0.271
Protein [10 E%]				
T0	48.88 (−28.19,125.95)	0.214	0.08 (−0.12,0.27)	0.439
T1	14.36 (−60.91,89.64)	0.708	0.08 (−0.11,0.27)	0.425
Fat [10 E%]				
T0	5.35 (−33.39,44.08)	0.787	−0.03 (−0.13,0.06)	0.489
T1	−17.00 (−55.49,21.50)	0.387	−0.04 (−0.14,0.06)	0.458
Alcohol [g]				
T0	−15.32 (−29.83,−0.80)	0.039	−0.01 (−0.05,0.02)	0.439
T1	−40.67 (−105.97,24.63)	0.222	−0.11 (−0.28,0.05)	0.182
Caffeine [100 mg]				
T0	−6.57 (−32.54,19.41)	0.620	−0.03 (−0.10,0.03)	0.313
T1	−12.20 (−40.04,15.64)	0.390	−0.05 (−0.13,0.02)	0.139
HEI [10 points]				
T0	39.26 (12.29,66.22)	0.004	0.06 (−0.01,0.13)	0.081
T1	42.76 (15.98,69.55)	0.002	0.10 (0.03,0.16)	0.006

Estimated is the regression coefficient describing the association between the intake of a certain amount or percentage and infant weight and BMI. [a] linear regression models adjusted for pre-pregnancy BMI, age, parity and group assignment. BMI: body mass index; HEI: Healthy Eating Index; T0: assessment before or in the 12th week of gestation; T1: assessment after the 29th week of gestation.

3.3. Diet Quality and Infant Weight Outcomes

Maternal dietary quality, measured with a HEI, was positively associated with birth weight in both early (39.26 g per 10 points (95% CI 12.29 to 66.22 g, $p = 0.004$)) and late pregnancy (42.76 g per 10 points (95% CI 15.98 to 69.55 g, $p = 0.002$)). Additionally, late pregnancy HEI was positively associated with the neonatal BMI ($p = 0.006$), whereas there was no evidence for such an association with early HEI ($p = 0.081$). These observations did not translate into increased odds of the offspring being LGA or having a birth weight above 4000 g (Table 5). Per 10 g maternal sugar consumption in early pregnancy, the odds of the offspring being born with a low birth weight were increased by 1.07 (95% CI 1.01 to 1.13, $p = 0.026$). Maternal energy intake, as well as macronutrient intake as percent of energy, did not show any further associations with the offspring's risk of being born with low or high birth weight, SGA or LGA (Table 5).

Table 5. Associations between maternal energy, macronutrient intake and dietary quality and neonatal weight-related parameters.

Energy and Macronutrient Intake	Low Birth Weight		High Birth Weight		SGA		LGA	
	Adjusted Odds Ratio [a] (95% CI)	Adjusted p Value [a]	Adjusted Odds Ratio [a] (95% CI)	Adjusted p Value [a]	Adjusted Odds Ratio [a] (95% CI)	Adjusted p Value [a]	Adjusted Odds Ratio [a] (95% CI)	Adjusted p Value [a]
Energy [100 kcal/day]								
T0	1.01 (0.98,1.05)	0.560	1.01 (0.98,1.04)	0.509	1.00 (0.97,1.03)	0.854	1.01 (0.98,1.04)	0.630
T1	0.99 (0.95,1.03)	0.594	1.01 (0.98,1.03)	0.659	0.98 (0.96,1.01)	0.267	0.99 (0.96,1.02)	0.604
Carbohydrates [10 E%]								
T0	0.96 (0.73,1.26)	0.761	0.94 (0.76,1.17)	0.587	0.92 (0.74,1.13)	0.408	1.03 (0.83,1.29)	0.780
T1	1.05 (0.76,1.45)	0.786	1.01 (0.79,1.27)	0.966	0.83 (0.65,1.06)	0.131	1.09 (0.85,1.39)	0.501
Saccharose [10 g/day]								
T0	1.07 (1.01,1.13)	0.026	0.97 (0.92,1.03)	0.358	1.01 (0.96,1.07)	0.627	0.99 (0.94,1.05)	0.702
T1	0.98 (0.90,1.07)	0.664	0.98 (0.92,1.04)	0.513	0.96 (0.90,1.02)	0.210	0.96 (0.90,1.03)	0.244
Protein [10 E%]								
T0	0.77 (0.38,1.55)	0.457	1.31 (0.76,2.23)	0.331	0.95 (0.56,1.61)	0.852	1.02 (0.58,1.81)	0.940
T1	1.11 (0.51,2.40)	0.802	1.32 (0.76,2.30)	0.329	0.98 (0.55,1.75)	0.948	1.49 (0.84,2.66)	0.173
Fat [10 E%]								
T0	1.14 (0.80,1.61)	0.467	1.05 (0.80,1.38)	0.735	1.14 (0.88,1.49)	0.329	0.94 (0.71,1.25)	0.673
T1	0.91 (0.61,1.36)	0.647	0.92 (0.69,1.23)	0.584	1.33 (0.99,1.79)	0.057	0.79 (0.58,1.07)	0.131
Alcohol [g]								
T0	1.01 (0.88,1.15)	0.905	0.77 (0.55,1.07)	0.115	1.05 (0.98,1.13)	0.181	1.03 (0.94,1.12)	0.555
T1	1.05 (0.53,2.07)	0.887	0.85 (0.46,1.58)	0.616	0.74 (0.35,1.58)	0.442	0.81 (0.42,1.59)	0.544
Caffeine [100 mg]								
T0	1.09 (0.88,1.34)	0.431	0.94 (0.77,1.14)	0.494	1.03 (0.86,1.24)	0.739	1.03 (0.87,1.22)	0.718
T1	0.93 (0.68,1.27)	0.638	0.84 (0.66,1.07)	0.154	1.13 (0.93,1.37)	0.210	0.87 (0.68,1.10)	0.245
HEI [10 points]								
T0	0.86 (0.68,1.09)	0.220	1.11(0.92,1.34)	0.290	0.84(0.70,1.02)	0.076	1.10(0.90,1.35)	0.363
T1	0.80 (0.61,1.06)	0.117	1.15(0.94,1.41)	0.171	0.85(0.69,1.04)	0.104	1.15(0.93,1.43)	0.188

Estimated is the regression coefficient describing the association between the intake of a certain amount or percentage and infant weight-related parameters. [a] linear regression models adjusted for pre-pregnancy BMI, age, parity and group assignment. BMI: body mass index; HEI: Healthy Eating Index; LGA: large for gestational age; SGA: small for gestational age; T0: assessment before or in the 12th week of gestation; T1: assessment after the 29th week of gestation.

4. Discussion

This secondary analysis of the GeliS trial shows associations between the maternal diet in early and late pregnancy and offspring weight parameters. Although no consistent associations between energy intake and macronutrient composition and neonatal birth weight and weight-derived parameters were shown, several aspects of maternal dietary behaviour were related to neonatal weight parameters.

Our analysis provides evidence that a healthy balanced antenatal diet, indicated by higher scores on the HEI, promotes birth weight within an adequate range and does not increase the risk of high birth weight or LGA. An increase in neonatal body weight with an increasing HEI has also been reported by others [25]. We could not confirm findings by investigators who observed that women with a healthier dietary pattern bore offspring with a reduced risk for low birth weight [26]. However, the latter study was performed in Ghana where the risk of low birth weight is much higher compared to developed countries [27]. Moreover, fruit and vegetable consumption were identified as factors that are positively associated with infant weight and BMI at birth. This observation is in line with findings of other studies reporting an increase in birth weight with increasing intake of fruits and vegetables [12,28]. While maternal vegetable intake did not modify the risk of being born SGA or LGA in our study, a high fruit intake in early pregnancy seemed to slightly increase the risk of LGA.

Our data did not indicate a beneficial association between the consumption of fruits and vegetables and the odds of being born SGA. In general, the data showing a protective effect of vegetable and fruit consumption on infants being born SGA is conflicting [12]. This may result from the heterogeneity in methods used for dietary assessment in the few studies. Moreover, effects may differ between high-

and low-income countries [12]. The observed effects of fruit and vegetable intake in our cohort may be a surrogate reflecting healthier dietary choices, as similar associations were observed regarding the HEI.

For instance, factors related to a lower neonatal body weight in the GeliS cohort included food parameters reflecting a rather unhealthy diet, such as soft drinks, sugar and alcohol intake. Soft drink and saccharose consumption were inversely associated with birth weight. An increase in sugar consumption in early pregnancy was additionally found to increase the risk of being born with a low birth weight. Both soft drinks and saccharose are energy-providing components of the diet that do not deliver any further nutrients of specific value. A high consumption may be accompanied by a lower consumption of nutritious foods and this could explain the negative association with birth weight. A negative effect of the intake of sugar and sugar-rich products on offspring birth weight has also been reported in other studies [28,29], whereas the role of soft drinks needs to be further elucidated. In the literature, the consumption of sugar-containing beverages has been suggested to have both an increasing [14] and a decreasing effect [30] on neonatal birth weight. Another factor, which we found to be negatively associated with birth weight, was alcohol consumption. This is consistent with evidence from a recent review and meta-analysis suggesting a relationship between low amounts of alcohol intake and the prevalence of children born SGA [31]. Although alcohol intake was found to be associated with a reduction in birth weight in the GeliS trial, there was no evidence for a modification of the SGA risk. However, reported alcohol consumption was generally low among our study population [32] and intake may be underreported, thus limiting the validity of our observations as well as those from others.

Fast food consumption was associated with an increased risk of the offspring being born with a high birth weight. This may be related to the high energy density of fast food which can generally increase overall energy intake [33]. A higher risk for delivering macrosomic infants in women eating a diet rich in energy-dense fast food has been suggested [34], but evidence is sparse. In our cohort, we found no evidence for an effect of energy and fat intake itself on birth weight and weight-related parameters. Likewise, although other maternal dietary factors, such as the intake of dairy products [11] or fish [13], have previously been shown to modify infant birth weight, we were not able to confirm these observations.

The presented cohort data have some limitations. Due to the high number of recruited pregnant women, maternal diet was assessed by means of a self-administered FFQ and energy and macronutrient intake were estimated based on the FFQ. More precise methods for the assessment of the maternal diet, such as weighted dietary records, were not feasible in the context of the large-scale GeliS study. However, they may have a greater potential to reveal significant effects of the maternal diet on neonatal weight and weight-related characteristics. In addition, maternal antenatal physical activity was not considered as a covariate in exploring associations between food intake and offspring weight data. We acknowledge that physical activity may be an additional modifying factor for food and energy intake and may likewise influence neonatal outcomes [35]. Due to the nature of the trial designed as a routine care study, offspring data were limited to reported body weight and weight-derived parameters. An additional assessment of infant body composition may provide a more comprehensive picture of the observed associations, as suggested for instance in the INFAT trial [36]. Moreover, infant weight was measured at different clinics, and it is possible that measurements may not have been conducted completely standardised.

The reported effects of the maternal diet on infant weight and weight-related parameters at birth were only modest and clinical relevance of the observed associations is thus questionable. Nonetheless, this secondary analysis of the GeliS cohort has some strengths that merit particular attention. A wide spectrum of dietary data was analysed with regard to offspring weight and weight-related data, including the consumption of particular foods and food groups, energy and macronutrient intake, as well as dietary quality measured with an HEI that was specifically developed for the FFQ used in this study [20,22]. Within the large-scale GeliS trial, we collected dietary and infant data directly in the setting of routine prenatal care. We were able to follow participants from early pregnancy through the postpartum period. In contrast to many other studies, dietary data were collected twice during pregnancy in the GeliS cohort, enabling separate analyses of potential effects of the antenatal diet on offspring outcomes in early and late pregnancy. Our cohort included both primi- and multiparous women from different BMI categories with varying educational levels. This offered a view on the impact of the maternal diet on offspring weight in a diverse target population which is, in many characteristics, representative for German women of childbearing age.

5. Conclusions

In conclusion, a healthy maternal diet characterised by a high intake of fruit and vegetables, as well as a high HEI, was shown to modestly increase birth weight within the adequate range without augmenting the risk for high birth weight or LGA. In contrast, intake of soft-drinks, saccharose and alcohol represented factors associated with a decrease in birth weight. Maternal intake of fast food in early pregnancy was related to a higher risk for infants to have a high birth weight. In the on-going follow-up of the GeliS cohort, the long-term effects of the maternal diet on offspring weight development during infancy will be evaluated.

Author Contributions: Conceptualization, H.H., K.R., J.G. and J.H.; methodology, H.H., K.R., J.G., J.H. and L.S.; formal analysis, J.G. and L.S.; investigation, J.G. and J.K.; resources, K.R., E.R., L.K., J.K. and J.G.; data curation, J.G. and L.S.; writing—original draft preparation, J.G.; writing—review and editing, J.H., K.R., L.S., J.K., M.S., D.M., E.R., L.K. and H.H.; visualization, J.G.; supervision, H.H.; project administration, H.H. and K.R.; funding acquisition, H.H.

Acknowledgments: We gratefully acknowledge the valuable contribution from the Munich Study Centre at the Technical University of Munich and project managers at the expert centres for nutrition/community catering at the regional offices (AELF) of the Bavarian State Ministry of Food, Agriculture and Forestry (StMELF) which have been coordinating the study on the regional level. We gratefully acknowledge the support of our colleague Christina Holzapfel, Institute for Nutritional Medicine. The support from Martin Wabitsch and Stefanie Brandt, Pediatric Endocrinology and Diabetes, Department of Pediatrics and Adolescent Medicine, University Medical Center Ulm, Kurt Ulm and Victoria Kehl, Institute of Medical Informatics, Statistics and Epidemiology, Klinikum rechts der Isar of the Technical University of Munich, the network "Healthy Start - Young Family Network", Federal Center for Nutrition (BZfE), Federal Office for Agriculture and Food (BLE), belonging to the national IN FORM initiative (Maria Flothkötter, Katharina Krüger), Bonn, Uta Engels, Sports Centre, University of Regensburg, Karl-Heinz Ladwig, Head of Research Group Mental Health at the Institute of Epidemiology, Helmholtz Centre Munich, K.T.M. Schneider, Division of Obstetrics and Perinatal Medicine, Technical University of Munich, Rüdiger von Kries, Institute of Social Paediatrics and Adolescent Medicine, Ludwig-Maximilians-University Munich, Regina Ensenauer, von Hauner Children's Hospital, Ludwig-Maximilians-University Munich and Heinrich Heine University Düsseldorf, Rolf Holle, Institute of Health Economics and Health Care Management, Institute of Epidemiology, Helmholtz Centre Munich, Gabi Pfeifer, Educational Center Nuremberg, and Eveline Rieg, Competence Centre for Nutrition, Freising/Kulmbach, are gratefully acknowledged. We gratefully acknowledge Gert Mensink, Robert Koch Institute, Berlin for guidance in the analysis of the FFQ including the Healthy Eating Index and the Max Rubner Institute, Karlsruhe for provision of reference data from the German National Consumption Survey II (NVS II). Finally, we would like to thank our colleagues Annie Naujoks, Kristina Geyer and Roxana Raab, Institute for Nutritional Medicine, for their support and all participating practices, gynecologists, medical personnel, midwives, participants and their families for their involvement.

References

1. Schellong, K.; Schulz, S.; Harder, T.; Plagemann, A. Birth weight and long-term overweight risk: Systematic review and a meta-analysis including 643,902 persons from 66 studies and 26 countries globally. *PLoS ONE* **2012**, *7*, e47776. [CrossRef]
2. Harder, T.; Rodekamp, E.; Schellong, K.; Dudenhausen, J.W.; Plagemann, A. Birth weight and subsequent risk of type 2 diabetes: A meta-analysis. *Am. J. Epidemiol.* **2007**, *165*, 849–857. [CrossRef]
3. Kim, S.Y.; Sharma, A.J.; Sappenfield, W.; Wilson, H.G.; Salihu, H.M. Association of maternal body mass index, excessive weight gain, and gestational diabetes mellitus with large-for-gestational-age births. *Obstet. Gynecol.* **2014**, *123*, 737–744. [CrossRef] [PubMed]

4. Lau, E.Y.; Liu, J.; Archer, E.; McDonald, S.M.; Liu, J. Maternal weight gain in pregnancy and risk of obesity among offspring: A systematic review. *J. Obes.* **2014**, *2014*, 524939. [CrossRef] [PubMed]
5. Mamun, A.A.; Mannan, M.; Doi, S.A.R. Gestational weight gain in relation to offspring obesity over the life course: A systematic review and bias-adjusted meta-analysis. *Obes. Rev.* **2014**, *15*, 338–347. [CrossRef] [PubMed]
6. Fraser, A.; Tilling, K.; Macdonald-Wallis, C.; Sattar, N.; Brion, M.-J.; Benfield, L.; Ness, A.; Deanfield, J.; Hingorani, A.; Nelson, S.M.; et al. Association of maternal weight gain in pregnancy with offspring obesity and metabolic and vascular traits in childhood. *Circulation* **2010**, *121*, 2557–2564. [CrossRef] [PubMed]
7. Pérez-Morales, M.E.; Bacardi-Gascon, M.; Jimenez-Cruz, A. Association of excessive GWG with adiposity indicators and metabolic diseases of their offspring: Systematic review. *Nutr. Hosp.* **2015**, *31*, 1473–1480. [CrossRef]
8. Grieger, J.A.; Clifton, V.L. A review of the impact of dietary intakes in human pregnancy on infant birthweight. *Nutrients* **2014**, *7*, 153–178. [CrossRef]
9. Abu-Saad, K.; Fraser, D. Maternal nutrition and birth outcomes. *Epidemiol. Rev.* **2010**, *32*, 5–25. [CrossRef]
10. Imdad, A.; Bhutta, Z.A. Effect of balanced protein energy supplementation during pregnancy on birth outcomes. *BMC Public Health* **2011**, *11* (Suppl. 3), S17. [CrossRef]
11. Brantsæter, A.L.; Olafsdottir, A.S.; Forsum, E.; Olsen, S.F.; Thorsdottir, I. Does milk and dairy consumption during pregnancy influence fetal growth and infant birthweight? A systematic literature review. *Food Nutr. Res.* **2012**, *56*. [CrossRef] [PubMed]
12. Murphy, M.M.; Stettler, N.; Smith, K.M.; Reiss, R. Associations of consumption of fruits and vegetables during pregnancy with infant birth weight or small for gestational age births: A systematic review of the literature. *Int. J. Womens Health* **2014**, *6*, 899–912. [CrossRef] [PubMed]
13. Leventakou, V.; Roumeliotaki, T.; Martinez, D.; Barros, H.; Brantsaeter, A.-L.; Casas, M.; Charles, M.-A.; Cordier, S.; Eggesbø, M.; van Eijsden, M.; et al. Fish intake during pregnancy, fetal growth, and gestational length in 19 European birth cohort studies. *Am. J. Clin. Nutr.* **2014**, *99*, 506–516. [CrossRef] [PubMed]
14. Phelan, S.; Hart, C.; Phipps, M.; Abrams, B.; Schaffner, A.; Adams, A.; Wing, R. Maternal behaviors during pregnancy impact offspring obesity risk. *Exp. Diabetes Res.* **2011**, *2011*, 985139. [CrossRef] [PubMed]
15. International Weight Management in Pregnancy (i-WIP) Collaborative Group. Effect of diet and physical activity based interventions in pregnancy on gestational weight gain and pregnancy outcomes: Meta-analysis of individual participant data from randomised trials. *BMJ* **2017**, *358*, j3119. [CrossRef]
16. Rauh, K.; Kunath, J.; Rosenfeld, E.; Kick, L.; Ulm, K.; Hauner, H. Healthy living in pregnancy: A cluster-randomized controlled trial to prevent excessive gestational weight gain—Rationale and design of the GeliS study. *BMC Pregnancy Childbirth* **2014**, *14*, 119. [CrossRef]
17. Kunath, J.; Günther, J.; Rauh, K.; Hoffmann, J.; Stecher, L.; Rosenfeld, E.; Kick, L.; Ulm, K.; Hauner, H. Effects of a lifestyle intervention during pregnancy to prevent excessive gestational weight gain in routine care—The cluster-randomised GeliS trial. *BMC Med.* **2019**, *17*, 5. [CrossRef] [PubMed]
18. Koletzko, B.; Bauer, C.-P.; Bung, P.; Cremer, M.; Flothkötter, M.; Hellmers, C.; Kersting, M.; Krawinkel, M.; Przyrembel, H.; Rasenack, R.; et al. Ernährung in der Schwangerschaft—Teil 2. Handlungsempfehlungen des Netzwerks "Gesund ins Leben—Netzwerk Junge Familie". *Deutsche Medizinische Wochenschrift* **2012**, *137*, 1366–1372. [CrossRef]
19. National Research Council. *Weight Gain during Pregnancy. Reexamining the Guidelines*; Rasmussen, K.M., Yaktine, A.L., Eds.; National Academies Press: Washington, DC, USA, 2009; ISBN 9780309131131.
20. Haftenberger, M.; Heuer, T.; Heidemann, C.; Kube, F.; Krems, C.; Mensink, G.B.M. Relative validation of a food frequency questionnaire for national health and nutrition monitoring. *Nutr. J.* **2010**, *9*, 36. [CrossRef]
21. Meltzer, H.M.; Brantsaeter, A.L.; Ydersbond, T.A.; Alexander, J.; Haugen, M. Methodological challenges when monitoring the diet of pregnant women in a large study: Experiences from the Norwegian Mother and Child Cohort Study (MoBa). *Matern. Child Nutr.* **2008**, *4*, 14–27. [CrossRef]
22. Kuhn, D.-A. Entwicklung eines Index zur Bewertung der Ernährungsqualität in der Studie zur Gesundheit Erwachsener in Deutschland (DEGS1), German ("Development of a dietary quality index in the German Health Examination Survey for Adults"). Master's Thesis, Robert Koch Institute, Berlin, Germany, 2017.

23. Kleinwechter, H.; Schäfer-Graf, U.; Bührer, C.; Hoesli, I.; Kainer, F.; Kautzky-Willer, A.; Pawlowski, B.; Schunck, K.; Somville, T.; Sorger, M. Gestationsdiabetes mellitus (GDM)—Diagnostik, Therapie und Nachsorge. *Diabetologie und Stoffwechsel* **2016**, *11*, S182–S194. [CrossRef]
24. Metzger, B.E.; Gabbe, S.G.; Persson, B.; Buchanan, T.A.; Catalano, P.A.; Damm, P.; Dyer, A.R.; de Leiva, A.; Hod, M.; Kitzmiler, J.L.; et al. International association of diabetes and pregnancy study groups recommendations on the diagnosis and classification of hyperglycemia in pregnancy. *Diabetes Care* **2010**, *33*, 676–682. [CrossRef] [PubMed]
25. Rodríguez-Bernal, C.L.; Rebagliato, M.; Iñiguez, C.; Vioque, J.; Navarrete-Muñoz, E.M.; Murcia, M.; Bolumar, F.; Marco, A.; Ballester, F. Diet quality in early pregnancy and its effects on fetal growth outcomes: The Infancia y Medio Ambiente (Childhood and Environment) Mother and Child Cohort Study in Spain. *Am. J. Clin. Nutr.* **2010**, *91*, 1659–1666. [CrossRef] [PubMed]
26. Abubakari, A.; Jahn, A. Maternal Dietary Patterns and Practices and Birth Weight in Northern Ghana. *PLoS ONE* **2016**, *11*, e0162285. [CrossRef] [PubMed]
27. He, Z.; Bishwajit, G.; Yaya, S.; Cheng, Z.; Zou, D.; Zhou, Y. Prevalence of low birth weight and its association with maternal body weight status in selected countries in Africa: A cross-sectional study. *BMJ Open* **2018**, *8*, e020410. [CrossRef] [PubMed]
28. Kjøllesdal, M.K.R.; Holmboe-Ottesen, G. Dietary Patterns and Birth Weight-a Review. *AIMS Public Health* **2014**, *1*, 211–225. [CrossRef] [PubMed]
29. Lenders, C.M.; Hediger, M.L.; Scholl, T.O.; Khoo, C.S.; Slap, G.B.; Stallings, V.A. Gestational age and infant size at birth are associated with dietary sugar intake among pregnant adolescents. *J. Nutr.* **1997**, *127*, 1113–1117. [CrossRef]
30. Grundt, J.H.; Eide, G.E.; Brantsaeter, A.-L.; Haugen, M.; Markestad, T. Is consumption of sugar-sweetened soft drinks during pregnancy associated with birth weight? *Matern. Child Nutr.* **2017**, *13*. [CrossRef]
31. Mamluk, L.; Edwards, H.B.; Savović, J.; Leach, V.; Jones, T.; Moore, T.H.M.; Ijaz, S.; Lewis, S.J.; Donovan, J.L.; Lawlor, D.; et al. Low alcohol consumption and pregnancy and childhood outcomes: Time to change guidelines indicating apparently 'safe' levels of alcohol during pregnancy? A systematic review and meta-analyses. *BMJ Open* **2017**, *7*, e015410. [CrossRef]
32. Günther, J.; Hoffmann, J.; Kunath, J.; Spies, M.; Meyer, D.; Stecher, L.; Rosenfeld, E.; Kick, L.; Rauh, K.; Hauner, H. Effects of a Lifestyle Intervention in Routine Care on Prenatal Dietary Behavior—Findings from the Cluster-Randomized GeliS Trial. *JCM* **2019**, *8*, 960. [CrossRef]
33. Ledikwe, J.H.; Blanck, H.M.; Kettel Khan, L.; Serdula, M.K.; Seymour, J.D.; Tohill, B.C.; Rolls, B.J. Dietary energy density is associated with energy intake and weight status in US adults. *Am. J. Clin. Nutr.* **2006**, *83*, 1362–1368. [CrossRef] [PubMed]
34. Wen, L.M.; Simpson, J.M.; Rissel, C.; Baur, L.A. Maternal "junk food" diet during pregnancy as a predictor of high birthweight: Findings from the healthy beginnings trial. *Birth* **2013**, *40*, 46–51. [CrossRef] [PubMed]
35. Hoffmann, J.; Günther, J.; Geyer, K.; Stecher, L.; Kunath, J.; Meyer, D.; Spies, M.; Rosenfeld, E.; Kick, L.; Rauh, K.; et al. Effects of prenatal physical activity on neonatal and obstetric outcomes—Findings from the cluster-randomised GeliS trial. *BMC Pregnancy Childbirth* **2019**, under review.
36. Brei, C.; Stecher, L.; Meyer, D.M.; Young, V.; Much, D.; Brunner, S.; Hauner, H. Impact of Dietary Macronutrient Intake during Early and Late Gestation on Offspring Body Composition at Birth, 1, 3, and 5 Years of Age. *Nutrients* **2018**, *10*, 579. [CrossRef] [PubMed]

11

Growth Patterns of Neonates Treated with Thermal Control in Neutral Environment and Nutrition Regulation to Meet Basal Metabolism

Shiro Kubota [1,2,†], Masayoshi Zaitsu [3,4,†] and Tatsuya Yoshihara [2,5,*]

1 Kubota Life Science Laboratory Co., Ltd., Saga 840-0535, Japan; kubotahp@gmail.com
2 Kubota Maternity Clinic, Fukuoka 810-0014, Japan
3 Department of Social and Behavioral Sciences, Harvard T.H. Chan School of Public Health, Boston, MA 02115, USA; m-zaitsu@m.u-tokyo.ac.jp
4 Department of Public Health, Graduate School of Medicine, The University of Tokyo, Tokyo 113-0033, Japan
5 Clinical Research Center, Fukuoka Mirai Hospital, Fukuoka 813-0017, Japan
* Correspondence: tatsuya@clipharm.med.kyushu-u.ac.jp
† These authors contributed equally to this work.

Abstract: Little is known about the growth patterns of low birth weight neonates (<2500 g) during standardized thermal control and nutrition regulation to meet basal metabolism requirements compared to those of non-low birth weight neonates (2500 g and above). We retrospectively identified 10,544 non-low birth weight and 681 low birth weight neonates placed in thermo-controlled incubators for up to 24 h after birth. All neonates were fed a 5% glucose solution 1 h after birth and breastfed every 3 h (with supplementary formula milk if applicable) to meet basal metabolism requirements. Maximum body-weight loss (%), percentage body-weight loss from birth to peak weight loss (%/day), and percentage body-weight gain from peak weight loss to day 4 (%/day) were assessed by multivariable linear regression. Overall, the growth curves showed a uniform J-shape across all birth weight categories, with a low mean maximum body-weight loss (1.9%) and incidence of neonatal jaundice (0.3%). The body-weight loss patterns did not differ between the two groups. However, low birth weight neonates showed significantly faster growth patterns for percentage body-weight gain: $\beta = 0.52$ (95% confidence interval, 0.46 to 0.58). Under thermal control and nutrition regulation, low birth weight neonates might not have disadvantages in clinical outcomes or growth patterns.

Keywords: growth chart; breastfeeding; physiological body-weight loss; thermal control; basal maintenance expenditure

---

1. Introduction

During the first days of life, infants show a physiological phenomenon of temporary body-weight loss. However, excess body-weight loss in the neonatal period tends to increase risks of hypoglycemia, hypernatremia, and hyperbilirubinemia, resulting in permanent neurological damage [1]. While the American Academy of Pediatrics criteria currently recommend a cut-off point of 7% for physiological body-weight loss [2], excess loss resulting from inadequate intake is an emerging concern among high-risk populations, such as (but not limited to) East-Asian neonates, even after controlling for genetic polymorphisms [3–6].

In a cohort of non-low birth weight (NLBW) neonates (birth weight 2500 g and above) in Japan not admitted to the neonatal intensive care unit (NICU), we previously reported a potential standardized neonatal regimen, a local neonatal protocol involving a combination of thermal control and nutrition regulation to meet basal metabolism requirements (~50 kcal/kg), in order to reduce the incidence of neonatal jaundice by preventing excess body-weight loss [7]. This combination method included a neutral thermal environment during the first hours after birth with an ambient room temperature of ~34 °C (93.2 °F) [8–10]. In contrast to ambient room temperature (~24 °C/75.2 °F), a neutral thermal environment maintained an optimal body temperature through circulatory stability and improved digestive function [8–10]. The combination method also included nutrition regulation to meet the basal metabolism requirement [11], in which neonates were fed a 5% glucose solution 1 h after birth, a convenient method to prevent hypoglycemia and neonatal jaundice [12], followed by breastfeeding every 3 h with supplementary formula milk if applicable. In previous findings, compared to either thermal control or nutrition regulation alone, the combination method had better safety profiles for neonatal growth (e.g., serum glucose levels, circulatory stability, digestive functions, and metabolism) [7,8].

In addition to gestational age and maternal factors (such as maternal smoking, preeclampsia, and gestational diabetes), birth weight plays a crucial role in neonatal body weight growth. Compared to NLBW neonates, low birth weight (LBW) neonates (birth weight <2500 g) are more likely to be at risk for disadvantages in clinical outcomes or growth patterns, such as excess body-weight loss, neonatal jaundice, and delayed body-weight growth [13–17]. However, few studies have focused on LBW neonates not admitted to the NICU, and little is known about the contribution of our combination method among LBW neonates.

Accordingly, the goal of the present study was to characterize the body-weight growth patterns and clinical outcomes in this population of neonates who had received the combination method. Using data from a cohort with NLBW and LBW neonates treated by the combination method, we examined the detailed patterns of body-weight growth among NLBW and LBW neonates during the first days of life. We also examined whether the body-weight growth pattern in LBW neonates differed from that in NLBW neonates under the combination method.

2. Materials and Methods

2.1. Study Settings

This retrospective, longitudinal study of neonates during the initial days of life used clinical data from a cohort of neonates born in Kubota Maternity Clinic in Fukuoka, Japan (1989 to 2017). The details of the database are described elsewhere [7]. Briefly, Kubota Maternity Clinic was a general obstetrics and gynecological hospital that provided general obstetrics care and closed in 2017. The characteristics of the population were similar to those reported in previous studies in Japan [3,18,19]. All neonates were treated with the combination method (standardized thermal control and nutrition regulation) and discharged by a physician on day 4 or later, when the serum bilirubin level was <15 mg/dL, body weight was recovered from its lowest level, and phototherapy was no longer required. Since the bilirubin level usually peaks at approximately day 4 among Japanese neonates [18,19], discharge on day 4 or later is the standard practice in Japan. Clinical information on all neonates and their mothers had been collected since 1989, except for those who had neonatal asphyxia, congenital heart failure or malformation, or were transferred to a tertiary hospital (such as a university hospital) for neonatal intensive care. We obtained a de-identified dataset through a research agreement with the hospital; the study was approved by the research ethics committees of Hakata Clinic and registered at UMIN-CTR (UMIN000030011).

We included all 11,445 eligible term and preterm neonates treated with the combination method who (1) had a birth weight 1700 g and greater, (2) had an Apgar score of 7 or higher, and (3) were not admitted to the NICU. We excluded 221 neonates with incomplete data (1.9%), yielding a study population of 11,224 neonates.

2.2. Thermal Control and Nutrition Regulation to Meet Basal Metabolism

The details of standardized thermal control and nutrition regulation to meet basal metabolism, a local neonatal regimen, have been described elsewhere [7,8]. Briefly, following delivery in a delivery room maintained at ~25 °C (77 °F), neonates were immediately wiped with cotton towels, administered intraoral suction on a warm bed at ~40 °C (104 °F), hugged by their mothers (skin-to-skin contact), and placed in a transparent thermo-controlled incubator (N-ideal H-2000, Nakamura Medical Industry, Tokyo, Japan) within 2 min of birth. Transparent thermo-controlled incubators were placed next to delivery beds in the delivery room (not placed in the NICU). Neonates remained visible and were continuously observed, not only by physicians and nurses (e.g., Apgar score), but also by their mothers. All neonates remained in incubators for at least 2 h. For the first hour, the incubators were set at 34 °C (93.2 °F); for the second hour, the temperature was turned down to 30 °C (86 °F) to help neonates adapt to normal room temperature. After the initial 2 h, NLBW neonates were transferred to a bed in a standard monitoring room set at ~24 to 26 °C (75.2 to 78.8 °F). LBW neonates with birth weights of 2000 to 2499 g stayed in incubators for an extra 2 to 12 h, while those with birth weights <2000 g stayed in incubators for an extra 12 to 24 h at 28 °C (82.4 °F) before transferring to a standard monitoring room. The optimal profiles of the neutral environment for thermogenesis, circulatory stability, and actual central/peripheral body temperatures have been validated in previous studies with human neonates [8–10].

For nutritional regulation, neonates were orally fed a 5% glucose solution (10 mL/kg) with 1 mL of vitamin K syrup containing 2 mg menatetrenone 1 h after birth and then breastfed every 3 h [7,12]. If breast milk production was insufficient, neonates were additionally bottle-fed formula milk until they were sated to maintain a 50 kcal/kg basal metabolism [11]. The oral 5% glucose solution has been shown to be a convenient method to prevent hypoglycemia, while allowing continuous breastfeeding [7,12]. In addition, supplemental bottle-feeding with formula milk was based on previous findings suggesting that the estimated calories provided by breast milk were below the basal metabolism a few days after birth among the study population and that nutrition regulation did not affect breastmilk production [7]. For NLBW neonates, high-calorie formula milk (16 kcal/20 mL) was administered for the first 48 h, followed by normal-calorie formula milk (13 kcal/20 mL) after 48 h. For LBW neonates, high-calorie formula milk was administered throughout the hospital stay.

2.3. Birth Weight Categories

Neonates, whose birth weights were normally distributed (Figure 1), were grouped into NLBW (2500 g and above; n = 10,544) and LBW (<2500 g; n = 680) neonates. Both groups were further categorized into a narrower range of birth weights: among LBW neonates, <2000 g (n = 20) and 2000 to 2499 g (n = 660); among NLBW neonates, 2500 to 2999 g (n = 5001), 3000 to 3499 g (n = 4752), 3,500 to 3999 g (n = 757), and 4000 g and above (n = 34).

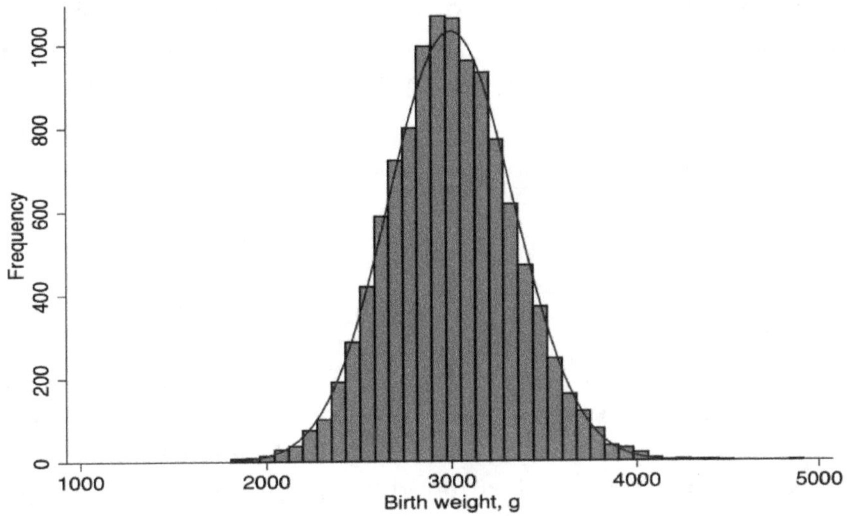

Figure 1. Distribution of birth weight among 11,224 neonates who received standardized thermal control and nutrition regulation to meet basal metabolism.

2.4. Assessment of Clinical Outcomes and Changes in Body Weight

Using body-weight measured at birth and every day during the first four days (SW-5200, Toitu, Tokyo, Japan), we determined the percentage body-weight growth every day [((weight each day − birth weight]/birth weight) × 100%) and maximum body-weight loss (([birth weight − minimum weight]/birth weight) × 100%). Excess body-weight loss was defined as a maximum body-weight loss of at least 7% [2]. The incidence of neonatal jaundice was defined as use of phototherapy, which was based on peak bilirubin levels ≥18 mg/dL along with other clinical findings [7].

Due to physiological body-weight loss, we divided the observation period into "decreasing" (before the day of peak weight loss) and "increasing" (after the day of peak weight loss) periods. For each period, we assessed the percentage body-weight change per day. During the first decreasing period from birth to peak weight loss, we determined the body-weight loss per day ((birth weight − minimum weight)/day of peak weight loss) and percentage body-weight loss per day (([birth weight − minimum weight]/birth weight) × (100%/day of peak weight loss)). During the latter increasing period, from peak weight loss to day 4, we determined the body-weight gain per day ((weight at day 4 − minimum weight)/(4 − day of peak weight loss)) and percentage body-weight gain per day ((weight at day 4 − minimum weight]/birth weight) × (100%/(4 − day of peak weight loss)).

2.5. Statistical Analysis

To produce growth curves in a growth chart among the 11,674 neonates, we plotted the mean body weights measured at birth and every day during the first four days separately by birth weight categories. We directly connected the mean values with lines, because fitted lines such as splines eliminated the initial drop of body weight in prior analyses (data not shown). We also drew a chart indicating the percentages of body-weight growth stratified by birth weight. In these charts, we additionally plotted the values measured at day 5 for neonates discharged at day 5 and later (10,336 neonates, 92%) and the values measured at one-month neonatal check-ups (approximately 30 days after birth; 8071 neonates, 72%).

The background demographics and clinical outcomes were then compared between the LBW and NLBW neonates by t- or chi-squared tests. In the decreasing period, the regression coefficient (β) and 95% confidence interval (CI) for the percentage body-weight loss per day against birth weight (referent group, NLBW neonates) were estimated by linear regression. Covariates included sex, gestational age, Apgar score, Cesarean delivery, maternal age, maternal body mass index, parity, hypertensive disorders of pregnancy, and birth year. In the increasing period, the same regression analysis was applied for the percentage body-weight gain per day. In stratified analyses using a continuous variable of birth weight, a linear regression model was applied for analysis among NLBW and NLBW neonates, respectively, to check the association between birth weight and percentage body-weight-growth.

The alpha value was set at 0.05 and all P-values were two-sided. Data were analyzed using STATA/MP 13.1 (Stata-Corp, College Station, TX, USA).

3. Results

Overall, the growth curves showed a uniform, J-shaped pattern across all birth weight categories (Figure 2). On average, the neonates started to recover their weights within two days of birth and the mean maximum body-weight loss (mean (SD)) was low (1.9% (1.5%)). The incidence of neonatal jaundice was 0.3% and the incidence of excess body-weight loss was 0.4% (Table 1). We did not observe any neonatal morbidity or mortality events, as well as readmission after discharge, during the study period. Most of the background distributions differed between the NLBW and LBW neonates, except for maternal age (Table 1).

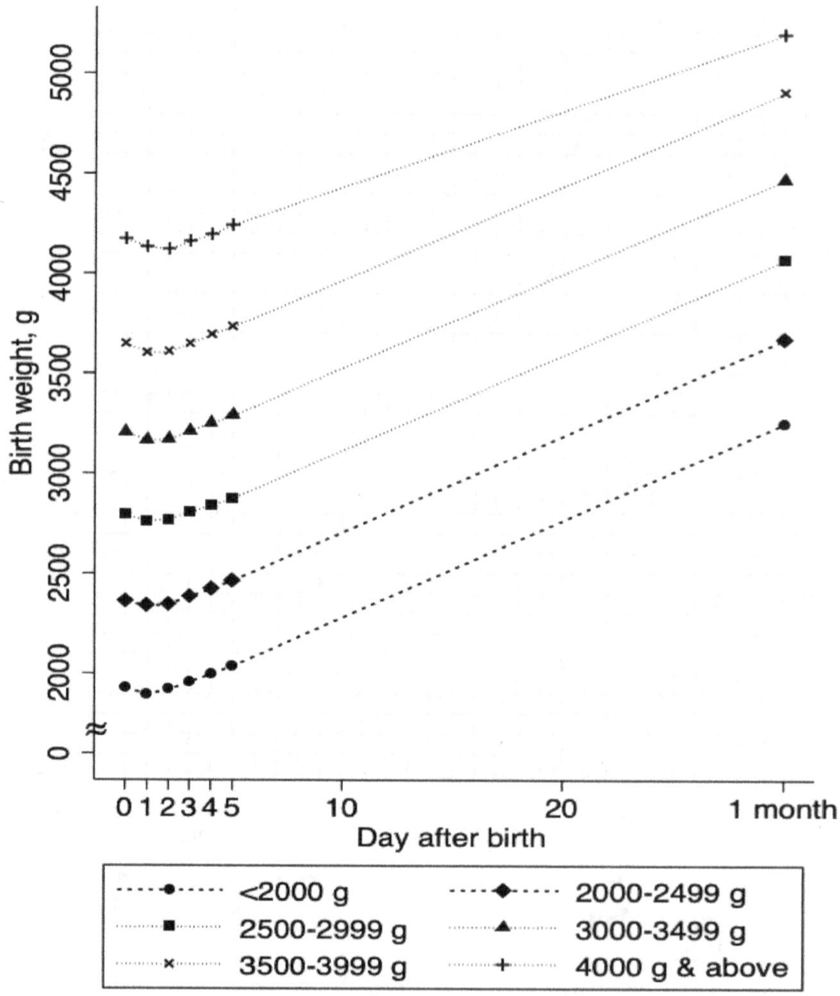

Figure 2. Body weight growth curves stratified by birth weights. The mean body weights are shown as connected lines stratified by birth weight categories. Values from day 0 through day 4 were estimated in 11,224 neonates; values at day 5 and 1 month (approximately 30 days of birth) were estimated in 10,336 neonates and 8071 neonates, respectively.

Table 1. Background and clinical characteristics of 11,224 neonates who received optimal thermal control with sufficient nutrition.

Characteristics	Mean (SD) or number (%)			p
	Total n = 11,224	NLBW Neonates (≥2500 g) n = 10,544	LBW Neonates (<2500 g) n = 680	
Background characteristics				
Female	5468 (49%)	5066 (48%)	402 (59%)	<0.001
Gestational age (weeks)	39.0 (1.2)	39.0 (1.1)	37.9 (1.4)	<0.001
Birth weight (g)	3000 (337)	3,043 (300)	2346 (136)	<0.001
Apgar score at 1 min	9.6 (0.6)	9.6 (0.6)	9.5 (0.6)	<0.001
Caesarean delivery	899 (8.0%)	810 (7.7%)	89 (13%)	<0.001
Maternal age (years)	31 (4)	31 (4)	31 (4)	0.58
Maternal BMI (kg/m^2)	20.0 (2.0)	20.1 (2.0)	19.7 (2.0)	<0.001
Multipara	5,256 (47%)	4,982 (47%)	274 (40%)	<0.001
Hypertensive disorders of pregnancy	43 (0.4%)	36 (0.3%)	7 (1.0%)	0.005
Birth year	2001 (8)	2001 (8)	2002 (8)	0.001
Clinical outcomes				
Maximum weight loss (%)	1.9 (1.5)	1.9 (1.5)	1.8 (1.5)	0.056
Excess weight loss 7% and above	44 (0.4%)	39 (0.4%)	5 (0.7%)	0.14
Day of peak weight loss	1.4 (0.9)	1.4 (0.9)	1.3 (0.9)	0.004
Body-weight loss per day (g)	40 (36)	41 (36)	31 (29)	<0.001
Percentage body-weight loss per day (%) [1]	1.3 (1.2)	1.3 (1.2)	1.3 (1.2)	0.52
Body-weight gain per day (g)	41 (24)	41 (25)	39 (21)	0.06
Percentage body-weight gain per day (%) [2]	1.4 (0.8)	1.4 (0.8)	1.7 (0.9)	<0.001
Peak bilirubin level at day 4 (mg/dL)	8.5 (2.7)	8.5 (2.7)	8.4 (2.7)	0.42
Phototherapy	30 (0.3%)	30 (0.3%)	0 (0.0%)	0.16

BMI, body mass index; NLBW, non-low birth weight; LBW, low birth weight. [1] Defined as ((birth weight − minimum weight)/birth weight) × (100%/day of peak weight loss). [2] Defined as ((weight at day 4 − minimum weight)/birth weight) × (100%/(4 − day of peak weight loss])).

Clinical outcomes, including maximum body-weight loss, bilirubin levels, and phototherapy, did not differ between NLBW and LBW neonates. Although the mean body-weight loss per day (grams) differed, the mean body-weight gain per day (grams) did not differ between groups (Table 1). Compared to those in NLBW neonates, the duration to peak weight loss was shorter (1.4 versus 1.3 days, $p < 0.003$) and the percentage of body-weight gain per day was higher (1.4 versus 1.7%, $p < 0.001$) in LBW neonates (Table 1). As birth weight decreased, the percentage body-weight gain increased (Figure 3).

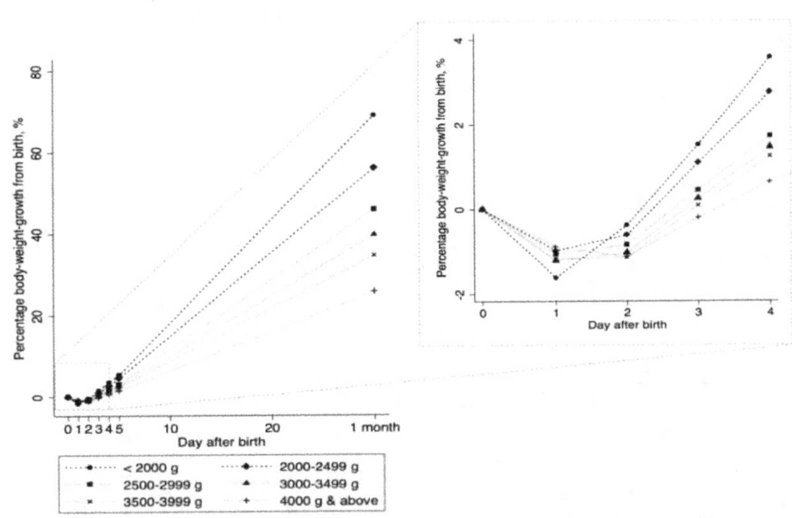

Figure 3. Daily percentages of bodyweight growth against birth weight. Each connected line shows the change in the percentage bodyweight growth from birth weight (([weight at every day − birth weight]/birth weight) × 100%), stratified by birth weight categories. Values from day 0 through day 4 were estimated in 11,224 neonates; values at day 5 and 1 month (approximately 30 days of birth) were estimated in 10,336 neonates and 8071 neonates, respectively.

Regression analyses in the decreasing period revealed that, compared to that in NLBW neonates, the percentage body-weight loss per day did not differ in LBW neonates (Table 2). In the increasing period, compared to that in NLBW neonates, the percentage body-weight gain per day was significantly higher in LBW neonates (Table 2): β = 0.52 (95% CI, 0.46 to 0.58). In stratified analyses in the decreasing period, a higher percentage of body-weight loss per day was only associated with higher birth weights in NLBW neonates (Table 3). In the increasing period, a higher percentage of body-weight gain per day was significantly associated with lower birth weights across all birth weight categories (Table 3).

Table 2. Body weight growth patterns against birth weight estimated by multivariable linear regression analysis.

Characteristics	Model 1 [3]		Model 2 [4]	
	β (95% CI)	*p*	β (95% CI)	*p*
Percentage body weight loss per day [1]				
LBW (<2500 g)	−0.03 (−0.12 to 0.06)	0.52	0.03 (−0.06 to 0.13)	0.48
Female			0.05 (0.004 to 0.09)	0.03
Gestational week			0.03 (0.01 to 0.05)	0.001
Apgar score			0.13 (0.09 to 0.17)	<0.001
Caesarean delivery			0.12 (0.03 to 0.20)	0.005
Maternal age			0.003 (−0.003 to 0.01)	0.34
Maternal body mass index			−0.03 (−0.04 to −0.01)	<0.001
Multipara			0.21 (0.16 to 0.26)	<0.001
Hypertensive disorders of pregnancy			0.24 (−0.11 to 0.59)	0.18
Birth year			−0.02 (−0.02 to −0.02)	<0.001
Percentage body weight gain per day [2]				
LBW (<2500 g)	0.33 (0.26 to 0.39)	<0.001	0.52 (0.46 to 0.58)	<0.001
Female			−0.12 (−0.15 to −0.10)	<0.001
Gestational week			0.15 (0.14 to 0.16)	<0.001
Apgar score			−0.02 (−0.04 to 0.01)	0.17
Caesarean delivery			0.001 (−0.05 to 0.05)	>0.99
Maternal age			−0.005 (−0.005 to 0.004)	0.82
Maternal body mass index			0.001 (−0.01 to 0.01)	0.97
Multipara			−0.08 (−0.11 to −0.05)	<0.001
Hypertensive disorders of pregnancy			0.05 (−0.18 to 0.29)	0.66
Birth year			−0.02 (−0.02 to −0.01)	<0.001

β, regression coefficient; CI, confidence interval; LBW, low birth weight. [1] Defined as ((birth weight − minimum weight)/birth weight) × (100%/day of peak weight loss). [2] Defined as ((weight at day 4 − minimum weight)/birth weight) × (100%/(4 − day of peak weight loss)). [3] Simple linear regression model for body-weight growth patterns against birth weight (referent group, NLBW neonates). Data were estimated in 10,544 non-low birth weight neonates and 680 low birth weight neonates. [4] Additionally adjusted for potential confounding variables of sex, gestational age, Apgar score, Cesarean delivery, maternal age, maternal body mass index, parity, hypertensive disorders of pregnancy, and birth year.

Table 3. Regression coefficients and 95% confidence intervals estimated with a continuous variable of birth weight in regression analyses, stratified by non-low birth weight and low birth weight neonates.

Characteristics	Percentage Body-Weight-Loss per Day [1]		Percentage Body-Weight-Gain per Day [2]	
	β (95% CI) [3]	*p*	β (95% CI)[3]	*p*
Overall (*n* = 11,224)				
Birth weight (per 100 g)	0.01 (−0.003 to 0.01)	0.06	−0.05 (−0.06 to −0.05)	<0.001
Non-LBW (2500 g and above, *n* = 10,544)				
Birth weight (per 100 g)	0.01 (0.001 to 0.02)	0.02	−0.04 (−0.05 to −0.03)	<0.001
LBW (<2500 g, *n* = 680)				
Birth weight (per 100 g)	0.003 (−0.07 to 0.08)	0.93	−0.16 (−0.21 to −0.11)	<0.001

Abbreviations: β, regression coefficient; CI, confidence interval; LBW, low birth weight. [1] Defined as ((birth weight − minimum weight)/birth weight) × (100%/day of peak weight loss). [2] Defined as ((weight at day 4 − minimum weight)/birth weight) × (100%/(4 − day of peak weight loss)). [3] Multivariable linear regression analysis for body-weight-growth patterns against birth weight, adjusted for sex, gestational age, Apgar score, cesarean delivery, maternal age, maternal body mass index, parity, hypertensive disorders of pregnancy, and birth year.

4. Discussion

Under a local neonatal regimen involving a standardized thermal control and nutrition regulation to meet basal metabolism, neonatal growth curves showed a uniform, J-shaped pattern with an initial physiological body-weight loss (~2% loss from birth weight), regardless of birth weight. The incidence of excess body-weight loss was low (<1%), with a short duration to peak weight loss (<2 days) and a low incidence of neonatal jaundice (0.3%). Compared to NLBW neonates, LBW neonates did not appear to have disadvantages in clinical outcomes, including excess body-weight loss and neonatal jaundice. LBW neonates also potentially showed faster body-weight gain patterns, with a trend suggesting that a higher percentage body-weight gain per day was associated with lower birth weight.

In the contemporary understanding of neonatal body-weight growth, the gradient of birth weight for the speed of body-weight gain is positive. That is, heavier birth weight neonates enjoy the advantages of faster body-weight gain and neonatal body-weight growth curves have continuously shown a divergent pattern across birth weight categories [13–17]. During the second half of the twentieth century, when perinatal and neonatal medicine and NICU were on the rise, this positive gradient in birth weight for neonatal body-weight gain was considered a rule of thumb and early illustrations of this positive gradient date as far back as Dancis et al. in 1948 [13]. Over the course of the twentieth century, this positive gradient persisted, reflecting larger insensible water loss in lower birth weight neonates (more premature neonates) [15,17,20]. Part of the reason for our observed pattern, which may potentially buck the contemporary trend, may be due to the neutral thermal environment that improves digestive function with circulatory stability, resulting in the neonatal capability to be fed sufficiently to meet basal metabolism and prolonged thermal regulation in LBW neonates [8–12]. Additionally, in a recent study with exclusively breastfed neonates, 50% of neonates recovered their weight around 10 days after birth [21]. By contrast, most of the neonates recovered their weight by 4 days after birth in our study, suggesting that our nutrition regulation with supplemental formula milk may successfully meet the basal metabolism in our high-risk population.

Body weight is a robust and straightforward anthropometric indicator to grow neonates. The criteria for body-weight-growth have been varied, which may partly due to differences in growth patterns of breastfeeding and formula-feeding based on calorific intakes. For example, in Western countries, studies suggest the potential cut-off point of ~5% to 12% for exclusively breastfed neonates and ~2% to 3% for formula-fed neonates [22–26], while the American Academy of Pediatrics recommends explicitly the cut-off point of 7% for excess body-weight loss among exclusively breastfed neonates [2]. By contrast, in Japan, although some studies suggest the potential cut-off point of ~4% to 10% [3,7], and other expert opinions even support the cut-off point of up to ~15%, any evidence-based clinical guidelines have yet to be established. Given the emerging concern for excess body-weight loss from inadequate intake in East-Asian countries including Japan [3–5], physiological body-weight loss would be a body-weight loss for neonates adequately fed to meet basal metabolism, at least in high-risk populations. Indeed, we observed an initial ~2% body-weight loss as the physiological loss with a low incidence of neonatal jaundice in our study population. Therefore, our growth chart may help not only healthcare providers but also mothers of neonates in that high-risk population.

Gestational age and maternal factors during pregnancy may affect neonatal growth pattern. In previous studies, gestational age $\leq$38 weeks was associated with an increased risk of neonatal jaundice [27]. Maternal smoking during pregnancy and preeclampsia were associated with decreased birth weight, whereas gestational diabetes was associated with increased birth weight [28–30]. In Finland, comprehensive screening of gestational diabetes was associated with decreased mean birth weight and macrosomia rates but was associated with an increased prevalence of neonatal hypoglycemia [30]. In our study, gestational age was consistently associated with neonatal growth pattern. However, significant effects of hypertensive disorders of pregnancy and maternal body mass index were inconsistent under the combination method (although we could not assess the impact of gestational diabetes due to the limitation of our data). Additionally, no hypoglycemia was observed in our high-risk population. Therefore, in addition to LBW neonates, neonates with gestational age $\leq$38 weeks, maternal smoking, preeclampsia, and gestational diabetes, might benefit the most from the combination method.

Some limitations should be noted. First, we did not have a control group with other nutrition treatments (exclusively breastfeeding and exclusively formula-feeding). In addition, we did not have hourly data of body weight and did not include sick infants who required intravenous infusion [13,25,31]. The thermal regulation also differed between birth weight categories, thereby introducing potential bias and limiting external generalizability. However, internal validity might be maintained for the comparison of NLBW and LBW neonates from the same source population. Second, other anthropometric parameters, such as body length and head circumference, and potential maternal confounding variables. such as diabetes, were not available [15–17,32]. However, body weight is a reliable indicator of neonatal growth [7,15]. Third, use of supplemental feeding is controversial due to the risk of breastfeeding failure, and excessive weight gain and the combination method might raise concerns for introducing unintended adverse events [1,33]. However, in previous studies, supplemental feeding did not affect breast milk production [7] and breastfeeding was not consistently associated with the reduction of obesity or body fat mass in children or adolescents [34]. In addition, a recent randomized clinical trial concluded that supplementing breastfeeding with early limited formula milk (10 mL) did not interfere with breastfeeding [35]. Fourth, we were not able to assess the impact of standardized early skin-to-skin contact on the incidence of hypothermia or hypoglycemia compared to our early skin-to-skin contact within 2 min. However, in previous studies, profiles of serum glucose levels and core/peripheral distribution of body temperature were likely better in neonates with thermal regulation compared with those without thermal regulation [7–9]. Therefore, future studies, including randomized controlled trials, are warranted to further understand how thermal control and nutrition regulation influence neonatal growth.

Lastly, in the era of early neonatal hospital discharge, standardized thermal regulation and nutrition regulation to meet basal metabolism (without NICU care) may reduce medical expenditures of readmission for phototherapy with costly NICU care among LBW neonates [1,36]. Even in our high-risk study population, we observed a very low incidence of neonatal jaundice (0.4%), which corresponds to the incidence in Western settings [27,37]. Given the very low incidence of neonatal jaundice, a potential reduction of medical expenditure would be expected by the combination method, in addition to improved education (clinicians, nurses, and parents) and systemic institutional and community-wide approaches [38,39]. Due to extra thermal regulation that might further stabilize cardiopulmonary circulation and improve digestive function, no phototherapy was required in NLBW neonates [8–10]. In addition, the combination method did not require intravenous infusion therapy and did not result in neonatal morbidity, mortality, or readmission after discharge, thereby potentially increasing the efficient use of NICU resources and potentially reducing clinical complications associated with intravenous infusion among LBW neonates. Furthermore, the initial 2 h spent in the incubator might help to avoid the substantially longer incubation required for phototherapy, thereby potentially increasing opportunities for physical contact between mothers and their babies.

In conclusion, neonatal body-weight growth patterns were characterized under standardized thermal control and nutrition regulation, with a low incidence of unfavorable clinical outcomes, regardless of birth weight category. Under this combination method, LBW neonates might not have disadvantages in clinical outcomes or growth patterns.

Author Contributions: Conceptualization, S.K.; data curation, S.K., M.Z., and T.Y.; formal analysis, M.Z. and T.Y.; investigation, S.K. and T.Y.; methodology, S.K., M.Z., and T.Y.; project administration, T.Y.; resources, S.K.; supervision, T.Y.; writing—original draft, M.Z.; writing—review and editing, S.K., M.Z., and T.Y.

Acknowledgments: We would like to thank Editage (www.editage.jp) for English language editing.

References

1. Maisels, M.J.; McDonagh, A.F. Phototherapy for neonatal jaundice. *N. Engl. J. Med.* **2008**, *358*, 920–928. [CrossRef] [PubMed]
2. Gartner, L.M.; Morton, J.; Lawrence, R.A.; Naylor, A.J.; O'Hare, D.; Schanler, R.J.; Eidelman, A.I. American Academy of Pediatrics Section on Breastfeeding. *Pediatrics* **2005**, *115*, 496–506. [PubMed]
3. Sato, H.; Uchida, T.; Toyota, K.; Kanno, M.; Hashimoto, T.; Watanabe, M.; Nakamura, T.; Tamiya, G.; Aoki, K.; Hayasaka, K. Association of breast-fed neonatal hyperbilirubinemia with UGT1A1 polymorphisms: 211G>A (G71R) mutation becomes a risk factor under inadequate feeding. *J. Hum. Genet.* **2013**, *58*, 7–10. [CrossRef] [PubMed]
4. Chen, Y.J.; Chen, W.C.; Chen, C.M. Risk factors for hyperbilirubinemia in breastfed term neonates. *Eur. J. Pediatr.* **2012**, *171*, 167–171. [CrossRef] [PubMed]
5. Chen, C.F.; Hsu, M.C.; Shen, C.H.; Wang, C.L.; Chang, S.C.; Wu, K.G.; Wu, S.C.; Chen, S.J. Influence of breast-feeding on weight loss, jaundice, and waste elimination in neonates. *Pediatr. Neonatol.* **2011**, *52*, 85–92. [CrossRef]
6. Seske, L.M.; Merhar, S.L.; Haberman, B.E. Late-onset hypoglycemia in term newborns with poor breastfeeding. *Hosp. Pediatr.* **2015**, *5*, 501–504. [CrossRef] [PubMed]
7. Zaitsu, M.; Yoshihara, T.; Nakai, H.; Kubota, S. Optimal thermal control with sufficient nutrition may reduce the incidence of neonatal jaundice by preventing body-weight loss among NLBW infants not admitted to neonatal intensive care unit. *Neonatology* **2018**, *114*, 348–354. [CrossRef] [PubMed]
8. Kubota, S.; Koyanagi, T.; Hori, E.; Hara, K.; Shimokawa, H.; Nakano, H. Homeothermal adjustment in the immediate post delivered infant monitored by continuous and simultaneous measurement of core and peripheral body temperatures. *Biol. Neonate* **1988**, *54*, 79–85. [CrossRef] [PubMed]
9. Yoshimura, T.; Tsukimori, K.; Wake, N.; Nakano, H. The influence of thermal environment on pulmonary hemodynamic acclimation to extrauterine life in normal full-term neonates. *J. Perinat. Med.* **2007**, *35*, 236–240. [CrossRef] [PubMed]
10. Hey, E.N.; Katz, G. The optimum thermal environment for naked babies. *Arch. Dis. Child* **1970**, *45*, 328–334. [CrossRef]
11. Gross, S.J.; David, R.J.; Bauman, L.; Tomarelli, R.M. Nutritional composition of milk produced by mothers delivering preterm. *J. Pediatr.* **1980**, *96*, 641–644. [CrossRef]
12. Aoshima, N.; Fujie, Y.; Itoh, T.; Tukey, R.H.; Fujiwara, R. Glucose induces intestinal human UDP-glucuronosyltransferase (UGT) 1A1 to prevent neonatal hyperbilirubinemia. *Sci. Rep.* **2014**, *4*, 6343. [CrossRef] [PubMed]
13. Dancis, J.; O'Connell, J.R.; Holt, L.E., Jr. A grid for recording the weight of premature infants. *J. Pediatr.* **1948**, *33*, 570–572. [CrossRef]
14. Brosius, K.K.; Ritter, D.A.; Kenny, J.D. Postnatal growth curve of the infant with extremely LBW who was fed enterally. *Pediatrics* **1984**, *74*, 778–782. [PubMed]
15. Itabashi, K.; Takeuchi, T.; Okuyama, K.; Kuriya, N.; Ohtani, Y. Postnatal growth curves of very LBW Japanese infants. *Acta Paediatr. Jpn.* **1992**, *34*, 648–655. [CrossRef] [PubMed]
16. Itabashi, K.; Takeuchi, T.; Hayashi, T.; Okuyama, K.; Kuriya, N.; Otani, Y. Postnatal reference growth curves for very LBW infants. *Early Hum. Dev.* **1994**, *37*, 151–160. [CrossRef]
17. Diekmann, M.; Genzel-Boroviczeny, O.; Zoppelli, L.; von Poblotzki, M. Postnatal growth curves for extremely LBW infants with early enteral nutrition. *Eur. J. Pediatr.* **2005**, *164*, 714–723. [CrossRef] [PubMed]
18. Kuboi, T.; Kusaka, T.; Kawada, K.; Koyano, K.; Nakamura, S.; Okubo, K.; Yasuda, S.; Isobe, K.; Itoh, S. Hour-specific nomogram for transcutaneous bilirubin in Japanese neonates. *Pediatr. Int.* **2013**, *55*, 608–611. [CrossRef] [PubMed]
19. Itoh, S.; Kondo, M.; Kusaka, T.; Isobe, K.; Onishi, S. Differences in transcutaneous bilirubin readings in Japanese term infants according to feeding method. *Pediatr. Int.* **2001**, *43*, 12–15. [CrossRef]
20. Hammarlund, K.; Sedin, G.; Stromberg, B. Transepidermal water loss in newborn infants. VIII. Relation to gestational age and post-natal age in appropriate and small for gestational age infants. *Acta Paediatr. Scand.* **1983**, *72*, 721–728. [CrossRef]
21. Paul, I.M.; Schaefer, E.W.; Miller, J.R.; Kuzniewicz, M.W.; Li, S.X.; Walsh, E.M.; Flaherman, V.J. Weight Change Nomograms for the First Month After Birth. *Pediatrics* **2016**, *138*. [CrossRef] [PubMed]

22. American Academy of Pediatrics Subcommittee on Hyperbilirubinemia. Management of hyperbilirubinemia in the newborn infant 35 or more weeks of gestation. *Pediatrics* **2004**, *114*, 297–316. [CrossRef]
23. Laing, I.A.; Wong, C.M. Hypernatraemia in the first few days: Is the incidence rising? *Arch. Dis. Child. Fetal Neonatal Ed.* **2002**, *87*, F158–F162. [CrossRef]
24. Academy of Breastfeeding Medicine Protocol Committee. ABM clinical protocol #3: Hospital guidelines for the use of supplementary feedings in the healthy term breastfed neonate, revised 2009. *Breastfeed Med.* **2009**, *4*, 175–182.
25. Miller, J.R.; Flaherman, V.J.; Schaefer, E.W.; Kuzniewicz, M.W.; Li, S.X.; Walsh, E.M.; Paul, I.M. Early weight loss nomograms for formula fed newborns. *Hosp. Pediatr.* **2015**, *5*, 263–268. [CrossRef] [PubMed]
26. Martens, P.J.; Romphf, L. Factors associated with newborn in-hospital weight loss: Comparisons by feeding method, demographics, and birthing procedures. *J. Hum. Lact.* **2007**, *23*, 233–241. [CrossRef] [PubMed]
27. Maisels, M.J.; Kring, E. Length of Stay, Jaundice, and Hospital Readmission. *Pediatrics* **1998**, *101*, 995–998. [CrossRef]
28. Inoue, S.; Naruse, H.; Yorifuji, T.; Kato, T.; Murakoshi, T.; Doi, H.; Subramanian, S.V. Impact of Maternal and Paternal Smoking on Birth Outcomes. *J. Public Health (Oxf.)* **2017**, *39*, 1–10. [CrossRef]
29. Hung, T.H.; Hsieh, T.T.; Chen, S.F. Risk of Abnormal Fetal Growth in Women with Early- and Late-Onset Preeclampsia. *Pregnancy Hypertens.* **2018**, *12*, 201–206. [CrossRef]
30. Koivunen, S.; Torkki, A.; Bloigu, A.; Gissler, M.; Pouta, A.; Kajantie, E.; Vaarasmaki, M. Towards National Comprehensive Gestational Diabetes Screening—Consequences for Neonatal Outcome and Care. *Acta Obstet. Gynecol. Scand.* **2017**, *96*, 106–113. [CrossRef]
31. Fonseca, M.J.; Severo, M.; Santos, A.C. A new approach to estimating weight change and its reference intervals during the first 96 hours of life. *Acta Paediatr.* **2015**, *104*, 1028–1034. [CrossRef]
32. Villar, J.; Giuliani, F.; Bhutta, Z.A.; Bertino, E.; Ohuma, E.O.; Ismail, L.C.; Barros, F.C.; Altman, D.G.; Victora, C.; Noble, J.A.; et al. Postnatal growth standards for preterm infants: The Preterm Postnatal Follow-up Study of the INTERGROWTH-21(st) Project. *Lancet Glob. Health* **2015**, *3*, e681–e691. [CrossRef]
33. Victora, C.G.; Bahl, R.; Barros, A.J.; Franca, G.V.; Horton, S.; Krasevec, J.; Murch, S.; Sankar, M.J.; Walker, N.; Rollins, N.C. Lancet Breastfeeding Series Group: Breastfeeding in the 21st century: Epidemiology, mechanisms, and lifelong effect. *Lancet* **2016**, *387*, 475–490. [CrossRef]
34. Moschonis, G.; de Lauzon-Guillain, B.; Jones, L.; Oliveira, A.; Lambrinou, C.P.; Damianidi, L.; Lioret, S.; Moreira, P.; Lopes, C.; Emmett, P.; et al. The effect of early feeding practices on growth indices and obesity at preschool children from four European countries and UK schoolchildren and adolescents. *Eur. J. Pediatr.* **2017**, *176*, 1181–1192. [CrossRef]
35. Flaherman, V.J.; Narayan, N.R.; Hartigan-O'Connor, D.; Cabana, M.D.; McCulloch, C.E.; Paul, I.M. The Effect of Early Limited Formula on Breastfeeding, Readmission, and Intestinal Microbiota: A Randomized Clinical Trial. *J. Pediatr.* **2018**, *196*, 84–90. [CrossRef]
36. Suresh, G.K.; Clark, R.E. Cost-effectiveness of strategies that are intended to prevent kernicterus in newborn infants. *Pediatrics* **2004**, *114*, 917–924. [CrossRef]
37. Eggert, L.D.; Wiedmeier, S.E.; Wilson, J.; Christensen, R.D. The Effect of Instituting a Prehospital-Discharge Newborn Bilirubin Screening Program in an 18-Hospital Health System. *Pediatrics* **2006**, *117*, e855–e862. [CrossRef]
38. Flaherman, V.; Schaefer, E.W.; Kuzniewicz, M.W.; Li, S.X.; Walsh, E.M.; Paul, I.M. Health Care Utilization in the First Month After Birth and its Relationship to Newborn Weight Loss and Method of Feeding. *Acad. Pediatr.* **2018**, *18*, 677–684. [CrossRef]
39. Bhutani, V.K.; Johnson, L.H.; Schwoebel, A.; Gennaro, S. A Systems Approach for Neonatal Hyperbilirubinemia in Term and Near-Term Newborns. *J. Obstet. Gynecol. Neonatal Nurs.* **2006**, *35*, 444–455. [CrossRef]

12

Impact of Maternal Nutrition and Perinatal Factors on Breast Milk Composition after Premature Delivery

Jean-Michel Hascoët [1,2,*], Martine Chauvin [3], Christine Pierret [3], Sébastien Skweres [1], Louis-Dominique Van Egroo [4], Carole Rougé [5] and Patricia Franck [6]

1 Department of Neonatology, Maternite Regionale, CHRU Nancy, 54035 Nancy, France; sebastienskweres@hotmail.fr
2 DevAH, Lorraine University, 54500 Vandoeuvre les Nancy, France
3 Dietetic and Nutrition Unit, CHRU Nancy, 54035 Nancy, France; m.chauvin@chru-nancy.fr (M.C.); c.pierret@chru-nancy.fr (C.P.)
4 Saint Cloud Hospital, 92210 Paris, France; louisdo.vanegroo@club-internet.fr
5 Bledina Limonest, 69410 Champagne-au-Mont-d'Or, France; carole.rouge@danone.com
6 Biology Laboratory, CHRU Nancy, 54035 Nancy, France; p.franck@chru-nancy.fr
* Correspondence: jean-michel.hascoet@univ-lorraine.fr

Abstract: (1) Background: Premature infants require mothers' milk fortification to meet nutrition needs, but breast milk composition may be variable, leading to the risk of inadequate nutrition. We aimed at determining the factors influencing mothers' milk macronutrients. (2) Methods: Milk samples were analyzed for the first five weeks after premature delivery by infrared spectroscopy. Mothers' nutritional intake data were obtained during standardized interviews with dieticians, and then analyzed with reference software. (3) Results: The composition of 367 milk samples from 81 mothers was (median (range) g/100 mL): carbohydrates 6.8 (4.4–7.3), lipids 3.4 (1.3–6.4), proteins 1.3 (0.1–3.1). There was a relationship between milk composition and mothers' carbohydrates intake only ($r = 0.164$; $p < 0.01$). Postnatal age was correlated with milk proteins ($r = -0.505$; $p < 0.001$) and carbohydrates ($r = +0.202$, $p < 0.001$). Multiple linear regression analyses showed (coefficient) a relationship between milk proteins $r = 0.547$ and postnatal age (−0.028), carbohydrate intake (+0.449), and the absence of maturation (−0.066); associations were also found among milk lipids $r = 0.295$, carbohydrate intake (+1.279), and smoking (−0.557). Finally, there was a relationship among the concentration of milk carbohydrates $r = 0.266$, postnatal age (+0.012), and smoking (−0.167). (4) Conclusions: The variability of mothers' milk composition is differentially associated for each macronutrient with maternal carbohydrate intake, antenatal steroids, smoking, and postnatal age. Improvement in milk composition could be achieved by the modification of these related factors.

Keywords: maternal nutrition; breast milk; premature delivery; milk composition

---

1. Introduction

Premature infants require mothers' milk fortification to meet their nutrition needs [1]. This fortification is usually standardized using an assumed macronutrient milk composition [2]. However, studies have suggested that breast milk composition variability may be much wider than expected [3,4], leading to inadequate newborn nutrition. McLeod et al. performed a survey of protein and energy intake by milk analysis within the first 28 days of life in 63 infants born before 33 weeks' gestation to assess their effect on growth [3]. Their results show that breast milk composition vary for all of the macronutrients with median protein concentrations of 16.6 g/L ranging from 13.4 g/L to 27.6 g/L, and median caloric intake of 73.3 Kcal/100 mL ranging from 63 Kcal/100 mL to 93 Kcal/100 mL. Of note, actual protein intake was correlated with infants' growth. The authors concluded that preterm milk composition is very variable, and routine fortification using assumed averaged composition may result in inadequate nutrition with slower weight gain, as observed in their study [3].

Inadequate nutrition could indeed explain in part the postnatal growth restriction observed in many premature infants [5,6]. We aimed at determining factors, including mothers' nutritional intake, which may be associated and explain breast milk macronutrient variability after premature delivery before 34 weeks' gestational age.

2. Materials and Methods

This is an observational study using milk bank data. In our level III Maternity Hospital, mothers' own milk is pasteurized for premature infants. After pasteurization, we routinely analyze breast milk composition to verify the appropriateness of standardized fortification. For the purpose of the study, we collected data for all of the milk batches that each mother provided to the milk bank regardless of the time of the milk collection to evaluate the milk composition variation throughout the first five weeks of lactation. Each batch is a pool of one to three days, depending on the volume collected and frozen by each mother at home. Once a volume of at least 500 mL was collected, the mother would hand over the frozen batch to the milk bank for pasteurization. Hand-over occurred daily to twice a week.

Mothers who delivered a premature infant before 34 weeks' gestation at our unit were enrolled within five days after delivery when they announced their choice for breastfeeding. Mothers' dietary preference and nutritional intake data were obtained during personalized interviews with experienced dieticians. They used standardized questionnaires based on validated documents in the National French survey. The dieticians recalled dietary intake information from the two weeks prior to the interview. Perinatal data were prospectively collected at the time of the interview and from the mothers' file. We analyzed maternal diet and macronutrient intake from the recall data averaged per day with appropriate software (Geni® V7.0, Micro6, Villers les Nancy-F, France).

For milk analysis, we used the same protocol as described in the literature [7,8] and advised by the manufacturer. In short, mothers milk pools over one to three days were delivered frozen (−20 °C) to the milk bank, thawed, pasteurized, aliquoted in bottles of 50 mL, and stored at −80 °C. Two samples of one mL from two different bottles of each batch were analyzed after homogenization by ultrasound to compensate for milk thawing and verify the quality of the homogenization. We used infrared spectroscopy pre-calibrated against a chemical reference with analytical accuracy <0.1 g/100 mL (Miris AB® V3, Uppsala, Sweden). Since it has been shown that mid-infrared analyzers may require calibration adjustment, we verified the calibration daily to ensure appropriate measures [9]. The samples were rejected if variability was over 10%; otherwise, the average of the two values was kept for further analysis.

We started our statistical analyses by power calculation relying upon McLeod [3]. We calculated that to demonstrate a significant relationship with a coefficient of at least $r = 0.550$, which is considered clinically significant, with an alpha risk of 0.016 (Bonferroni correction for the three nutrients) and a power of 0.90, 78 mothers with at least two samples would be needed (Power and Precision™ V4, Biostat Inc., Englewood, NJ, USA, 2001). Normally distributed data, assessed by a Shapiro–Wilk test of normality, are presented as mean values with standard deviation (SD), the median, and the interquartile range (IQR); non-normally distributed data are presented as medians with IQR only. To evaluate the differences between groups, we used the Student *t*-test for continuous variables and the Chi-squared test or Fisher exact test when appropriate for categorical variables. For continuous variables not normally distributed, we used the Mann–Whitney U test. To determine which variables were associated with milk composition, we performed a bivariate analysis, and then a stepwise multiple linear regression, including all of the variables associated with milk composition in bivariate analysis, with a tolerance set at 10^{-5} with the probability to remove the set at 0.15 and a confidence interval of 0.95. Observed differences were considered statistically significant if $p < 0.05$. Statistical analysis was performed with SYSTAT 12 software (2007, Systat Software Inc., San Jose, CA, USA).

The study has been approved by our Institutional Ethics and Review Board on 9 March 2013 (Number: MRU13-02).

3. Results

3.1. Description of the Studied Population

From August 2013 to January 2014, 367 milk samples were obtained from 81 mothers (Figure 1). Two to 10 batches were collected from the mothers (median (IQR): three (two to six)).

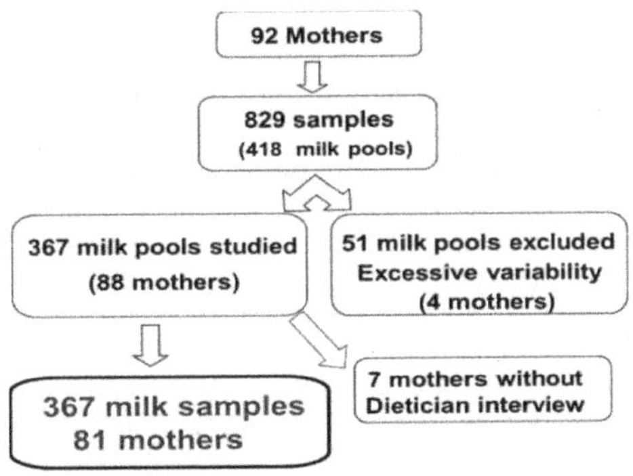

Figure 1. flow chart.

The mothers involved in the study were 29 years old (19–42) (median (range)). Their average height was 1.64 m (1.53–1.85) for a weight of 63 kg (42–110) and a body mass index (BMI) of 23.2 (16.4–43). Weight gain during pregnancy ranged from 0 to 30 kg (mean 10.2 kg). The age of delivery was 31 weeks' gestational age (24–34). Twenty (25%) mothers smoked during pregnancy; 63 (78%) were single pregnancies, and 19 (23%) presented with toxemia. Prenatal maturation with corticosteroids was achieved in 37 (46%) mothers and partial maturation in 33 (41%). Vaginal delivery occurred in 42 mothers (52%) and cesarean section occurred in 39 (48%).

Forty-nine (60%) newborns were males; neonatal adaptation was good with an Apgar score above six at one and five minutes for all infants. Their mean birth weight was 1523 ± 512 g (median (range) = 1460 (600–2500) g).

3.2. Maternal Nutritional Intake and Milk Composition

Maternal nutritional intake was 2169 ± 562 Kcal/day (2146 (1197–3628)) with 88 ± 28 g/day (88 (40–213)) of fat intake, 86 ± 20 g/day (87 (40–160)) of protein intake, and 257 ± 81 g/day (247 (103–533)) of overall carbohydrate intake.

The global milk sample composition was (median [range]/100 mL): carbohydrates 6.8 g (4.4–7.3), lipids 3.4 g (1.3–6.4), proteins 1.3 g (0.1–3.1). The correlation between mothers' food intake and milk composition is shown in Table 1.

Table 1. Linear regression between mothers' food intake and milk composition (coefficient r).

Nutrients Intake	Milk Calories	Milk Proteins	Milk Lipids	Milk Carbohydrates
Log Energy	0.110 *	0.094	0.106 *	0.034
Protein	0.01	0.03	0.01	0.04
Fat	0.03	0.04	0.03	0.03
Carbohydrates	0.131 **	0.109 *	0.127 *	0.035

* $p < 0.05$; ** $p < 0.01$.

3.3. *Perinatal Factors' Effect on Milk Composition*

3.3.1. Postnatal Age Effect on Milk Composition

Weekly mean protein content significantly decreased for the first four weeks post-delivery, and then remained stable at week five. We observed a comparable but inverse evolution for carbohydrates, and there was no significant difference over the first five weeks after delivery for the fat content of mothers' milk (Table 2).

Table 2. Average milk composition per postnatal week.

Week	1 (n = 52)	2 (n = 125)	3 (n = 91)	4 (n = 68)	5 (n = 31)
Protein	1.78 ± 0.39 *	1.40 ± 0.40 *	1.26 ± 0.34 *	1.08 ± 0.36 *	1.05 ± 0.40
Lipids	3.23 ± 0.80	3.58 ± 0.98	3.59 ± 0.97	3.41 ± 0.96	3.40 ± 1.06
CHO	6.50 ± 0.43 *	6.66 ± 0.38 *	6.70 ± 0.46 *	6.81 ± 0.44 *	6.75 ± 0.44

* $p < 0.01$.

We observed a significant linear regression for carbohydrate and an inverse correlation for protein contents, as shown in Figure 2.

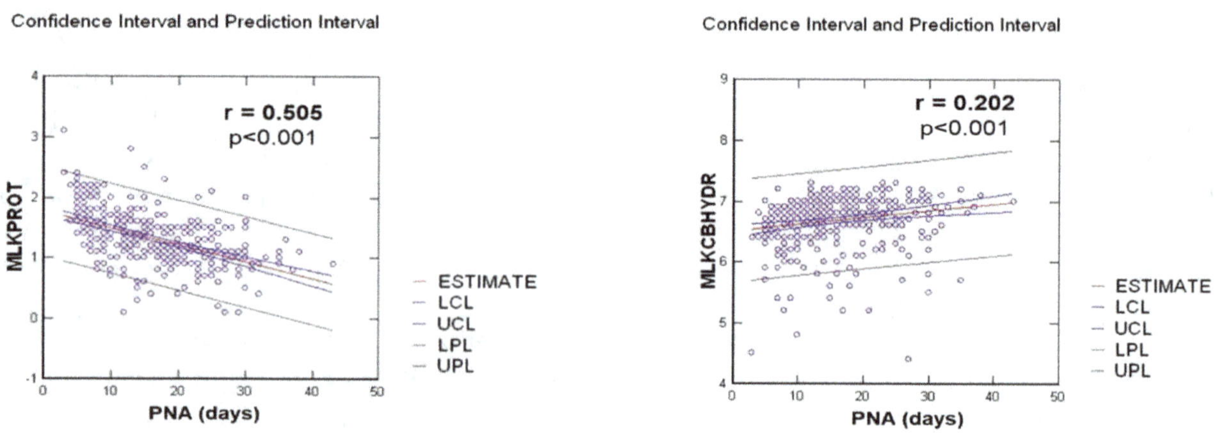

(**a**) (**b**)

Figure 2. Linear regression between milk composition in g/100 mL and postnatal age (PNA) in days, for: (**a**) Protein milk content (MLKPROT); (**b**) Carbohydrate milk content (MLKCBHYD).

3.3.2. Perinatal Factors' Impact on Milk Composition in Bivariate Analysis

There was no relationship between the milk composition and the mothers' age, weight, height, or BMI before pregnancy. There was no relationship either for the mode of delivery, multiple pregnancies, toxemia, or gestational age at delivery. We observed a weak association between weight gain during pregnancy and milk lipid content ($r = 0.117$, $p = 0.026$). Finally, we observed a significant correlation between milk composition and antenatal steroid maturation, smoking during pregnancy, and an inverse relationship with the infants' birth weight. Detailed data are shown in Table 3.

Table 3. Confounding perinatal factors for milk composition.

Milk Content (Mean, g/100 mL)	Smoking		Antenatal Steroids		Birth Weight (Linear Regression: r)
	Yes	No	Yes	No	
Lipids	3.10	3.59 *	3.6 *	3.1	0.082
Carbohydrates	6.57	6.71 *	6.7	6.6	−0.259 *
Protein	1.34	1.33	1.3	1.2	−0.318 *
Calories	62.8	67.8 *	67.6 *	61.9	−0.106

* $p < 0.05$.

3.3.3. Stepwise Multivariate Regression Analysis of Factors Associated with Milk Composition in Bivariate Analysis

All of the factors showing a significant association with mothers' milk content in bivariate analysis were included in the model presented in Table 4.

Table 4. Multivariate analysis of factors associated with mothers' milk content.

Milk Content	Postnatal Age	Carbohydrate Intake	Smoking	No Steroids	Weight Gain
Lipids ($r^2 = 0.087$)	NS	1.279 *	−0.557 *	NS	NS
Carbohydrates ($r^2 = 0.071$)	0.012 *	NS	−0.167 *	NS	NS
Protein ($r^2 = 0.299$)	−0.028 *	0.449 *	NS	−0.066 *	NS
Calories ($r^2 = 0.101$)	NS	14.053 *	−5.901 *	NS	NS

* $p < 0.05$; NS: non-significant.

4. Discussion

Our study confirms that breast milk composition in macronutrients has a large variability, as suggested in previous studies [3,4]. Therefore, fortification of the assumed averaged macronutrient in milk leads to inadequate nutritional intake for most premature infants. Our data show that indeed, maternal nutrition may influence breast milk macronutrient composition in mothers who delivered prematurely. Our data also show that only overall carbohydrate is positively correlated with protein, fat, and caloric density. To our knowledge, this observation has not been yet reported. In their study comparing the breast milk nitrogen content of mothers from two different Chinese areas, Zhao et al. found no significant difference in 18 studied amino acids, despite significant lower protein intake in one of the studied areas [10]. This is consistent with our results. Likewise, in their study on maternal supplementation with omega-3 precursors, Mazurier et al. showed a qualitative alteration with increased alpha-linoleic acid content, but no significant modification of the overall lipid concentration [11]. This observation also recalls that a true difference in the secretory activity of the mammary gland is not merely a difference in concentration. In a recent survey on food and nutrient intake of women in France, Hebel et al. showed that few lactating mothers met the nutritional guidelines, and may therefore be at risk of food and nutrient inadequacies [12]. One could speculate that improving the maternal nutritional balance, especially an appropriate overall carbohydrate intake, might contribute to improved milk composition for preterm infant feeding.

Longitudinal analysis of milk composition showed a significant decrease in milk protein content with an inverse correlation for carbohydrate and a stable lipid concentration over the first four weeks after delivery. These data are consistent with the publication of Maly et al. [8], who found the same evolution for the three macronutrients and Mahakan et al. [4], who found a 50% decrease in protein concentrations with a 30% increase in carbohydrate concentrations over the first 28 days after delivery. From his review analysis on human milk in premature infants [13], which included the studies Charpak et al. [14] and Bauer et al. [15], Underwood evaluated the changes in milk composition over eight weeks from delivery, and found the same results as in our study over this longer assessment period. Yoneyama et al. suggested that there may be a negative correlation between protein content and milk volume and between early and mature milk [16]. This observation may explain why breastfeeding infants adjust their volume intake in relation with milk caloric density and protein content. However, when feeding premature neonates, the amount of milk is usually fixed to a target volume [17]. Therefore, protein content evolution is important to take into account when considering the fortification of human milk for premature infants.

Few data are available for the impact of perinatal factors on milk composition. In our study, we did not find any significant association among the mothers' age, weight, height, or BMI before pregnancy. In their study on maternal nutrition and body composition during breast feeding, Bzikowska-Jura et al. [7] found a variance in milk fat content related to BMI. However, they studied the actual BMI at three time points, while we differentiated between BMI before pregnancy and weight gain during pregnancy, which was indeed associated with milk fat content. Thus, our results are consistent with published data, but suggest that it is not BMI per se, but rather weight gain during pregnancy that may be associated with milk composition. Also, there was no relationship for the mode of delivery, multiple pregnancies, or toxemia. As in our study, Maly et al. [8] showed no effect of the degree of prematurity at delivery on milk composition. However, we found a moderate effect of birth weight in bivariate analysis, but not after adjusting for other confounding factors in multivariate analysis (data not shown). Finally, we showed that breast milk protein concentrations were positively correlated with mothers' overall carbohydrate intake, and negatively correlated with the duration of lactation from birth onwards, and the absence of steroid maturation; breast milk carbohydrate concentrations were positively correlated with the duration of lactation, and negatively correlated with smoking, as shown in the study of Bachour et al. [18], whereas breast milk lipid concentrations were positively correlated with mothers' carbohydrate intake and negatively correlated with smoking.

Our study has strength and limitations. Our strength relies upon the number of samples, the blinded collection of the data, and the reproducibility of milk content measurements with a rejection when the control variability was above 0.10. Also, the dietary questionnaire over two weeks recall, which was given by experienced dieticians with an illustrated standardized catalog for the amount of food, allowed an appropriate evaluation of the averaged usual diet of the mothers. However, this questionnaire was given two weeks from the interview, and may not strictly reflect the diet of the lactating mother at the time of milk collection. Anyhow, one may speculate that the level of macronutrients intake would be only slightly modified from the routine diet of the patients. We did not find a significant difference from the results with sugar, fibers, or overall carbohydrate; therefore, we presented only the results with overall carbohydrate, but this would be confirmed by further targeting the study. Finally, because this is an observational study, we were not able to standardize the time that the mothers would hand over their milk collected at home to the milk bank, nor the number of collection days within each pool. However, this would only vary from one to three days, and we longitudinally evaluated the results over five weeks. Thus, even though this study does not really present an individual longitudinal analysis, the linear regressions that were observed for the overall population and the multivariate analysis, taking time as a confounding factor, are likely to allow a good reliability for our findings.

In conclusion, our study confirms that human milk macronutrients composition has a wide variability. This variability is differentially associated for each macronutrient, and associated with maternal carbohydrates intake, antenatal steroids, smoking, and the delay from delivery. To improve mothers' milk composition to values closer to the one needed for achieving infants' nutrition needs [19], one could aim for improving the prenatal nutritional balance in pregnant women, particularly for carbohydrate intake, supporting an appropriate weight gain during pregnancy, and advising stopping smoking. In the case of expected prematurity, steroid maturation is also needed to improve milk composition. Ideally, breast milk composition would be regularly measured for individualized fortification to achieve the appropriate growth of preterm infants. However, when it is only possible to apply standard fortification, at least human milk composition in relation to lactation duration from birth should be taken into account. Targeting investigation should be performed and confirm the observed data.

Author Contributions: All of the authors made significant contributions to the study: "conceptualization, J.-M.H., S.S. and L.-D.V.E.; methodology, mothers' interviews M.C. and C.P.; methodology, milk analysis with quality assessment and validation P.F.; validation, J.-M.H., S.S. and P.F.; formal analysis, J.-M.H.; investigation, M.C., C.P. and S.S.; writing—original draft preparation, J.-M.H.; writing—review and editing P.F., S.S., C.R. and L.-D.V.E.; supervision, J.-M.H.; funding acquisition, C.R. and L.-D.V.E.; finally, all authors read and approved the final version of the manuscript".

Acknowledgments: We thank Inga C Teller, PhD, Nutricia Research, Utrecht, The Netherlands, for her significant help in reviewing and editing the manuscript.

References

1. Agostoni, C.; Buonocore, G.; Carnielli, V.; De Curtis, M.; Darmaun, D.; Decsi, T.; Domellöf, M.; Embleton, N.; Fusch, C.; Genzel-Boroviczeny, O.; et al. Enteral Nutrient Supply for Preterm Infants: Commentary from the European Society of Paediatric Gastroenterology, Hepatology and Nutrition Committee on Nutrition. *J. Pediatr. Gastroenterol. Nutr.* **2010**, *50*, 85–91. [CrossRef] [PubMed]
2. Martin, C.R.; Brown, Y.F.; Ehrenkranz, R.A.; O'Shea, T.M.; Allred, E.N.; Belfort, M.B.; McCormick, M.C.; Leviton, A. Nutritional Practices and Growth Velocity in the First Month of Life in Extremely Premature Infants. *Pediatrics* **2009**, *124*, 649–657. [CrossRef] [PubMed]
3. McLeod, G.; Sherriff, J.; Nathan, E.; E Hartmann, P.; Simmer, K. Four-week nutritional audit of preterm infants born < 33 weeks gestation. *J. Paediatr. Child Health* **2013**, *49*, E332–E339. [PubMed]
4. Mahajan, S.; Chawla, D.; Kaur, J.; Jain, S. Macronutrients in breastmilk of mothers of preterm infants. *Indian Pediatr.* **2017**, *54*, 635–637. [CrossRef] [PubMed]
5. Embleton, N.E.; Pang, N.; Cooke, R.J. Postnatal Malnutrition and Growth Retardation: An Inevitable Consequence of Current Recommendations in Preterm Infants? *Pediatrics* **2001**, *107*, 270–273. [CrossRef] [PubMed]
6. Cooke, R.J.; Ainsworth, S.B.; Fenton, A.C. Postnatal growth retardation: A universal problem in preterm infants. *Arch. Dis. Child.-Fetal Neonatal Ed.* **2004**, *89*, 428–430. [CrossRef] [PubMed]
7. Bzikowska-Jura, A.; Czerwonogrodzka-Senczyna, A.; Olędzka, G.; Szostak-Węgierek, D.; Weker, H.; Wesołowska, A. Maternal Nutrition and Body Composition During Breastfeeding: Association with Human Milk Composition. *Nutrients* **2018**, *10*, 1379. [CrossRef] [PubMed]
8. Malý, J.; Burianova, I.; Vitkova, V.; Ticha, E.; Navratilova, M.; Cermáková, E. Preterm human milk macronutrient concentration is independent of gestational age at birth. *Arch. Dis. Child. Fetal Neonatal Ed.* **2018**, *104*, F50–F56. [CrossRef] [PubMed]
9. Buffin, R.; Decullier, E.; Loys, C.-M.; Hays, S.; Studzinsky, F.; Jourdes, E.; Picaud, J.-C.; De Halleux, V.; Rigo, J. Assessment of human milk composition using mid-infrared analyzers requires calibration adjustment. *Am. J. Perinatol.* **2017**, *37*, 552–557. [CrossRef] [PubMed]
10. Zhao, X.; Xu, Z.; Wang, Y.; Sun, Y. Studies of the relation between the nutritional status of lactating mothers and milk composition as well as the milk intake and growth of their infants in Beijing. Pt. 4. The protein and amino acid content of breast milk. *Ying Yang Xue Bao* **1989**, *11*, 227–332. [PubMed]
11. Mazurier, E.; Rigourd, V.; Perez, P.; Buffin, R.; Couedelo, L.; Vaysse, C.; Belcadi, W.; Sitta, R.; Nacka, F.; Lamireau, D.; et al. Effects of Maternal Supplementation with Omega-3 Precursors on Human Milk Composition. *J. Hum. Lact.* **2017**, *33*, 319–328. [CrossRef] [PubMed]
12. Hebel, P.; Francou, A.; Van Egroo, L.D.; Rougé, C.; Mares, P. Consommation alimentaire et apports nutritionnels chez les femmes allaitantes, en France. *Cah. Nutr. Diét.* **2018**, *25*, 303.
13. Underwood, M.A. Human Milk for the Premature Infant. *Pediatr. Clin. N. Am.* **2013**, *60*, 189–207. [CrossRef] [PubMed]
14. Charpak, N.; Ruiz, J.; M Med Sci on behalf of the KMC Team. M Med Sci on behalf of the KMC Team. Breast milk composition in a cohort of pre-term infants' mothers followed in an ambulatory programme in Colombia. *Acta Paediatr.* **2007**, *96*, 1755–1759.
15. Bauer, J.; Gerss, J. Longitudinal analysis of macronutrients and minerals in human milk produced by mothers of preterm infants. *Clin. Nutr.* **2011**, *30*, 215–220. [CrossRef] [PubMed]
16. Yoneyama, K.; Goto, I.; Nagata, H. Relationship between volume and concentrations of various components of breast milk in early and 2-6 months lactation. *Nihon Koshu Eisei Zasshi* **1994**, *41*, 157–164. [PubMed]

17. Rochow, N.; Fusch, G.; Choi, A.; Chessell, L.; Elliott, L.; McDonald, K.; Kuiper, E.; Purcha, M.; Turner, S.; Chan, E.; et al. Target Fortification of Breast Milk with Fat, Protein, and Carbohydrates for Preterm Infants. *J. Pediatr.* **2013**, *163*, 1001–1007. [CrossRef] [PubMed]
18. Bachour, P.; Yafawi, R.; Jaber, F.; Choueiri, E.; Abdel-Razzak, Z. Effects of Smoking, Mother's Age, Body Mass Index, and Parity Number on Lipid, Protein, and Secretory Immunoglobulin A Concentrations of Human Milk. *Breastfeed. Med.* **2012**, *7*, 179–188. [CrossRef] [PubMed]
19. Gidrewicz, D.A.; Fenton, T.R. A systematic review and meta-analysis of the nutrient content of preterm and term breast milk. *BMC Pediatr.* **2014**, *14*, 216. [CrossRef] [PubMed]

13

Blind Analysis of Food-Related IgG Identifies Five Possible Nutritional Clusters for the Italian Population: Future Implications for Pregnancy and Lactation

Gabriele Piuri [1], Enrico Ferrazzi [1,2] and Attilio Francesco Speciani [1,*]

[1] Inflammation Society, 18 Woodlands Park, Bexley DA52EL, UK; gabriele.piuri@me.com (G.P.); enrico.ferrazzi@unimi.it (E.F.)
[2] Fondazione IRCCS Cà Granda, Ospedale Maggiore Policlinico, Department of Clinical Sciences and Community Health, University of Milan, 20122 Milan, Italy
* Correspondence: attilio.speciani@me.com

Abstract: Background: The influence of diet in pregnant women on the immune tolerance process is intricate. Food-specific immunoglobulin G (IgG) was associated with exposure to particular food antigens. The IgG antibodies can cross the placental barrier and enter into the colostrum, and maternal IgG is amply present in breast milk. This justifies studying the immunological connection between food-specific IgG antibodies and the mother–fetus relationship. This study was designed to analyze food-specific IgG concentrations and possible food-specific IgG concentration clusters in a large cohort of subjects with a common food culture. Methods: Food-specific IgG antibody concentrations were detected in 18,012 Caucasian or Southern European subjects over 18 years of age. We used an unsupervised hierarchical clustering algorithm to explore varying degrees of similarity among food-specific IgG antibodies. Results: We identified five food groups by the evaluation of food-specific IgG values: one includes foods with a high nickel content, the second cluster is associated with gluten, the third cluster includes dairy products, the fourth one is connected to fermented foods, and the last group is correlated with cooked oils. Discussion: The knowledge derived from studying a large sample allows us to determine food-specific IgG values from a single pregnant woman, compare it to an epidemic standard, and establish modifications required in her lifestyle to modulate her nutritional habits.

Keywords: pregnancy; lactation; weaning; food-related IgG; food clusters; non-IgE-mediated food reactions

---

1. Introduction

Recently published reviews support the biological association of food-specific immunoglobulin G (IgG) with exposure to particular food antigens [1,2]. IgG antibodies, especially IgG4, are highly related to the immune tolerance of food antigens, and IgG can be responsible for the attenuation of the immunological response. These protective antibodies might regulate the immune response by avoiding the binding of the antigen to the IgE already present on the surface, or by inhibiting the maturation of the dendritic cells, preventing the activation of possible allergic pathways [3]. IgG4 antibodies have diverse anti-inflammatory actions compared to other IgG subclasses. One of these differences is the reduced capacity to induce complement activation due to a low affinity for the C1q and Fc receptors. Due to their ability to bind different antigens in diverse sites, these antibodies do not precipitate antigens [4].

The relationship between IgE-mediated anaphylaxis and more subtle hyper-immune responses associated with high IgG titer is being increasingly studied and has now been precisely defined. Antigens can cause systemic anaphylaxis through the classical pathway by cross-linking IgE bound to mast cell FcεRI or through the alternative path by forming complexes with IgG. New studies have shown an IgG-dependent mechanism of anaphylaxis that involves IgG, FcγRs on macrophages, basophils and neutrophils, complement-derived peptides C3a and C5a, B-cell activating factor (BAFF), and platelet-activating factor (PAF) [5]. According to Finkelman [6–8] and Muñoz-Cano et al. [9], IgG, macrophages, basophils, and neutrophils may even be involved in human anaphylaxis. This delicate blinding of food antigens can be dysregulated by an excess of these specific food antigens related to IgG and activate inflammatory processes [8].

This fine-tuned immune equilibrium permits alien food antigens to land safely on the gut mucosa as they are processed and allowed to pass through the mucosal surface and become nutritional elements for the microbiota, becoming accepted as "legal aliens". This complex recognition occurs on the most notable large external surface in the human body, which is 200 times wider than skin. The repetitive and continuous consumption of a particular food that corresponds to a higher production of specific antibodies can fracture the equilibrium, increase inflammatory mediators [8], and damage the delicate gap junctions in the gut mucosa [10].

High concentrations of food-specific IgG antibodies have been successfully identified as foes in non-IgE-mediated food reactions. Bentz et al. reported significantly higher food-specific IgG antibodies in patients with Crohn's disease in contrast with healthy controls [11]. The same patients showed significant clinical improvement in inflammatory bowel disease (IBD) symptoms when the foods associated with highly specific IgG were removed from the diet [11]. In agreement with these findings, Cai et al. observed high levels of IgG antibodies to specific food antigens in patients affected by IBD [12]. Alpay et al. evaluated the effect of a personalized nutritional approach based on food-specific IgG in sequences of migraine attacks in a randomized, double-blind, cross-over, headache-diary-based trial on patients diagnosed with migraines without auras [13]. A similar double-blind, placebo-controlled, dietary re-challenge trial was performed by Biesiekierski [14] to prove that the symptoms of irritable bowel syndrome (IBS) could be reduced in patients without proven celiac disease and with clinical sensitivity to gluten. A similar study demonstrated that clinical symptoms of IBS were significantly reduced in patients affected by Sjogren's syndrome who underwent a diet characterized by high concentrations of food-specific IgG [15]. IBS is a less-defined pathological condition, yet increased gastrointestinal permeability and gut inflammation were observed by Shulman in children [16]. Similar patterns of food-specific IgG and IgG4 were observed in eosinophilic esophagitis [17], and such deposits of IgG4 may even distinguish patients with gastro-esophageal reflux disease versus eosinophilic esophagitis.

The Western diet is prone to causing this imbalance [18] and is characterized by a lack of variety and seasonality that could elicit excessive antibody production against food antigen clusters. In parallel, the lack of fiber in a diet produces a poor prebiotic environment, directly affecting the gut microbiota. These conditions might convert the role of the microbiota from an anti-inflammatory partner of dendritic cells in the intestinal mucosa into an aggressive collection of pro-inflammatory bacteria.

We hypothesized that high food-specific IgG concentrations in subjects suffering from organ or systemic inflammation might be critical in a pro-inflammatory scenario. This study was designed to analyze food-specific IgG concentrations and possible food-specific IgG concentration clusters in a large cohort of subjects with a common food culture and affected by gastroenteric inflammatory symptoms and/or other tissue or systemic inflammations.

2. Materials and Methods

2.1. Subjects

All of 18,012 patients suspected a relationship between food intake and symptoms such as bloating, constipation, diarrhea, heartburn, gastritis, or other signs and symptoms of possible gastroenteric inflammation. They were all Caucasian or Southern European subjects over 18 years of age. Written consent to this observational study was obtained by all participants who self-enrolled in the study, according to privacy regulations. Sample collection was performed by finger pricks using a nylon swab for the storage of dried blood (Copan Diagnostics, Inc., Murrieta, CA, USA). Blood samples were delivered to a laboratory (Diagnostica Spire S.r.l. Reggio Emilia, Italy) and analyzed within less than seven days from sample collection to ensure the data accuracy. Food-specific IgG antibody concentrations were detected by employing ELISA plates produced by Immunolab GmbH (Kassel, Germany) customized for 44 common Italian food antigens. Lower and upper detection limits for IgG antibodies were 0.0 U/mL and 100 U/mL, respectively.

2.2. Statistical Methods

The frequency distribution of food-specific IgG concentrations in this population was determined for each food antigen tested. Non-parametric descriptive statistics (median and interquartile range) were adopted for non-normal (D'Agostino and Pearson normality test) or bimodal distributions.

We used an unsupervised hierarchical clustering algorithm to explore varying degrees of similarity among food-specific IgG, adapting the statistical methods used by Eisen et al. [19]. The object of using this algorithm was to compute a dendrogram that assembled all food-specific IgG into a single tree. For any food-specific IgG, an upper-diagonal similarity matrix containing similarity scores for all pairs of food-specific IgG was calculated. The matrix was scanned to identify the highest value, representing the most similar pair of food-specific IgG. A node was created joining these two foods, and a new food-specific IgG level was computed for the node by averaging observations for the joined elements. The similarity matrix was then updated with this new node, replacing the two joined elements, and the process was repeated (n − 1) times until only a single element remained. The algorithm initially had 44 food-specific IgG antibodies (one for each antigen), which were gradually grouped together into higher-degree clusters according to their similarities. The algorithm stopped when all food-specific IgG antibodies were grouped into the same cluster. The bar on the left side of the dendrogram indicates the dissimilarity (1 − Correlation) for every node. A lower dissimilarity suggests a higher correlation between the foods, or the clusters of foods, linked together by a node and can be useful to better understand the relationship between the different foods.

3. Results

Food-specific IgG values were measured in 18,012 Italian patients (74.1% women, mean age 44.5 ± 15.5 years). Table 1 shows the IgG concentration for each of the 44 food antigens tested in alphabetical order and the type of distribution observed. Most IgG distributions were asymmetrical. For food-specific IgG with a bimodal distribution, we indicate medians with an interquartile range of both modes. Due to exposure to different food antigens, the IgG concentrations were very low for foods that showed levels of IgG <1 U/mL, such as olives, peaches, tea, honey, red grapes, and zucchini. High levels were found for foods that showed concentrations of IgG >20 U/mL, such as processed cheese, cow milk, and common wheat. Notably, the IgG values with a bimodal distribution were higher compared with IgG values with an asymmetrical distribution.

Table 1. List of tested foods, median and interquartile range of corresponding immunoglobulin G (IgG) values, and type of frequency distribution. For food-related IgG with a bimodal distribution, the interquartile range of both modes is indicated.

Food–Antigen	IgG Levels U/mL	Distribution
Almonds	8.35 (4.55–14.25)	Asymmetrical
Aspergillus fumigatus	3.95 (1.63–10.75)	Asymmetrical
Barley	9.16 (5.06–15.36)	Asymmetrical
Barley malt	1.17 (0.55–2.54)	Asymmetrical
Buckwheat	6.99 (3.43–12.49)	Asymmetrical
Candida albicans	2.48 (0.97–7.00)	Asymmetrical
Canned tuna	3.24 (1.42–6.21)	Asymmetrical
Champignon mushrooms	4.05 (1.38–9.60)	Asymmetrical
Chicken	0.78 (0.29–1.60)	Asymmetrical
Corn	1.32 (0.67–2.51)	Asymmetrical
Eggs	8.63 (3.01–21.58)	Asymmetrical
Goat milk	8.18 (3.92–17.39)	Asymmetrical
Hazelnuts	5.19 (2.46–9.5)	Asymmetrical
Honey	0.07 (0.00–0.41)	Asymmetrical
Kamut	6.47 (3.87–11.27)	Asymmetrical
Kiwis	3.16 (1.55–6.72)	Asymmetrical
Lentils	0.65 (0.25–1.51)	Asymmetrical
Mozzarella cheese	8.71 (4.7–15.56)	Asymmetrical
Oats	1.97 (0.99–4.28)	Asymmetrical
Olives	0.01 (0.00–0.16)	Asymmetrical
Onion	0.71 (0.32–1.40)	Asymmetrical
Oranges	0.19 (0.02–0.79)	Asymmetrical
Parmesan cheese	8.77 (3.45–18.72)	Asymmetrical
Peaches	0.01 (0.00–0.16)	Asymmetrical
Peanuts	7.83 (4.28–13.71)	Asymmetrical
Porcini mushrooms	2.83 (1.1–7.08)	Asymmetrical
Potato	3.34 (1.56–6.30)	Asymmetrical
Red grapes	0.08 (0.00–0.50)	Asymmetrical
Rice	0.52 (0.10–1.48)	Asymmetrical
Ricotta cheese	13.71 (7.32–28.15)	Asymmetrical
Rye	1.28 (0.61–2.65)	Asymmetrical
Soy	0.97 (0.45–2.05)	Asymmetrical
Spinach	0.20 (0.01–0.97)	Asymmetrical
Tea	0.02 (0.00–0.19)	Asymmetrical
Tomato	3.94 (1.20–9.10)	Asymmetrical
Walnuts	0.41 (0.07–1.19)	Asymmetrical
Zucchini	0.08 (0.00–0.60)	Asymmetrical
Beer yeast	3.80 (1.87–6.81) 17.92 (9.01–30.36)	Bimodal
Common wheat	11.07 (7.95–14.61) 32.53 (24.83–41.21)	Bimodal
Cow milk	8.54 (4.68–13.10) 37.55 (27.60–49.70)	Bimodal
Durum wheat	12.04 (7.86–16.47) 34.64 (28.39–42.74)	Bimodal
Pork	1.17 (0.53–2.75) 10.74 (6.05–18.16)	Bimodal
Processed cheese	14.72 (8.86–21.90) 47.19 (38.76–58.96)	Bimodal
Spelt	6.42 (3.71–9.89) 23.46 (18.01–30.26)	Bimodal

Figure 1 shows four models with both asymmetrical and bimodal frequency distribution. We provide diagrams of food-specific IgG values of all 44 foods tested in the Supplementary Materials (Figure S1). Figure 2 shows the dendrogram produced from the results of the clustering algorithm, which identifies five food groups by the evaluation of food-specific IgG values (for every node $p < 0.001$). The first group includes foods with a high nickel content, such as tomato, kiwi fruit, peanuts, almonds, and buckwheat. Inside this group, a second cluster can be identified that includes wheat and associated grains such as Kamut, spelt, and barley. The third cluster includes dairy products (such as cow's and goat's milk as well as Parmesan, mozzarella, and ricotta cheese). The fourth one includes yeasts such as *Candida albicans* and *Saccharomyces cerevisiae* and porcini and champignon mushrooms. This cluster is likely connected to fermented foods. The last group contains roasted nuts (peanuts and almonds) and is probably correlated with heated and cooked oils.

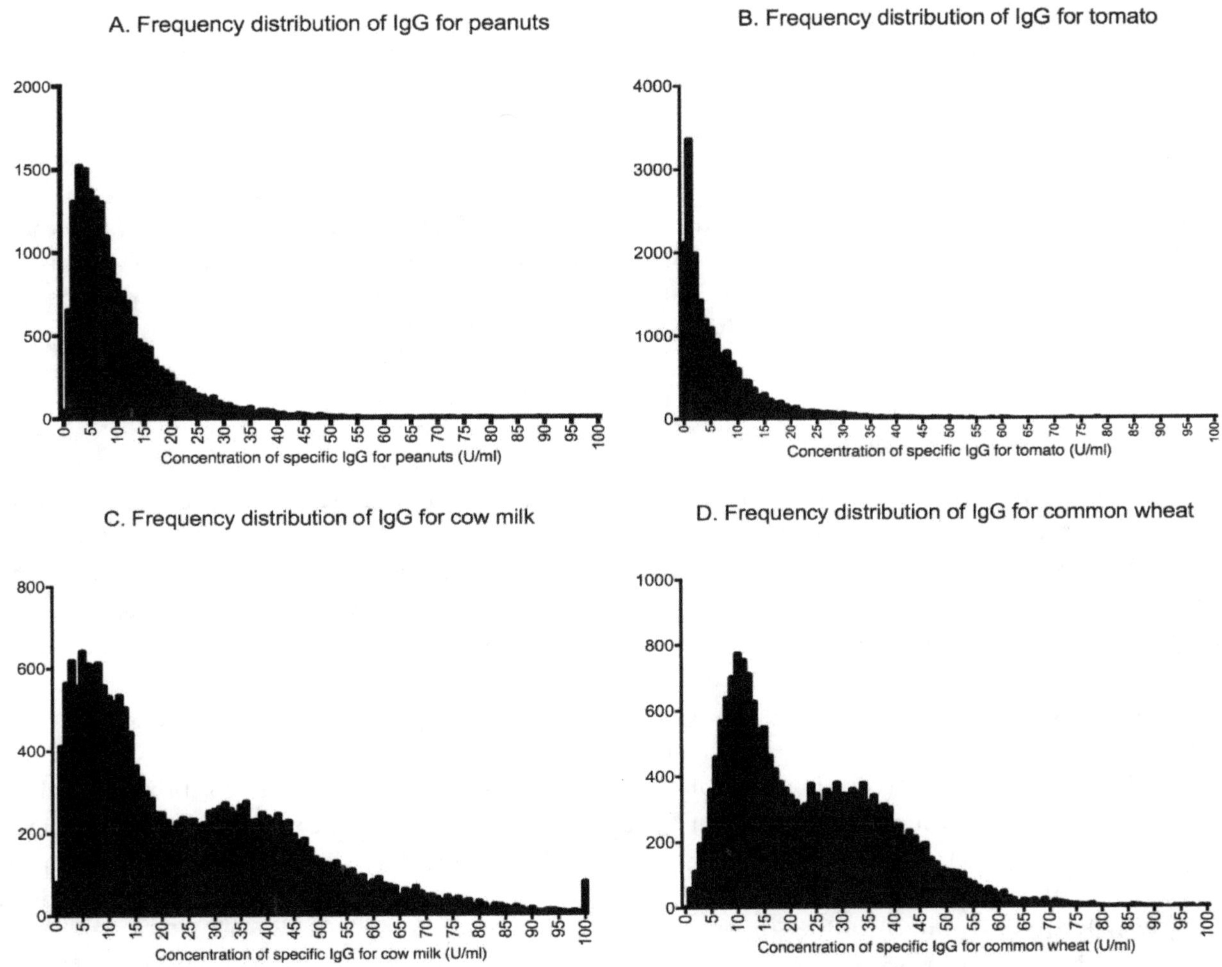

Figure 1. Examples of asymmetrical and bimodal distribution of frequencies for food-specific IgG. (**A**,**B**) Graphs showing two examples (for peanuts and tomato, respectively) of asymmetrical distribution of IgG. (**C**,**D**) Graphs showing two examples (for cow's milk and common wheat, respectively) of bimodal distribution of IgG.

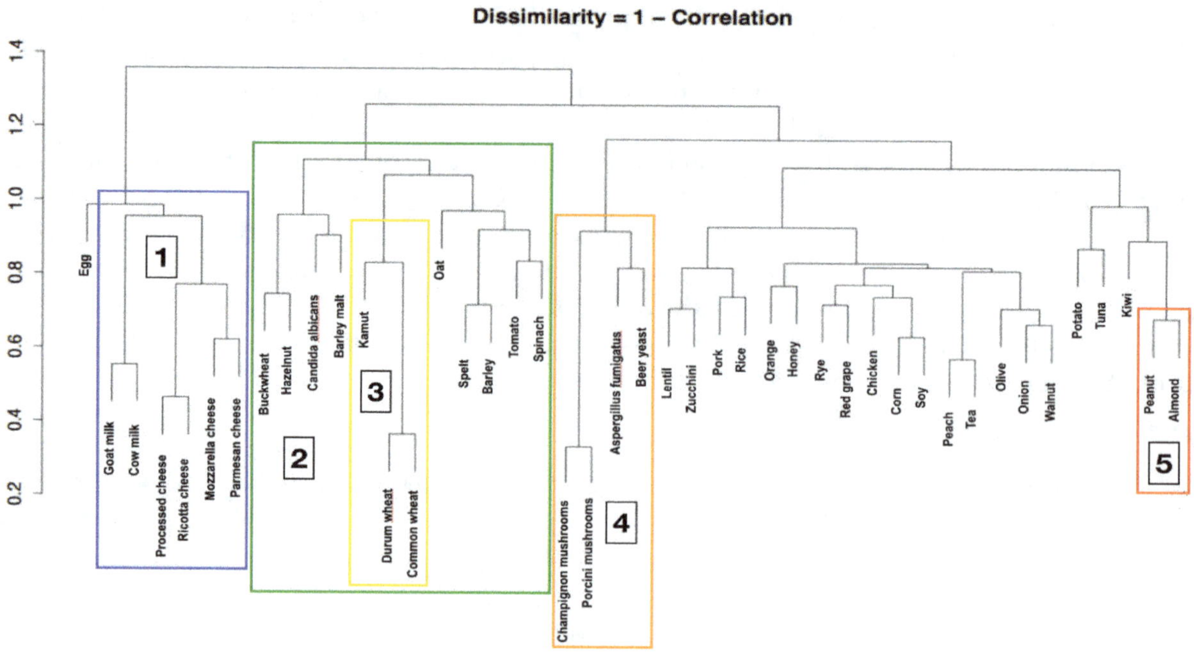

Figure 2. Dendrogram resulting from the clustering algorithm. It is possible to identify five large food clusters: (1) milk and dairy products, (2) foods with high content of nickel, (3) wheat-related grains, (4) fermented foods, and (5) roasted nuts and cooked oils (for every node $p < 0.001$). The bar on the left side of the dendrogram indicates the dissimilarity (1 – Correlation) for every node.

4. Discussion

4.1. Main Findings and Interpretation

The dendrogram obtained by the blind post-hoc matrix, correlated by similarity, allowed us to observe significant correlations between food-specific IgG antibodies that seem to correspond to typical Italian food habits [20–22]. Goat's and cow's milk, processed cheese, and mozzarella and Parmesan cheese were strongly correlated. The first node between processed cheese and ricotta cheese had the highest similarity. The second highest similarities were found via the dendrogram algorithm and were between mozzarella and Parmesan cheese and between goat's and cow's milk. These strict statistical similarities between IgG concentrations were found within dairy products. Such strict correlations, apparently biologically based, were also observed in yeasts (yeast and mushrooms) and in cereals containing gluten. The latter group is probably part of a larger cluster of foods containing nickel. The dendrogram algorithm also segregated a larger group of less strict correlations ranging at a dissimilarity level of 0.8 instead of the 0.3–0.5 dissimilarity level of the previously described clusters. A possible common denominator of these food-specific IgG could be represented by roasted nuts (peanuts and almonds), which are correlated with cooked oils.

The second relevant finding of this large cohort is represented by the distribution of the 44 food-specific IgG levels measured. As expected, the vast majority showed a modal distribution with a marked skewness toward lower concentrations. In eight of the food-specific IgG antibodies, the distribution was bimodal. These latter IgG levels showed significantly higher concentrations compared with IgG concentrations with mono-modal asymmetrical distribution. IgG levels for milk in this Italian population were among these bimodal distributions. The first Gaussian likely represents occasional consumers of milk and dairy products, whereas the second Gaussian reflects daily consumers. Although the use of dairy products is widespread in Italy, a large part of the adult Italian population does not consume milk regularly due to actual or suspected lactase non-persistence [23]. In contrast, the low concentration of specific IgG antibodies for peanuts reflects the nutritional habits of Italians, the vast majority of whom eat peanuts only occasionally.

The differences between IgG levels for different foods could be explained either by eating behaviors connected with increased or reduced intake or by the immunogenicity of the specific food antigen [1,2]. According to these tenets, the difference in the absolute values of IgG for consumers of large amounts of wheat (median concentration 18.22 U/mL) and for consumers of large amounts of honey (median concentration 0.07 U/mL) could be explained by intrinsic antigenic properties.

The production of food-specific IgG antibodies is directly related to the recurrent or prevalent intake of specific foods and can cause an immune reaction inducing, under specific conditions, an increase in inflammatory mediators [8]. The immune system does not specifically recognize foods by IgG, as in the case of IgE, but rather with an approach of similarity, identifying food antigen clusters that reflect the eating habits within different populations. According to this knowledge, the evaluation of the different distribution curves of IgG levels in the Italian population allows us to better understand the possible role of IgG production and how these antibodies can highlight a specific nutritional excess of a food cluster, suggesting a different dietary approach to inflammatory diseases. In agreement with Finkelman [6–8], the increased amount of contact with antigenic foods leads to the production of food-specific IgG for a large number of different foods, thus avoiding an absolute prevalence of a single specific antibody to a specific food group. With this information, the activation of a reasonable inflammatory response can be possibly prevented or modulated.

4.2. *Speculations and Further Hypothesis for Future Implications in Pregnancy and Lactation*

The influence of diet in pregnant women on the immune tolerance process is intricate. Thus, diet must be analyzed, not only from a compositional standpoint but also from an evolutionary point of view. Pregnancy symptoms, such as nausea and vomiting in the first trimester, might protect both the pregnant woman and the embryo from potentially harmful substances present in food [24], while, in the last trimester, cravings for food expose the fetus to a higher number of antigens and increase immune contact with the outside environment, yielding an immune imprinting. The fetus' immune knowledge of the outer world is guaranteed by the IgG produced by the mother. The IgG antibodies can cross the placental barrier and enter into the colostrum, and maternal IgG is amply present in breast milk. This justifies studying the immunological connection between food-specific IgG antibodies and the mother–fetus relationship [5]. This intrauterine information has allowed mammals to regard specific foods as sources of energy. The body knows if the food is sufficient for intimate contact with the organism and uses it as a nutrient.

4.3. *Strength and Limitations*

To the best of our knowledge, this is the first study of food-specific IgG involving thousands of subjects who have the same macro-ethnicity—Caucasians of Southern European ancestry—and who self-enrolled based on common gastro-enteric symptoms. Data on over 18,000 subjects were blindly analyzed by an independent third party that was unaware of the meaning of the codes attributed to each food-specific IgG. A major limitation of the statistical evidence observed is represented by the heterogeneity of the population recruited and by the fact that a direct correlation with different signs and symptoms was not available post hoc. However, the coherence of the distribution of IgG concentrations and the coherence of the clusters identified by the dendrogram algorithm with respect to the Italian food consumption profile allowed us to consider our findings genuine in the ongoing debate on food antigens and gastro-enteric IgG production, immune tolerance, and inflammation.

5. Conclusions

The dendrogram algorithm appeared to operate in a process resembling the immune system recognition of food antigens and similar related antigens. This finding allowed us to observe, confirm, and better specify the existence of five large clusters of different foods that appear to react in the same way to IgG antibodies.

Author Contributions: Conceptualization, G.P., E.F. and A.F.S.; Methodology, G.P. and A.F.S.; Software, G.P.; Validation, G.P., E.F. and A.F.S.; Formal Analysis, G.P.; Investigation, G.P., E.F. and A.F.S.; Resources, G.P.; Data Curation, G.P.; Writing—Original Draft Preparation, G.P. and A.F.S.; Writing—Review & Editing, G.P., E.F. and A.F.S.; Visualization, G.P.; Supervision, A.F.S.; Project Administration, G.P.; Funding Acquisition, A.F.S.

References

1. Ligaarden, S.C.; Lydersen, S.; Farup, P.G. IgG and IgG4 Antibodies in Subjects with Irritable Bowel Syndrome: A Case Control Study in the General Population. *BMC Gastroenterol.* **2012**, *12*, 166. [CrossRef]
2. Speciani, A.F.; Piuri, G.; Ferrazzi, E. IgG Levels to Food Correlate with Nutritional Exposure to Food Antigens but a Methodological Weakness of this Research Prevents the Recognition of Yeast-Related Foods as a Possible Cause of Irritable Bowel Syndrome (IBS). Comment to IgG and IgG4 Antibodies in Subjects with Irritable Bowel Syndrome: A Case Control Study in the General Population Solveig C Ligaarden*, Stian Lydersen and Per G Farup BMC Gastroenterology 2012, 12:166. *BMC Gastroenterol.* **2012**, *12*, 166.
3. Wisniewski, J.; Agrawal, R.; Woodfolk, J.A. Mechanisms of Tolerance Induction in Allergic Disease: Integrating Current and Emerging Concepts. *Clin. Exp. Allergy* **2013**, *43*, 164–176. [CrossRef]
4. Kolfschoten, M.V.D.N.; Schuurman, J.; Losen, M.; Bleeker, W.K.; Martinez, P.M.; Vermeulen, E.; Bleker, T.H.D.; Wiegman, L.; Vink, T.; Aarden, L.A.; et al. Anti-Inflammatory Activity of Human IgG4 Antibodies by Dynamic Fab Arm Exchange. *Science* **2007**, *317*, 1554–1557. [CrossRef] [PubMed]
5. Piuri, G. Individual Food Clusters Excess and Low-Grade Inflammation in Pregnancy. In *Metabolic Syndrome and Complications of Pregnancy*, 1st ed.; Ferrazzi, E., Sears, B., Eds.; Springer Science Publisher: New York, NY, USA; Heidelberg, Germany, 2015; pp. 23–33.
6. Finkelman, F.D. Anaphylaxis: Lessons from Mouse Models. *J. Allergy Clin. Immunol.* **2007**, *120*, 506–515. [CrossRef]
7. Khodoun, M.V.; Strait, R.; Armstrong, L.; Yanase, N.; Finkelman, F.D. Identification of Markers that Distinguish IgE-From IgG-Mediated Anaphylaxis. *Proc. Natl. Acad. Sci. USA* **2011**, *108*, 12413–12418. [CrossRef]
8. Finkelman, F.D.; Khodoun, M.V.; Strait, R. Human IgE-Independent Systemic Anaphylaxis. *J. Allergy Clin. Immunol.* **2016**, *137*, 1674–1680. [CrossRef] [PubMed]
9. Muñoz-Cano, R.; Picado, C.; Valero, A.; Bartra, J. Mechanisms of Anaphylaxis Beyond IgE. *J. Investig. Allergol. Clin. Immunol.* **2016**, *26*, 73–82. [CrossRef]
10. Fritscher-Ravens, A.; Schuppan, D.; Ellrichmann, M.; Schoch, S.; Röcken, C.; Brasch, J.; Bethge, J.; Böttner, M.; Klose, J.; Milla, P.J. Confocal Endomicroscopy Shows Food-Associated Changes in the Intestinal Mucosa of Patients with Irritable Bowel Syndrome. *Gastroenterology* **2014**, *147*, 1012–1020.e4. [CrossRef]
11. Bentz, S.; Hausmann, M.; Piberger, H.; Kellermeier, S.; Paul, S.; Held, L.; Falk, W.; Obermeier, F.; Fried, M.; Schölmerich, J.; et al. Clinical Relevance of IgG Antibodies against Food Antigens in Crohn's Disease: A Double-Blind Cross-Over Diet Intervention Study. *Digestion* **2010**, *81*, 252–264. [CrossRef]
12. Cai, C.; Shen, J.; Zhao, D.; Qiao, Y.; Xu, A.; Jin, S.; Ran, Z.; Zheng, Q. Serological Investigation of Food Specific Immunoglobulin G Antibodies in Patients with Inflammatory Bowel Diseases. *PLoS ONE* **2014**, *9*, e112154. [CrossRef] [PubMed]
13. Alpay, K.; Ertaş, M.; Orhan, E.K.; Üstay, D.K.; Lieners, C.; Baykan, B. Diet Restriction in Migraine, Based on IgG against Foods: A Clinical Double-Blind, Randomised, Cross-Over Trial. *Cephalalgia* **2010**, *30*, 829–837. [CrossRef]
14. Biesiekierski, J.R.; Newnham, E.D.; Irving, P.M.; Barrett, J.S.; Haines, M.; Doecke, J.D.; Shepherd, S.J.; Muir, J.G.; Gibson, P.R. Gluten Causes Gastrointestinal Symptoms in Subjects without Celiac Disease: A Double-Blind Randomized Placebo-Controlled Trial. *Am. J. Gastroenterol.* **2011**, *106*, 508–514. [CrossRef]
15. Kim-Lee, C.; Suresh, L.; Ambrus, J.L. Gastrointestinal Disease in Sjogren's Syndrome: Related to Food Hypersensitivities. *Springerplus* **2015**, *4*, 766. [CrossRef]
16. Shulman, R.J.; Eakin, M.N.; Czyzewski, D.I.; Jarrett, M.; Ou, C.-N. Increased Gastrointestinal Permeability and Gut Inflammation in Children with Functional Abdominal Pain and Irritable Bowel Syndrome. *J. Pediatr.* **2008**, *153*, 646–650. [CrossRef]
17. Clayton, F.; Fang, J.C.; Gleich, G.J.; Lucendo, A.J.; Olalla, J.M.; Vinson, L.A.; Lowichik, A.; Chen, X.;

Emerson, L.; Cox, K.; et al. Eosinophilic Esophagitis in Adults is Associated with IgG4 and not Mediated by IgE. *Gastroenterology* **2014**, *147*, 602–609. [CrossRef] [PubMed]

18. Thorburn, A.N.; Macia, L.; Mackay, C.R. Diet, Metabolites, and "Western-Lifestyle" Inflammatory Diseases. *Immunity* **2014**, *40*, 833–842. [CrossRef]
19. Eisen, M.B.; Spellman, P.T.; Brown, P.O.; Botstein, D. Cluster Analysis and Display of Genome-Wide Expression Patterns. *Proc. Natl. Acad. Sci. USA* **1998**, *95*, 14863–14868. [CrossRef] [PubMed]
20. Fatati, G. [Italian eating behavior: Survey 2011]. *Recenti Prog. Med.* **2012**, *103*, 225–233.
21. Pala, V.; Sieri, S.; Palli, D.; Salvini, S.; Berrino, F.; Bellegotti, M.; Frasca, G.; Tumino, R.; Sacerdote, C.; Fiorini, L.; et al. Diet in the Italian EPIC Cohorts: Presentation of Data and Methodological Issues. *Tumori J.* **2003**, *89*, 594–607. [CrossRef]
22. Riccioni, G.; Menna, V.; Di Ilio, C.; D'Orazio, N. Food-Intake and Nutrients Pattern in Italian Adult Male Subjects. *Clin. Ther.* **2004**, *155*, 283–286.
23. Hjartåker, A.; Lagiou, A.; Slimani, N.; Lund, E.; Chirlaque, M.D.; Vasilopoulou, E.; Zavitsanos, X.; Berrino, F.; Sacerdote, C.; Ocké, M.C.; et al. Consumption of Dairy Products in the European Prospective Investigation into Cancer and Nutrition (EPIC) Cohort: Data from 35 955 24-h Dietary Recalls in 10 European countries. *Public Health Nutr.* **2002**, *5*, 1259–1271. [CrossRef] [PubMed]
24. Sherman, P.W.; Flaxman, S.M. Nausea and Vomiting of Pregnancy in an Evolutionary Perspective. *Am. J. Obstet. Gynecol.* **2002**, *186*, S190–S197. [CrossRef] [PubMed]

14

Preconception and Prenatal Nutrition and Neurodevelopmental Disorders

Mengying Li, Ellen Francis, Stefanie N. Hinkle, Aparna S. Ajjarapu and Cuilin Zhang *

Division of Intramural Population Health Research, *Eunice Kennedy Shriver* National Institute of Child Health and Human Development, National Institutes of Health, Bethesda, MD 20817, USA

* Correspondence: zhangcu@mail.nih.gov

Abstract: Preconception and prenatal nutrition is critical for fetal brain development. However, its associations with offspring neurodevelopmental disorders are not well understood. This study aims to systematically review the associations of preconception and prenatal nutrition with offspring risk of neurodevelopmental disorders. We searched the PubMed and Embase for articles published through March 2019. Nutritional exposures included nutrient intake or status, food intake, or dietary patterns. Neurodevelopmental outcomes included autism spectrum disorders (ASD), attention deficit disorder-hyperactivity (ADHD) and intellectual disabilities. A total of 2169 articles were screened, and 20 articles on ASD and 17 on ADHD were eventually reviewed. We found an overall inverse association between maternal folic acid or multivitamin supplementation and children's risk of ASD; a meta-analysis including six prospective cohort studies estimated an RR of ASD of 0.64 (95% CI: 0.46, 0.90). Data on associations of other dietary factors and ASD, ADHD and related outcomes were inconclusive and warrant future investigation. Future studies should integrate comprehensive and more objective methods to quantify the nutritional exposures and explore alternative study design such as Mendelian randomization to evaluate potential causal effects.

Keywords: pregnancy nutrition; neurodevelopmental disorders; autism spectrum disorder; attention deficit disorder with hyperactivity; developmental origins of health and disease; systematic review; meta-analysis

---

1. Introduction

Maternal nutrition is critical for fetal brain development. Maternal diet prior to pregnancy is important for optimizing nutritional status which plays a vital role in maintaining a healthy pregnancy and supporting the developing fetus [1]. Nutrition around the time of conception is important for gamete function and placental development [2]. Starting 2–3 weeks after fertilization, the embryo undergoes orchestrated processes of neuronal proliferation and migration, synapse formation, myelination, and apoptosis to develop the fetal brain [3]. In this period of rapid development, the brain has heightened sensitivity to the environment, where perturbation may predispose the fetus to postnatal neurodevelopmental disorders [4,5]. Overall, supply of nutrients during the preconception and prenatal periods not only provides the basic building blocks for the brain [6], but may also "program" the brain through epigenetic mechanisms to confer risk or resilience to neurological conditions later in life [7]. The modifiable nature of maternal nutrition during sensitive periods potentially offers opportunities for intervention.

Several nutrients have previously been identified to have a critical role in prenatal neurodevelopment. For example, folate is an essential co-factor in one-carbon metabolism responsible for DNA and RNA synthesis and DNA methylation—processes that are particularly important during periods of rapid growth and development. Inadequate folate intake has been linked to altered DNA methylation [8,9] and compromised fetal brain development [10,11], particularly in animal studies. Preconception and early pregnancy supplementation of folic acid—the synthetic form of folate—was found effective in preventing neural tube defects [12]. In addition to folate, polyunsaturated fatty acids (PUFAs), particularly arachidonic acid (AA) of the omega-6 (n-6) family and docosahexaenoic acid (DHA) of the omega-3 (n-3) family, are structural components of neuronal membrane phospholipids and the myelin sheath insulating the neuronal axons [13]. PUFAs accumulate rapidly in the brain starting in the third trimester and continuing into early postnatal life [14], and the membrane PUFA composition is mainly dependent on maternal dietary supply of DHA [15]. Restriction of DHA and its precursors in the perinatal period negatively impact cognitive and behavioral outcomes in animal studies [16,17].

Some minerals are also known to play important roles in prenatal neurodevelopment. For example, iron is essential for the regulation of neuronal energy metabolism during development; deficiency affects the structure and function of fetal hippocampus, compromising learning and memory [18]. Similarly, iodine is necessary to produce thyroid hormones which regulate brain growth and development; deficiency during the prenatal period results in cognitive deficit [19]. While not a nutrient, caffeine, a psychoactive substance widely consumed through coffee and tea, improves alertness by blocking adenosine receptors in the brain. Prenatal and early postnatal exposure to caffeine alters brain neurochemistry and behavior in animal studies [20]. In addition to individual nutrients and substance, foods and dietary patterns may capture the combined and interactive effects of nutrients in prenatal neurodevelopment.

In the past decade, accumulating evidence from human epidemiological studies support the link between maternal nutrition and offspring cognitive and behavioral abilities [21–25]. Yet, it is unclear whether maternal nutrition is relevant to the risk of clinically defined neurodevelopmental disorders, which are characterized by deficits that produce impairments in daily functioning. A comprehensive and critical review of the evidence may shed light on the question. Limited studies previously reviewed evidence on maternal folic acid intake and offspring autism spectrum disorder (ASD) risk [26,27]; however, an updated review with a comprehensive critique of the evidence is needed. Furthermore, much of the evidence on maternal nutrition and offspring attention-deficit/hyperactivity disorder (ADHD) risk has not been reviewed. Lastly, critical questions regarding the most sensitive time windows (i.e., before vs. during pregnancy) for nutritional exposures remain unanswered. To address these critical knowledge gaps, we conducted a systematic review of epidemiologic studies examining the association of maternal nutrition before and during pregnancy with the risk of offspring neurodevelopmental disorders; we focused on dietary factors including supplements to inform potential public health interventions specific to maternal diet. To provide quantitative syntheses of evidence, we also performed meta-analyses whenever the data were available. A summary of proposed mechanisms in which preconception and prenatal nutrition affects risks of ASD and ADHD and relevant sensitive windows are presented in a schematic figure (Figure 1).

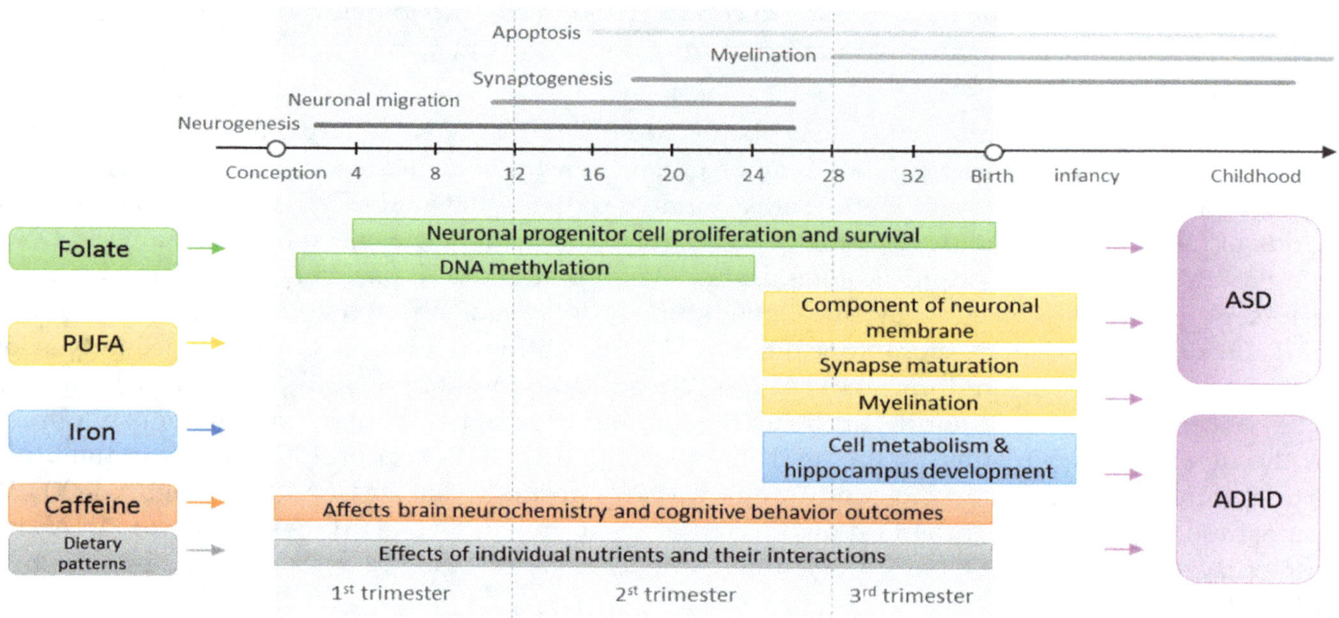

Figure 1. Proposed mechanisms in which preconception and prenatal nutrition affects the risk of autism spectrum disorder (ASD) and attention-deficit/hyperactivity disorder (ADHD). The neurodevelopmental timelines were adapted from the previous publications [3,28]. PUFA, polyunsaturated fatty acids.

2. Materials and Methods

2.1. Eligibility Criteria

The systematic review included studies investigating associations of nutrition before or during pregnancy with offspring major neurodevelopmental disorders, including ASD, ADHD, and intellectual disability (ID). Maternal nutrition was evaluated at multiple levels: nutrient intake, food intake, or dietary patterns. Clinical diagnosis, a positive screening outcome, or a continuous measure of the traits or symptoms of the disorder were considered as outcomes. The studies were conducted in human populations, of case-control, cohort, or experimental design, and published in the English language. Studies were excluded if the exposures were not reflective of maternal dietary intake, such as teratogens (e.g., alcohol), chemicals, certain circulating biomarkers that are not directly reflective of maternal intake (e.g., 25-hydroxyvitamin D and ferritin), biomarkers in umbilical cord blood, or dietary counseling without quantification of actual maternal diet. We also excluded studies where outcomes were not reflective of neurodevelopmental disorders (continuous measures of Intelligence quotient (IQ), or suboptimal IQ defined by a non-clinical cutoff), outcomes were secondary to structural birth defects (e.g., neural tube defect) or chromosomal disorders (e.g., Down Syndrome), relevant associations were not reported, or full-texts were not available. Other neurodevelopmental disorders (i.e., communication disorders, motor disorders, and specific learning disorders) were not covered in this review, as a pilot search found very few epidemiologic studies investigating these disorders in association with maternal nutrition.

2.2. Literature Search, Screening and Abstraction

We searched PubMed and Embase on 27 March 2019. Search strategies were developed a priori for each database with assistance from a librarian. The search targeted title, abstract, and subject headings. Search terms consisted of neurodevelopmental disorders (either the general term or specific terms for ASD, ID, or ADHD), nutrition (nutrients, foods, or dietary patterns), prenatal or preconception periods, and observational or experimental design, combined using the Boolean Operator "AND";

additional search terms were used to exclude animal studies. The search strategy and search history are presented in Table S1.

After the systematic search, we screened the title and abstract of the records for eligibility, and then assessed the full-text of the retained records for final inclusion decisions. We also examined the bibliographies of existing literature reviews on maternal nutrition and neurodevelopmental disorders to identify additional articles not covered in the systematic search. We abstracted relevant data in the included articles using a standardized form.

2.3. Meta-Analysis

We conducted meta-analyses of associations between specific nutritional exposures and neurodevelopmental outcomes whenever three or more relevant independent estimates were available. The analysis pooled relative risks (RRs) and odds ratios (ORs) estimated from cohort studies; OR is a reasonable approximation of RR in these studies as both ASD (prevalence 1–5%) [29] and ADHD (prevalence 5–10%) [30] are relatively rare. Estimates from case-control studies were not pooled with those from cohort studies due to differences in study design and retrospective recall of the nutritional exposures in these studies (all the case-control studies are retrospective); sensitivity analysis including estimates from the case-control studies did not change the findings substantively. Estimates of hazard ratio were not pooled with the RRs, as it is a conceptually different measure [31]. Pooled effect sizes were estimated using DerSimonian and Laird random-effects model. Studies reporting the diagnosis and the screening outcomes of neurodevelopmental disorders were meta-analyzed separately. Attempts were made to separate the effects of specific nutrients from multivitamins, and between exposures at different time periods (e.g., before pregnancy and during pregnancy), whenever possible. The meta-analysis was performed in Stata version 14 (StataCorp LLC, College Station, TX, USA) [32].

2.4. Quality Assessment

While generic tools to evaluate the quality of observational studies exists, these tools may not sufficiently address the methodological concerns important for the topic of interest and the type of studies included. As such, we critiqued the methodological quality of the included studies throughout the narrative review whenever relevant. We also discussed common issues across exposures and outcomes in a separate section following the reviews, with an emphasis for future directions.

3. Results and Commentary

A total of 2167 unique records were obtained from the systematic literature search. After screening the titles and abstracts, 102 relevant records remained. After the full-text review, 36 articles were included. Two additional articles were identified from the bibliographies of existing literature reviews, resulting in a total of 38 studies. Overall, 20 studies reported outcomes related to ASD, 17 ADHD, and 1 ID (Figure 2). The following review focuses on ASD and ADHD. Exposures in these studies included vitamins and minerals (i.e., folate, iron, calcium, and iodine), fatty acids (i.e., PUFA), foods (i.e., fish, fruits), supplements (i.e., multivitamins), and dietary patterns. Nutrients intake or status were grouped together with relevant food sources (e.g., folate with multivitamins, PUFA with seafood) to facilitate the interpretation of the findings. Nutrients or foods reported only in a single study were not reviewed below.

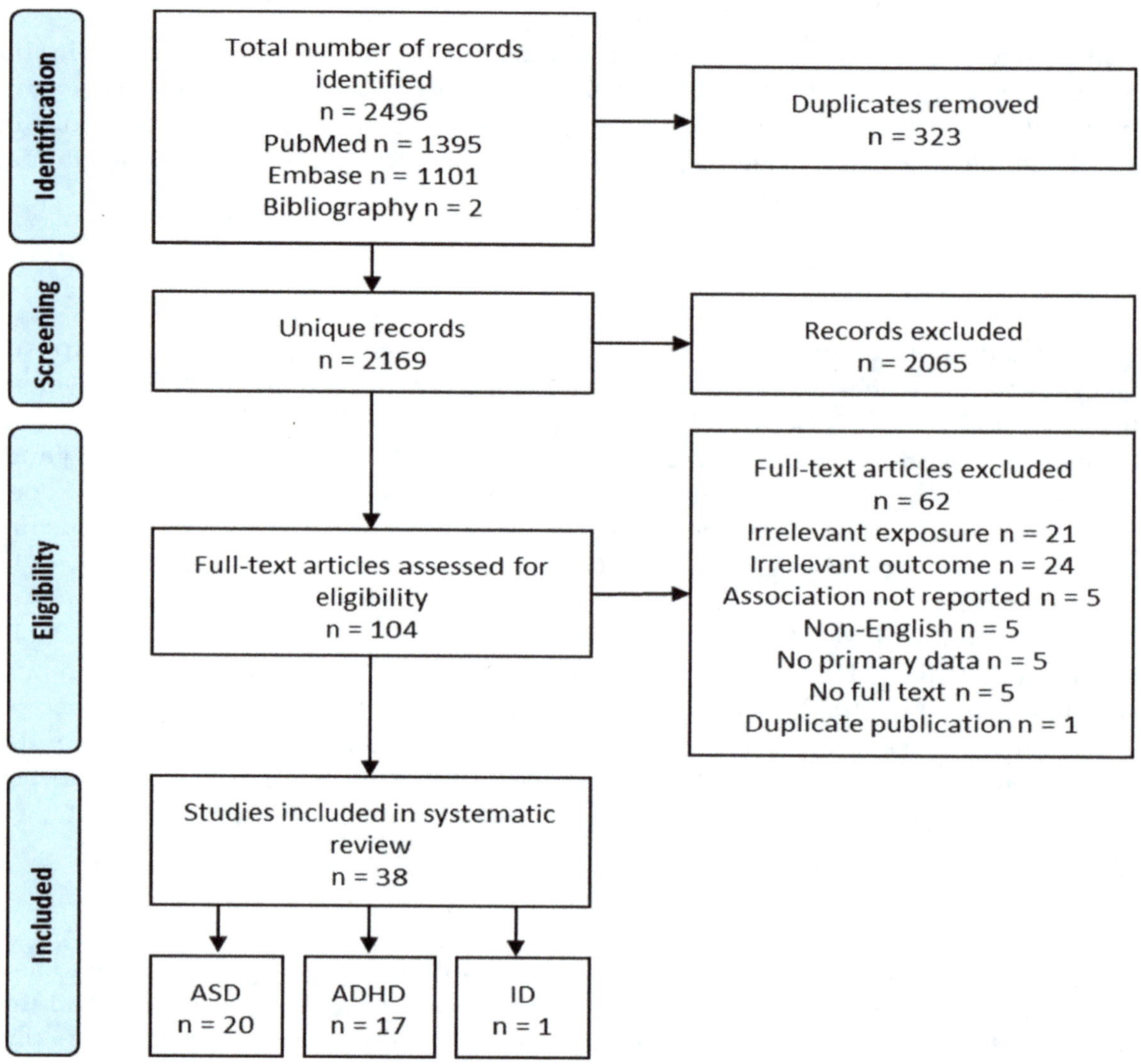

Figure 2. Flow diagram of study selection process, intellectual disability (ID).

3.1. Maternal Nutrition and ASD Risk

The characteristics and main findings of the studies on the associations between maternal nutrition and ASD are presented in Table 1. Of the 20 studies, 14 are prospective study and 6 are retrospective studies. These studies were conducted in the USA, Denmark, Norway, Sweden, The Netherlands, Spain, Israel, and China.

Table 1. Studies on maternal nutrition and offspring ASD risk or traits.

Source (Country)	Design & Sample	Maternal Exposures	Offspring Outcomes	Findings	Covariates
Vitamins and Minerals					
Folate and Multivitamin-ASD Diagnosis or Cutoff					
Schmidt et al. 2019 (USA) [33]	Prospective cohort; 332 children who were younger sibling of children with ASD in the MARBLES study	Vitamin and supplement use for the 6 months preconception and each month during the pregnancy assessed in interviews in the first and second halves of pregnancy and after birth	ASD assessed by ADOS at 3 years of age	Prenatal vitamin in the first month of pregnancy was associated with lower ASD risk (RR = 0.50, 95% CI: 0.30 to 0.81) *. Folic acid supplement ≥600 mcg/day in the first month of pregnancy was associated with lower ASD risk (RR = 0.38, 95% CI: 0.16, 0.90) *	Maternal education. The folic acid model further adjusted for iron intake
Levine et al. 2018 (Israel) [34]	Prospective cohort; 45,300 children	Intake of folic acid and multivitamin supplements before and during pregnancy was coded using ATC from the prescription registry	ASD diagnosis identified from health care registers from the Meuhedet health care organization; children were 10 years old	Folic acid and/or multivitamin both before (RR = 0.39, 95% CI: 0.30, 0.50) * and during (RR = 0.27, 95% CI: 0.22, 0.33) * pregnancy were associated with lower risk of ASD. Results on folic acid supplements and multivitamin as two separate exposures were consistent with the main findings	sex, birth year, socioeconomic status, a maternal and paternal psychiatric diagnosis by childbirth, maternal and paternal age at childbirth, and parity
Li et al. 2018 (China) [35]	Retrospective case-control; 374 ASD and 354 TD in the ACED	Food preference and supplement use preconception and during pregnancy assessed 3–6 years after delivery	ASD identified from special education schools; TD identified from ordinary schools; children were 3–6 years of age	Maternal folic acid supplementation before pregnancy was not associated with ASD risk (OR = 0.95, 95% CI: 0.61, 1.50); Maternal folic acid supplementation during pregnancy was associated with lower ASD risk (OR = 0.64, 95% CI: 0.41, 1.00) *	Child's and parental age, child's gender, parental education, maternal BMI before conception and delivery, premature delivery, and intake of other supplements

Table 1. *Cont.*

Source (Country)	Design & Sample	Maternal Exposures	Offspring Outcomes	Findings	Covariates
Raghavan et al. 2018 (USA) [36]	Prospective cohort; 1257 children in the Boston Birth Cohort	Multivitamin supplement intake before pregnancy and in each trimester assessed 1–3 days after delivery; plasma folate and vitamin B12 levels measured 1–3 days after delivery	ASD identified from electronic medical records in Boston Medical Center	Before pregnancy, multivitamin supplement was not associated with ASD risk (HR = 0.5, 95% CI: 0.1, 2.1). In the first trimester, ≤2 (HR = 3.4, 95% CI: 1.6, 7.2) * and >5 (HR = 2.3, 95% CI: 1.2, 3.6) * times/week of multivitamin supplement were both associated with higher risk of ASD compared to 3–5 times/day. Findings are similar at second and third trimester. Very high serum folate (HRs [95% CI] for decile 1 and 10 vs. the rest were 1.2 [0.5, 2.8] and 2.5 [1.3, 4.6]) * and vitamin B12 (HRs [95% CI] for decile 1 and 10 vs. the rest were 0.7 [0.3, 1.7] and 2.5 [1.4, 4.5]) * concentrations were both associate with higher ASD risk.	Maternal age, education, parity, BMI, smoking status, diabetes status, race, and *MTHFR* genotype, offspring gestational age, sex, and year of birth
Strom et al. 2018 (Denmark) [37]	Prospective cohort; 92,676 children in the DNBC	Folic acid supplementation and folate intake from food in the previous 4 weeks assessed by FFQ at GW 25	ASD cases identified in Danish Central Psychiatric Research Registry and the Danish National Patients Registry	Folic acid supplement at GW −4 to 8 was not associated with ASD risk (HR = 1.04, 95% CI: 0.94, 1.19). Folic acid supplement in mid pregnancy was not associated with ASD risk (HRs [95% CI] for <400 and ≥400 mcg/day vs. no intake was 1.01 [0.76, 1.34] and 0.98 [0.75, 1.29]). Folate from food was not associated with SD risk (HRs [95% CI] for quintile 2–5 were 0.82 [0.67, 1.01], 0.96 [0.78, 1.17], 0.85 [0.69, 1.04] and 0.94 [0.77, 1.16])	Maternal age, paternal age, parity, maternal smoking during pregnancy, maternal education, family socioeconomic status, whether the pregnancy was planned, maternal prepregnancy BMI and sex of the child

Table 1. *Cont.*

Source (Country)	Design & Sample	Maternal Exposures	Offspring Outcomes	Findings	Covariates
DeVilbiss et al. 2017 (Sweden) [38]	Prospective cohort; 273,107 children in the Stockholm youth cohort	Supplement use at the first antenatal visit coded in ATC from medical birth registry	ASD identified from computerized registers covering all pathways of ASD diagnosis and care in Stockholm County; children were 4–15 years old	Multivitamin supplement was associated with lower risk of ASD compared to no vitamin/mineral supplement (OR = 0.89, 95% CI: 0.82, 0.97) *. Folic acid supplement alone (OR = 1.27, 95% CI: 1.01, 1.60), iron supplement alone (0.96, 95% CI: 0.90, 1.03) and combined folic acid and iron supplement (OR = 0.92, 0.83 to 1.02) were not associated with ASD risk	Child characteristics (sex, birth year, and years resided in Stockholm County), socioeconomic indicators (education, family income, and maternal birth country), maternal characteristics (age, BMI, parity, smoking status), medication use during pregnancy (antidepressants or antiepileptics), and maternal neuropsychiatric conditions (anxiety disorders, autism, bipolar disorder, depression, epilepsy, intellectual disability, non-affective psychotic disorders, and stress disorders)
Virk et al. 2016 (Denmark) [39]	Prospective cohort; 35,059 children in the DNBC	Folic acid and multivitamin supplementations from 4 weeks preconception to GW 8 assessed by questionnaire at GW 12	ASD identified from National Hospital Register; children were 10 years of age	Folic acid supplement at GW −4 to 8 was not associated with ASD risk (RR = 1.06, 95% CI: 0.82, 1.36). Multivitamin supplement was not associated with ASD risk (RR = 1.00, 95% CI: 0.82, 1.22)	Maternal age; maternal smoking and alcohol consumption during pregnancy; household socioeconomic status-examined more but none changed estimates more than 5%
Braun et al. 2014 (USA) [40]	Prospective cohort; 209 children in the HOMA study	Current vitamin supplementation assessed by interviews at GW 14–39; whole blood folate concentrations measured at GW 11–21	Autistic-behaviors assessed by SRS at 4–5 years of age; scores >60 were defined as abnormal	Vitamin supplementation was associated with lower risk of failed SRS test (weekly/daily vs. never/rare intake: OR = 0.26, 95% CI: 0.08, 0.89) *. Whole blood folate concentrations were not associated with ASD risk (OR per SD = 1.42, 95% CI: 0.81, 2.49)	Whole blood folate concentration, maternal age, race, education, household income, marital status, employment during pregnancy, insurance status, depressive symptoms, serum cotinine concentrations, food security, and fresh fruit/vegetable intake
Nilsen et al. 2013 (Norway) [41]	Prospective cohort; 89,836 children in the MoBa	Folic acid intake before and/or during pregnancy recorded in Medical Birth Registry of Norway	ASD identified in Norwegian Patient Registry; all children were 3 years of older	Folic acid supplement was associated with lower ASD risk (OR = 0.86, 95% CI: 0.78, 0.95) *	Year of birth, maternal age, paternal age, marital status, and parity, hospital size

Table 1. *Cont.*

Source (Country)	Design & Sample	Maternal Exposures	Offspring Outcomes	Findings	Covariates
Suren et al. 2013 (Norway) [42]	Prospective cohort; 85,176 children in the MoBa	Folic acid and other supplementations from 4 weeks preconception to GW 8 assessed by questionnaire at GW 12	ASD identified through questionnaire screening at 3, 5 and 7 years, professional and parental referral, and the Norwegian Patient Registry when children were 3–10 years of age	Folic acid supplement was associated with lower ASD risk (OR = 0.61, 95% CI: 0.41, 0.90) *. Supplements with folic acid were associated with lower ASD risk, supplements without folic acid were not	Adjusted for year of birth, maternal education level, and parity
DeSoto et al. 2012 (USA) [43]	Retrospective case-control; 256 ASD and 752 TD in the Vaccine Safety Datalink project	Folic acid intake from prenatal vitamins	ASD identified based on medical record	Folic acid supplement/prenatal multivitamin was associated with higher ASD risk (OR = 2.34, 95% CI: 1.14, 4.82) *	Child and family characteristics (e.g., maternal age, birth weight, poverty ratio, birth order, breast feeding duration), maternal prenatal health care/seeking behavior (e.g., adequacy of prenatal care, cholesterol screen, pap smear, prenatal alcohol use, prenatal viral infections), and child medical conditions (e.g., anemia, pica)
Schmidt et al. 2012 (USA) [44]	Retrospective case-control; 429 ASD and 278 TD in CHARGE study	Folic acid intake from supplements and fortified cereals in each month from 3 months before conception to delivery assessed by interviews at 2–5 years after delivery	ASD identified from the California Regional Center System; matched TD identified from state birth files; children were 2 to 5 years old	Higher folic acid intake in the first trimester was associated with lower ASD risk (ORs [95% CI] for <500, 500–799, 800–1000 and >1000 mcg/day vs. no intake were 0.35 [0.10 1.24], 0.27 [0.06 1.36], 0.25 [0.05 1.22] and 0.18 [0.04 0.94]) *	Adjusted for maternal educational level, child's birth year, and log-transformed total iron and vitamin E from supplements and cereals; estimates were not substantially different when further adjusted for log-transformed vitamin B-12, vitamin B-6, vitamin C, vitamin D, or calcium from supplements and cereals or when adjusted for prenatal vitamin use in the first month of pregnancy
Schmidt et al. 2011 (USA) [45]	Retrospective case-control; 288 Autism and 278 TD in CHARGE study	Vitamin use in each month from 3 months before conception to delivery assessed by interviews at 2–5 years after delivery	Autism identified from the California Regional Center System; matched TD identified from state birth files; children were 2 to 5 years old	Prenatal vitamin supplement was associated with lower autism risk (OR [95% CI] for any use was 0.61 [0.39, 0.97]; ORs [95% CI] for irregular or <4 days/week, 4 days/week-daily, and > daily vs. no use were 0.96 [0.18–5.0], 0.61 [0.38–0.98] and 0.51 [0.19–1.4], p-trend = 0.002) * Multivitamin supplement was not associated with ASD risk [OR 1.2, 95% CI [0.51, 2.60]).	Maternal education and the child's year of birth

Table 1. *Cont.*

Source (Country)	Design & Sample	Maternal Exposures	Offspring Outcomes	Findings	Covariates
		Folate and multivitamin-ASD traits			
Steenweg-de Graaff et al. 2015 (The Netherlands) [46]	Prospective cohort; 3893 children in the Generation R study	Plasma folate concentrations at GW 10–17; folic acid supplementation from preconception to early pregnancy assessed by questionnaire early in pregnancy	Autistic traits using the SRS short form at 6 years of age; scores >95th percentile defined as abnormality	Folic acid supplement starting before pregnancy (beta per SD = −0.042, 95% CI: −0.068, −0.017) *, before GW 10 (beta per SD = −0.041, 95% CI: −0.066, -0.016) *, and after GW 10 (beta per SD = −0.057, 95% CI: −0.089, −0.025) * in pregnancy were all associated with fewer autistic traits. Higher serum folate concentration was not associated with fewer autistic traits (beta per SD = −0.007, 95% CI: −0.016, 0.001), nor the risk of being a probable ASD case (OR per SD = 1.03, 95% CI: 0.76, 1.39).	Gestational age at venipuncture, gender and age of the child, maternal psychopathology, education and family income
		Iron-ASD diagnosis or cutoff			
Schmidt et al. 2019 (USA) [33]	Prospective cohort; 332 children who were younger sibling of children with ASD in the MARBLES	Vitamin and supplement use for the 6 months preconception and each month during the pregnancy assessed in interviews in the first and second halves of pregnancy and after birth	ASD assessed by ADOS at 3 years of age	Iron supplement in the first month of pregnancy was not associated with ASD risk (RR = 1.47, 95% CI: 0.61, 3.55)	Maternal education and folic acid supplement
DeVilbiss et al. 2017 (Sweden) [38]	Prospective cohort; 273,107 children in the Stockholm Youth Cohort	Supplement use at the first antenatal visit coded in ATC from medical birth registry	ASD identified from computerized registers covering all pathways of ASD diagnosis and care in Stockholm County; children were 4–15 years old	Folic acid supplement alone (OR = 1.27, 95% CI: 1.01, 1.60), iron supplement alone (OR = 0.96, 95% CI: 0.90 to 1.03) and combined folic acid and iron supplement (OR = 0.92, 95% CI: 0.83, 1.02) were not associated with ASD risk	Child characteristics (sex, birth year, and years resided in Stockholm County), socioeconomic indicators (education, family income, and maternal birth country), maternal characteristics (age, body mass index, parity, smoking status), medication use during pregnancy (antidepressants or antiepileptics), and maternal neuropsychiatric conditions (anxiety disorders, autism, bipolar disorder, depression, epilepsy, intellectual disability, non-affective psychotic disorders, and stress disorders)

Table 1. *Cont.*

Source (Country)	Design & Sample	Maternal Exposures	Offspring Outcomes	Findings	Covariates
Schmidt et al. 2014 (USA) [47]	Retrospective case-control; 520 ASD and 346 TD in CHARGE study	Iron supplementation in each month from 3 months before conception to delivery assessed by interviews at 2–5 years after delivery	ASD identified from the California Regional Center System; matched TD identified from state birth files; children were 2 to 5 years old	Iron-specific supplement before and during pregnancy was not associated with ASD risk (ORs [95% CI] for gestational months −3 to 9 were 0.89 [0.19, 4.13], 0.89 [0.19, 4.13], and 0.78 [0.21, 2.84], 0.67 [0.29, 1.55], 0.72 [0.37, 1.39], 0.71 [0.40, 1.27], 0.64 [0.39, 1.04], 0.65 [0.41, 1.04], 0.66 [0.43, 1.02], 0.73 [0.48, 1.13], 0.77 [0.49, 1.20] and 0.64 [0.39, 1.03]). Total iron supplement before and during pregnancy were not associated with ASD risk	Maternal folic acid intake, home ownership, child's birth year. The model on total iron supplement was adjusted for folic acid
Calcium-ASD diagnosis or cutoff					
Li et al. 2018 (China) [35]	Retrospective case-control; 374 ASD and 354 TD in the ACED	food preference and supplement use preconception and during pregnancy assessed 3–6 years after delivery	ASD identified from special education schools; TD identified from ordinary schools; children were 3–6 years of age	Maternal calcium supplementation before pregnancy was associated with lower ASD risk (OR = 0.48, 95% CI: 0.28, 0.84) *; during pregnancy, it was not associated with ASD risk (OR = 1.11, 95% CI: 0.70, 1.75)	Child's and parental age, child's gender, parental education, maternal BMI before conception and delivery, premature delivery, and intake of other supplement
PUFA and seafood					
PUFA-ASD diagnosis or cutoff					
Lyall et al. 2013 (USA) [48]	Prospective cohort; 18,045 children in NHSII	Fat intake before pregnancy reported in the year assessed by FFQ after delivery	Autism, Asperger Syndrome, or PDD diagnosis reported by mothers at 4 years of age	Higher total PUFA from food (RRs [95% CI] for quartile 2–4 were 0.74 [0.55, 1.00], 0.73 [0.54, 0.99] and 0.77 [0.47, 1.26], *p*-trend = 0.05) * was associated with lower ASD risk. Total n-3 PUFA (0.98 [0.73, 1.32], 0.78 [0.57, 1.06] and 0.90 [0.66, 1.22], *p*-trend = 0.12), ALA (0.91 [0.67, 1.23], 0.86 [0.64, 1.16] and 0.80 [0.58, 1.08], *p*-trend = 0.14), EPA (1.11 [0.80, 1.54], 1.13 [0.79, 1.61] and 1.07 [0.76, 1.51], p-trend = 0.97), and DHA (1.05 [0.78, 1.42], 0.95 [0.69, 1.31] and 1.07 [0.79, 1.45], *p*-trend = 0.74) from food were not associated with ASD risk. Total n-6 PUFA (1.01 [0.75, 1.36], 1.01 [0.75, 1.36] and 0.66 [0.47, 0.92], *p*-trend = 0.01) * and LA (1.01 [0.76, 1.35], 0.86 [0.64, 1.16], 0.86 [0.64, 1.16] and 0.66 [0.48, 0.92], *p*-trend = 0.008) * from food were associated with lower ASD risk; AA (0.98 [0.73, 1.32], 0.78 [0.57, 1.06] and 0.79 [0.58, 1.09], *p*-trend = 0.09) were not associated with ASD risk	Adjusted for total energy intake, maternal age, child's year of birth, income level, race, body mass index, and prepregnancy smoking status. Removal of adjustment for smoking did not affect results. Additional adjustment for intake of protein, whole grains, alcohol, fruit, and vegetables, as well as for multivitamin use, physical activity, child birth order, and maternal pregnancy complications did not materially alter the results

Table 1. *Cont.*

Source (Country)	Design & Sample	Maternal Exposures	Offspring Outcomes	Findings	Covariates
			PUFA-ASD traits		
Steenweg-De Graaff et al. 2016 (The Netherlands) [49]	Prospective cohort; 4624 children in the Generation R study	Plasma fatty acid profiles measured before GW 25	Autistic traits assessed by SRS at 6 years of age	N-3 PUFA percentage was not associated with autistic trait (beta per SD = −0.002, 95% CI: −0.011, 0.006). Higher n-6 PUFA percentage was associated with fewer autistic traits (beta per SD = 0.011, 95% CI: 0.002, 0.020) *. Higher n-3 to n-6 ratio was associated with fewer autistic traits (beta per SD = −0.009, 95% CI: −0.017, −0.001) *	Gestational age at venipuncture, sex, and age of the child at assessment, maternal IQ, prepregnancy body mass index, educational level, national origin, age at enrollment, psychopathology score in mid-pregnancy, smoking, alcohol consumption, and folic acid supplement use during pregnancy, family income, child day-care attendance, and paternal educational level, national origin, and psychopathology score
			Seafood-ASD diagnosis or cutoff		
Gao et al. 2016 (China) [50]	Retrospective case-control; 108 ASD and 108 TD	Fish intake 6 months before pregnancy until delivery, assessed by FFQ 4–17 years after delivery	ASD identified from the registry of special education schools; matched TD identified from ordinary schools; children were 4–17 years old	Maternal no habit of eating grass carp was associated with higher risk of ASD (OR = 3.59, 95% CI: 1.22, 10.51) *	Maternal habit of eating grass carp, parental habit of eating hairtail, income level at childbirth, current income level. Paternal education, maternal education; matched on child age and sex
Lyall et al. 2013 (USA) [48]	Prospective cohort; 18,045 children in NHSII	Fish intake before pregnancy reported in the year assessed by FFQ after delivery	Autism, Asperger Syndrome, or PDD diagnosis reported by mothers at 4 years of age	Fish intake was not associated with ASD risk (RR [95% CI] for <1, 1 and >1 time/week were 1.10 [0.73, 1.66], 0.99 [0.65, 1.50] and 1.02 [0.59, 1.75])	Adjusted for total energy intake, maternal age, child's year of birth, income level, race, body mass index, and prepregnancy smoking status. Removal of adjustment for smoking did not affect results. Additional adjustment for intake of protein, whole grains, alcohol, fruit, and vegetables, as well as for multivitamin use, physical activity, child birth order, and maternal pregnancy complications did not materially alter the results

Table 1. *Cont.*

Source (Country)	Design & Sample	Maternal Exposures	Offspring Outcomes	Findings	Covariates
			Seafood-ASD traits		
Julvez et al. 2016 (Spain) [51]	Prospective cohort; 1589 children in the INMA study	Seafood intake in the first trimester assessed by interviews with FFQ at GW 10–13	Autism spectrum traits assessed by the Childhood Asperger Syndrome Test based on parent report at 5 years of age	Higher total seafood intake was associated with fewer autistic traits (beta [95% CI] for quintile 2–5 vs. 1 were −0.42 [−0.90, 0.07], −0.45 [−0.95, 0.05], -0.61 [−1.12, −0.11], and −0.55 [−1.06, −0.04], *p*-trend = 0.04) *. Large fatty fish and lean fish were both associated with fewer autistic traits, whereas small fatty fish and shellfish were not associated	Sex of the child, age during testing, cohort, quality of the test, and maternal energy intake during pregnancy, child's birth weight, gestational age, duration of breastfeeding, maternal age, educational level, social class, prepregnancy body mass index, parity, and country of origin/birth
Steenweg-De Graaff et al. 2016 (The Netherlands) [49]	Prospective cohort; 4624 children in the Generation R study	Fish intake in the past 3 months assessed by FFQ in early pregnancy	Autistic traits assessed by SRS at 6 years of age	Fish intake was not associated with autistic trait (beta = −0.022, 95% CI: −0.055, 0.010)	Gestational age at venipuncture, sex, and age of the child at assessment, maternal IQ, prepregnancy body mass index, educational level, national origin, age at enrollment, psychopathology score in mid-pregnancy, smoking, alcohol consumption, and folic acid supplement use during pregnancy, family income, child day-care attendance, and paternal educational level, national origin, and psychopathology score
			Fish oil-ASD diagnosis or cutoff		
Suren et al. 2013 (Norway) [42]	Prospective cohort; 85,176 children in the MoBa	Folic acid and other supplementations from GW −4 to 8 weeks assessed by questionnaire at GW 12	ASD identified through questionnaire screening at 3, 5 and 7 years, professional and parental referral, and the Norwegian Patient Registry when children were 3–10 years of age	Fish oil supplement at GW −4 to 8 was not associated with ASD risk (OR = 1.29, 95% CI: 0.88, 1.89)	Adjusted for year of birth, maternal education level, and parity

Table 1. *Cont.*

Source (Country)	Design & Sample	Maternal Exposures	Offspring Outcomes	Findings	Covariates
Fruit					
Fruit-ASD diagnosis or cutoff					
Gao et al. 2016 (China) [50]	Retrospective case-control; 108 ASD and 108 TD	Fruit intake 6 months before pregnancy until delivery, assessed by FFQ 4–17 years after delivery	ASD identified from the registry of special education schools; matched TD identified from ordinary schools; children were 4–17 years old	Maternal no habit of eating fruits was associated with higher risk of ASD (OR = 2.42, 95% CI: 1.24, 4.73) *	maternal habit of eating grass carp, parental habit of eating hairtail, income level at childbirth, current income level. Paternal education, maternal education; frequency matched on child age and sex
Dietary patterns					
Dietary patterns-ASD diagnosis or cutoff					
House et al. 2018 (USA) [52]	Prospective cohort; 325 children in the NEST study	adherence to Mediterranean diet periconception assessed by FFQ in the first trimester of pregnancy or at enrollment	ASD index from ITSEA administered by a parent, caregiver or staff at 1–2 years of age	Adherence to Mediterranean diet was associated with lower ASD risk (ORs [95% CI] for tertile 2 and 3 vs. 1 were 0.46 [0.23, 0.90] and 0.35 [0.15, 0.80]) *. However, the trend was not significant after FDA adjustment ($p = 0.09$)	Breastfeeding at least 3 months, age of child at behavioral assessment, maternal fiber intake, total calories, folate, education, diabetes, obesity, smoking, and age, as well as paternal age and child parity, premature birth, weight, race, and child sex
Li et al. 2018 (China) [35]	Retrospective case-control; 374 ASD and 354 TD in the ACED	"Mostly meat", "mostly vegetable" or "both meat and vegetable" dietary patterns assessed in questionnaires 3–6 years after delivery	ASD identified from special education schools; TD identified from ordinary schools; children were 3–6 years of age	Before pregnancy, maternal mostly meat (OR = 4.01, 95% CI:1.08, 14.89) * and mostly vegetable dietary pattern (OR = 2.23, 95% CI: 1.01, 4.95) * were both associated with higher ASD risk compared to both meat and vegetable dietary pattern. During pregnancy, they were not associated with ASD risk (ORs [95% CI] were 1.36 [0.29, 6.32] and 1.20 [0.53, 2.68])	Child's and parental age, child's gender, parental education, maternal BMI before conception and delivery, premature delivery, and other maternal dietary patterns

* Statistically significant findings (p-Value < 0.05). Abbreviates of research studies: ACED—Autism Clinical and Environmental Database; CHARGE—Childhood Autism Risks from Genetics and the Environment; DNBC—Danish National Birth Cohort; HOME—Health Outcomes and Measures of the Environment; INMA—INfancia y Medio Ambiente; ITSEA—Infant Toddler Social Emotional Assessment; MARBLES—Markers of Autism Risk in Babies—Learning Early Signs; NHSII—Nurses' Health Study II; MoBa—Norwegian Mother and Child Cohort Study. Other abbreviates: ADOS—the Autism Diagnostic Observation Schedule; ASD—autism spectrum disorder; ATC—Anatomical Therapeutic Chemical; BMI—body mass index; CI—confidence interval; FFQ—food frequency questionnaire; GW—gestational week; HR—hazard ratio; MTHFR—methylenetetrahydrofolate reductase; OR—odds ratio; PDD—pervasive developmental disorders; RR—relative risk; SD—standard deviation; SRS—social response scale; TD—typically developing.

3.1.1. Maternal Folate Intake/Status, Multivitamin Intake and Offspring ASD Risk

Fourteen studies examined the association of folic acid supplementation, folate status, or multivitamin intake in relation to offspring ASD risk. Among them, ten are prospective cohort studies [33,34,36–42], and four are retrospective case-control studies [35,43,45,53]. Studies on folate and multivitamins were combined as it is difficult to separate the two exposures. Among the 12 independent studies [33–38,40–43,53] including 594,229 children (8851 ASD cases), nine found a significant inverse association between maternal folic acid or multivitamin intake during pregnancy (with or without pre-pregnancy use) and offspring ASD risk [33–35,37,38,40–42,44–46], one a null association [37], one a significant positive association [43], and one a curve-linear association with modest intake/status associated with lowest ASD risk [36].

Of the nine studies reporting an inverse association between maternal folic acid or multivitamin intake/status during pregnancy and offspring ASD risk [33–35,37,38,40–42,45], four were large prospective cohort studies which identified ASD cases through population-based patient registries [38,41,42] or medical records of large health care organizations [34]; the ASD cases were either confirmed by specialist providers [34,41] or independently validated [38,42]. These studies included very large sample sizes (45,000–270,000 participants) and contributed the greatest weight to the overall evidence. Three were smaller cohort studies which assessed ASD risk within the study using validated instruments for ASD diagnosis [33] or screening [40,46]. Two were retrospective case-control studies where ASD cases were identified from service registries [35,44].

There are two common methodological concerns about these studies. First, there is potential measurement error in folic acid or multivitamin intake, which were generally assessed by self-report [33,35,42] or administrative records [34,38,41]. Of note, two studies with additional data on whole blood/plasma folate levels found the self-reported measure, but not the biomarker measure, to be associated with lower ASD risk [40,46]. The inconsistent findings may be due to measurement error in either measure, or differences in measurement timing. Second, there is potential bias due to residual confounding. Women who took folic acid supplements generally had higher socioeconomic status, healthier lifestyle, and lower BMI [33,37,38,42]; some of these factors, such as a lower BMI, may contribute to lower risk of ASD [54]. These factors were not always adjusted for, making the results subject to residual confounding.

Despite the methodological concerns, additional data support an inverse association between maternal folate status and ASD risk. For example, the *methylenetetrahydrofolate reductase* (*MTHFR*) gene encodes the methylenetetrahydrofolate reductase, a rate-limiting enzyme responsible for converting folate to its bioactive form for methylation reactions [55]; the minor T allele at loci *MTHFR* 677 is known to confer higher susceptibility to inadequate folate status [55]. In one study, maternal folic acid supplementation was associated with a much greater reduction of children's ASD risk when the mother and/or the child had at least one T allele, but the association was null when neither had a T allele [44]. Furthermore, two studies found maternal folic acid supplementation to be specifically associated with a lower risk of ASD, but not associated with the risk of developmental disorders other than ASD [33,44]. If maternal folic acid supplementation was spuriously associated with ASD due to residual confounding, it is likely that it would also show an association with other developmental disorders. Similarly, one study also found the risk of ASD to be specifically associated with folic acid intake, but not fish oil intake [42].

In contrast to the overall finding of an inverse association between folic acid or multivitamin intake/status and ASD risk, a study among 92,676 children in the Danish National Birth Cohort (DNBC) did not find a significant association between folic acid supplementation and ASD risk [37]. Possible explanations include better folate status without supplementation, lower frequency of T alleles at *MTHFR* 677, and insufficient doses of folic acid in the supplements [37,39]. In addition, a study including 1257 children in the Boston Birth Cohort found both low (<2 times/week) and high (>5 times/week) frequencies of multivitamin intake were associated with an elevated risk of ASD, compared to moderate intake (3–5 times/week) [36]. The increased risk associated with high frequencies of folic acid intake may be a result of the above normal level of folate in the study sample [36].

In the meta-analysis including six cohort studies reporting a linear relationship between maternal folic acid/multivitamin intake with offspring ASD diagnosis, maternal folic acid/multivitamin intake was significantly associated with a 36% reduction in offspring ASD risk (Figure 3. RR = 0.64, 95% CI: 0.46, 0.90). The heterogeneity across studies was highly significant ($I^2 = 96.1\%$, $p < 0.001$). To further explore the effect of timing on the association, we conducted additional meta-analyses including four studies examining folic acid/multivitamin supplementation during pregnancy only [33,34,38,39], and three studies examining supplementation before pregnancy only [34,36,39]. The overall effect estimates had a similar direction and magnitude compared to the main analysis. However, the confidence intervals were wider, and the associations were not significant for either analyses, likely due to fewer included studies (Figure 4). Of note, most studies that investigated folic acid/multivitamin supplementation during pregnancy were specific to early pregnancy [33,38,39]. Furthermore, studies that investigated supplementation at multiple times during pregnancy consistently found that supplementation in the first or second months of pregnancy, but not later in pregnancy, was associated with lower ASD risk [33,42,44]. We also separately performed meta-analyses for multivitamin or prenatal vitamins and folic acid-specific supplements. The overall effect estimates in both groups were similar to the main analysis, but not significant (Figure S1).

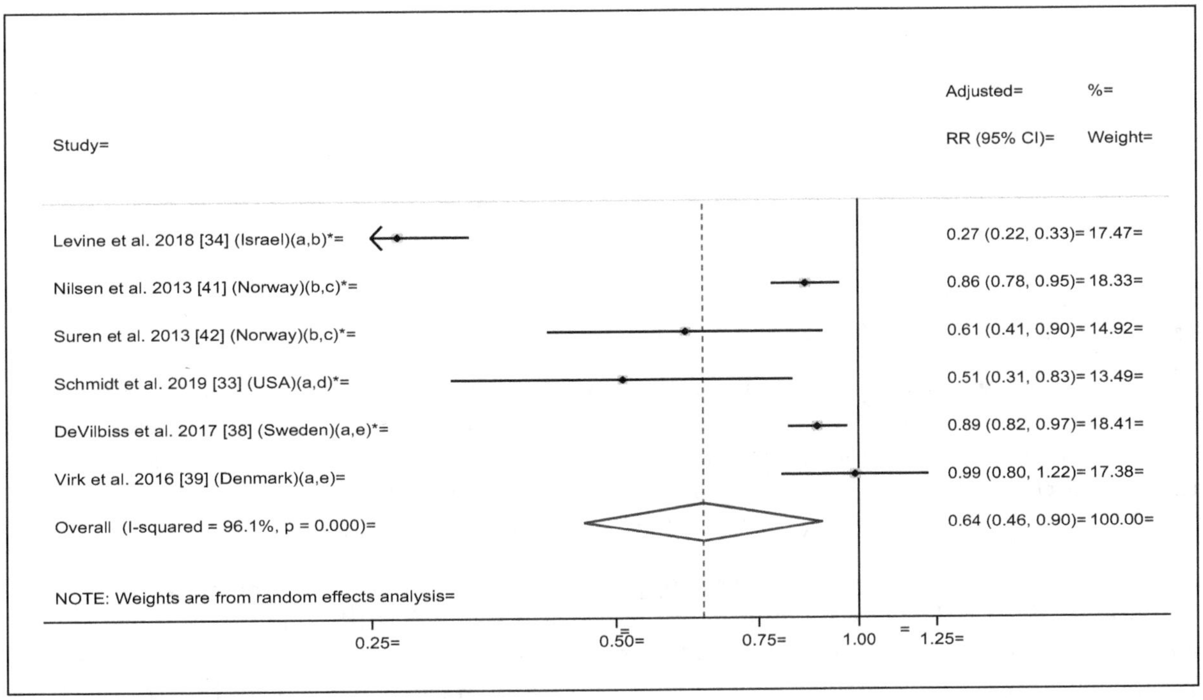

Figure 3. Adjusted relative risk (RRs) of offspring ASD risk associated with maternal intake of supplement containing folic acid, multivitamin or prenatal vitamin during pregnancy (with or without pre-pregnancy use). The overall effect size was estimated using random effects models weighted by inverse variance of each study. One data point was included for each study. Estimates covering any period during pregnancy were included. When estimates for folic acid and multivitamin were both available, the one for folic acid were selected. Notes: (a) Exposure during pregnancy; (b) Intake of supplement containing folic acid vs. no; (c) Exposure before and during pregnancy; (d) Folic acid intake ≥600 mcg/day vs. <600 mcg/day; (e) Intake of multivitamin vs. never/rarely. * $p < 0.05$.

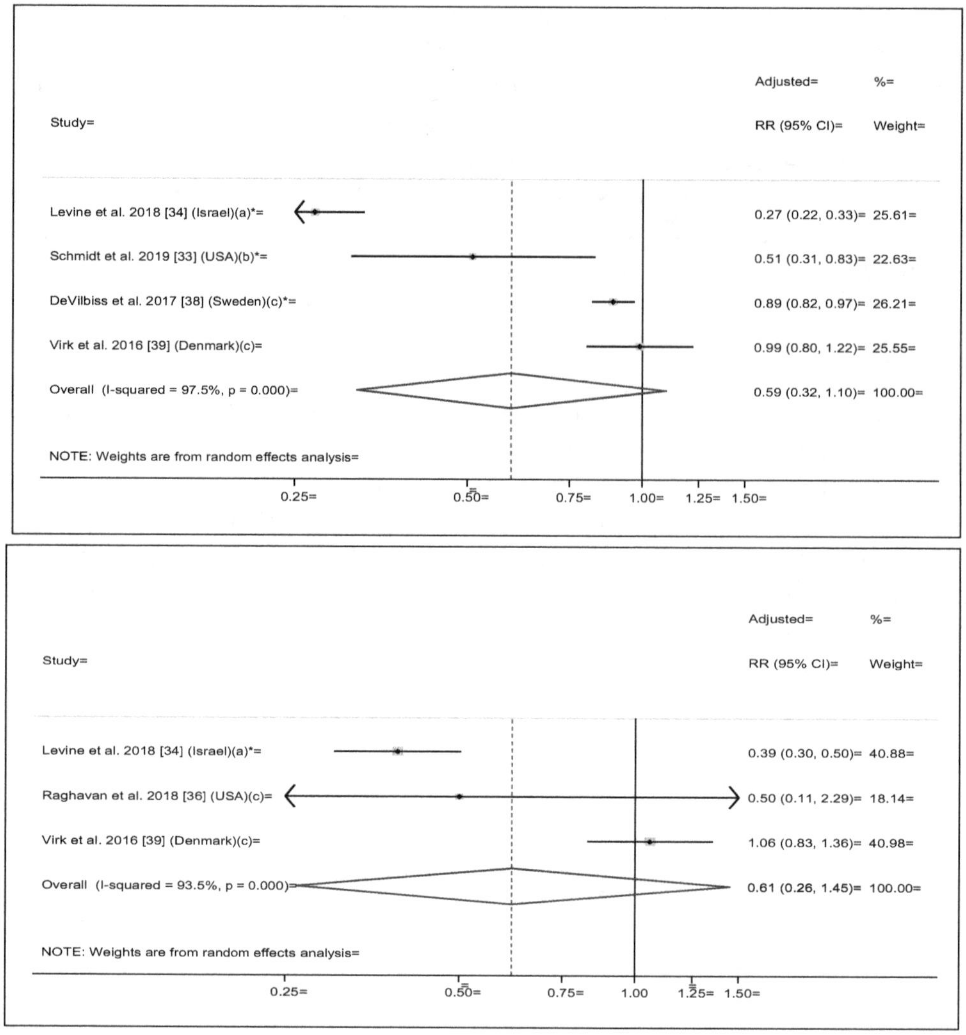

Figure 4. Adjusted relative risk (RRs) of offspring risk of ASD associated with maternal intake of supplement containing folic acid, multivitamin or prenatal vitamin during (top) and before (bottom) pregnancy. The overall effect size was estimated using random effects models weighted by inverse variance of each study. Notes: (a) Intake of supplement containing folic acid vs. no; (b) Folic acid intake ≥600 mcg/day vs. <600 mcg/day; (c) Intake of multivitamin vs. never/rarely. * $p < 0.05$.

Although folic acid is the most widely hypothesized ingredient in multivitamin related to the risk of offspring ASD risk in existing studies, it cannot be explicitly concluded that folic acid was responsible for the observed association yet. Several biological mechanisms support the potential effect of folic acid on reducing offspring ASD risk though. Changes in maternal folate intake result in altered DNA methylation of some genes such as *IGF2* in offspring [8,9], which has been implicated in neurodevelopmental disorders [56,57]. Furthermore, inadequate folate intake affects offspring brain development in animal models through decreasing progenitor cell proliferation [10] and increasing apoptosis [10,11], leading to impaired short-term memory [11]. On the other hand, more than 50 prenatal multivitamins that include folic acid also contain PUFAs [58], for example, and PUFAs are also known to affect prenatal neurodevelopment (see a summary in the introduction section).

In summary, data from the systematic review suggested an overall inverse association between prenatal folic acid/multivitamin supplementation and ASD risk. We also observed large heterogeneity in the association between folic acid/multivitamin intake and ASD risk across studies, which may reflect differences in background nutrient status [59], supplementation dose [39], and genetic polymorphism in nutrient metabolism [60]. Compared with the two earlier reviews [26,27], the present review included six additional recently published articles, thus, providing more conclusive findings. Future studies should simultaneously examine folic acid and other nutrients contained in multivitamins in order to identify the putative nutrients associated with offspring ASD risk; they should also utilize dietary folate intakes in conjunction with folate biomarkers which are more objective.

3.1.2. Maternal Iron Intake and Offspring ASD Risk

Three studies reported maternal iron supplementation and offspring ASD risk—a in large cohort of 273,107 children in Sweden [38], a small cohort of 332 children who had siblings with ASD in the US [33], and 520 ASD cases and 346 typically developing controls in the US [47]. These studies did not find an association between early pregnancy iron supplementation and ASD, regardless of the specific exposure (iron-specific supplementation, any iron supplementation, total iron supplementation). Only the retrospective study in the US examined iron supplementation later in pregnancy, and it found suggestive evidence of an association between total iron supplementation and iron-specific supplementation in the second and third trimester and a lower ASD risk, which did not reach significance. In addition, it also found a significant association between the exposures during breastfeeding and a lower ASD risk. In summary, studies on iron supplementation intakes in pregnancy and offspring ASD risk are limited. Available data do not suggest an association between prenatal iron supplementation and ASD risk.

3.1.3. Maternal PUFA Intake or Status, Seafood Intake and Offspring ASD Risk

Two studies examined maternal PUFA intake or status in relation to offspring ASD risk or traits. Among 18,045 children in the Nurses' Health Study II (NHSII) in the US, total and n-6 PUFA intake before pregnancy were all significantly and inversely associated with children's risk of ASD diagnosis as reported by mothers, whereas n-3 PUFA was not significantly associated with ASD risk [48]. In contrast, among 4624 children in the generation R study in The Netherlands, plasma n-6 PUFA levels in mid-pregnancy were significantly and positively associated with children's ASD traits measured by Social Response Scale (SRS), the ratio of n-3 to n-6 PUFA was inversely associated with the outcome. Similar to NHSII study, plasma n-3 PUFA levels were not associated with the outcome [49]. Both studies controlled for a comprehensive set of potential confounders including other aspects of diet [48] and dietary supplements [48,49]. Both n-3 and n-6 PUFA are necessary for prenatal brain development [13]; however, an elevated n-6 to n-3 PUFA ratio—characteristic of modern western diet [61]—could potentiate inflammatory processes [62]. Discrepant findings from the two studies may be due to the use of absolute versus relative concentrations of n-3 and n-6 PUFA levels, or differences in the timing of the exposure (before pregnancy vs. mid-pregnancy) and outcome measures (clinical diagnosis vs. trait).

Fish is the main dietary source of DHA—the n-3 PUFA most relevant for brain development [15]. In secondary analysis of the above-mentioned studies on PUFA intake/status, maternal fish intake was not associated with ASD diagnosis/traits [48,49]. In contrast, two other studies suggested a potential inverse association between maternal fish intake and offspring ASD risk [42,51]. Among 1589 children in the Spanish INMA study [51], maternal total seafood intake in the first trimester was associated with lower autistic traits measured by Childhood Asperger Syndrome Test; similar associations were observed for large fatty fish and lean fish. Another study of 108 ASD cases and 108 typically developing controls in China [50] found maternal "habit" (>3 times/week) of eating grass carp reported four to 17 years after delivery to be associated with a lower risk of ASD. However, the validity of the food frequency questionnaire in recalling diet after many years was not reported. Lastly, in one study among 85,176 children in the Norwegian Mother and Child Cohort Study (MoBa) [42], fish oil supplementation before and in early pregnancy was not associated with ASD risk.

In conclusion, findings of the associations between maternal PUFA or fish intake and ASD risk are inconclusive. Heterogeneity in the PUFA measurement or assessment (i.e., absolute vs. relative concentrations, intake vs. status) and ASD (i.e., clinical diagnosis vs. traits, intake vs. status) made it difficult to compare findings across studies. Furthermore, recall bias and potential residual confounding are also of concern.

3.1.4. Maternal Dietary Patterns and Offspring risk of ASD

Two studies reported associations between maternal dietary patterns and ASD risk. Among 325 children in the Newborn Epigenetics Study in the US [52], higher periconception Adherence to the Mediterranean diet was associated with a lower risk of ASD assessed by the Infant Toddler Social Emotional Assessment; the association became non-significant after adjusting for multiple comparisons. Among 374 ASD cases and 354 typically developing controls in the Autism Clinical and Environmental Database in China, maternal recall three to six years after delivery of a "mostly meat" and a "mostly vegetable" dietary pattern during pregnancy were both associated with a higher risk of ASD in children compared to a "both meat and vegetable" dietary pattern [35]. However, it appears that the dietary pattern was only assessed using a single question, and a specific definition of each dietary pattern was not given. Thus, it remains inconclusive if maternal dietary patterns are associated with offspring risk of ASD. More studies on this topic are needed in the future.

3.2. Maternal Nutrition and ADHD Risk

Characteristics and main findings of studies assessing the association between maternal nutrition and ADHD are presented in Table 2. Of the 17 studies, 16 are prospective observational study, and one was a randomized controlled trial. These studies were conducted in the UK, France, Spain, The Netherlands, Norway, Denmark, New Zealand, Japan, Brazil, and Mexico.

3.2.1. Maternal Folate Intake/Status, Multivitamin Intake and Offspring ADHD Risk

Three studies examined maternal folic acid supplementation in relation to offspring ADHD risk or symptoms [63–67], with most reporting null findings. Specifically, maternal folic acid-specific supplementation before and in early pregnancy was not associated with clinical diagnosis of hyperkinetic disorders or ADHD medication use in a large study of 35,059 children in the DNBC [65], although it was associated with a lower risk of hyperactivity-inattention problems as measured by the Strength and Difficulties Questionnaire (SDQ) among a subgroup of children followed to age seven. Similarly, maternal intake of any folic acid supplementation before or in early pregnancy was not associated with the risk of the hyperactivity-inattention problem among 6247 children in the Growing Up in New Zealand Study [63] and 420 children in the Menorca cohort in Spain [66].

One study examined maternal folate intake from food in relation to offspring ADHD risk. In the Japanese study including 1199 children in the Kyushu Okinawa Maternal and Child Health Study (KOMCHS) [64], higher intake of folate from food during pregnancy was associated with a non-significant reduction in children's risk of the hyperactivity-inattention problems (p-trend = 0.10), but folic acid supplementation was not accounted for. Lastly, one study examined folate status and total folate intake in relation to ADHD risk. In this small study including 136 children in the UK [67], early pregnancy red blood cell folate concentration and total folate intake from food and supplements, but not late pregnancy intake, were inversely associated with hyperactivity-inattention score. However, unlike the larger studies above, this study only adjusted for a limited set of covariates; residual confounding from maternal lifestyle factors was possible. In summary, no convincing evidence supports an association between folate intake from food or supplements and ADHD risk.

Among the studies previously mentioned, three also assessed the association between maternal multivitamin intake and child ADHD risk [63,65,66]. Overall, the findings are inconsistent. Maternal multivitamin intake was associated with a lower risk of hyperkinetic disorders and ADHD medication in the DNBC [65], but it was not associated with the hyperactivity-inattention problems in the Growing up in New Zealand Study [63]. Maternal intake of multivitamins containing no folic acid was associated with a non-significant reduction in risk of the hyperactivity-inattention problem in the Spanish Menorca cohort (OR = 0.24, 95% CI: 0.05, 1.31) [66]. However, the composition of such multivitamins was not clear. More studies are needed to assess this association further and to examine nutrients other than folate that may be related to ADHD risk.

Table 2. Studies on maternal nutrition and offspring ADHD risk or symptoms.

Source (Country)	Design & Sample	Maternal Exposures	Offspring Outcomes	Findings	Covariates
			Vitamins and Minerals		
			Folate and Multivitamin-ADHD Diagnosis or Cutoff		
D'Souza et al. 2019 (New Zealand) [63]	Prospective cohort; 6246 children in the Growing Up in New Zealand Study	Folic acid and multivitamin supplementation before pregnancy, during the first trimester, and after the first trimester assessed in interviews in late pregnancy	Hyperactivity-inattention symptoms assessed by SDQ using mothers' report at 2 years of age; clinical cutoff was used to define abnormality	Folic acid intake was not associated with ADHD risk (ORs [95% CI] for first trimester only and no intake vs. intake both before pregnancy and at first trimester were 0.98 [0.74, 1.31] and 0.88 [0.57, 1.34]). Multivitamin was not associated with ADHD risk (OR = 0.97, 95% CI: 0.75, 1.24)	Mother's ethnicity, mother's education, mother's age when pregnant, child's gestational age, child's birth weight, child's gender, parity, planned pregnancy, mother in paid employment, area-level deprivation, and rurality
Miyake et al. 2018 (Japan) [64]	Prospective cohort; 1199 children in the KOMCHS	Folate and other B-vitamin intake from food in the past month assessed by FFQ at GW 5 to 39	Hyperactivity-inattention symptoms assessed by SDQ using mothers' report at 5 years of age; clinical cutoff was used to define abnormality	Folate from food was not associated with hyperactivity-inattention problem (ORs [95% CI] for quartile 2–4 were 0.75 [0.46, 1.21], 0.66 [0.40, 1.07], and 0.69 [0.42, 1.12], p-trend = 0.10). Vitamin B12 (ORs [95% CI] for quartile 2–4 were 0.80 [0.49, 1.29], 0.99 [0.61, 1.61] and 0.81 [0.50, 1.32], p-trend = 0.60) and B2 (ORs for quartile 2–4 were 1.09 [0.68, 1.75], 1.03 [0.64, 1.66] and 0.61 [0.36, 1.03], p-trend = 0.08) from food were not associated hyperactivity-inattention problem. Higher vitamin B6 from food was associated with lower risk of hyperactivity-inattention problem (ORs for quartile 2–4 were 0.76 [0.48, 1.21], 0.58 [0.36, 0.94] and 0.57 [0.34, 0.94], p-trend = 0.01) *	Maternal age, gestation at baseline, region of residence at baseline, number of children at baseline, maternal and paternal education, household income, maternal depressive symptoms during pregnancy, maternal alcohol intake during pregnancy, maternal vitamin B complex supplement use during pregnancy, maternal smoking during pregnancy, child's birth weight, child's sex, breastfeeding duration, and smoking in the household during the first year of life.

Table 2. *Cont.*

Source (Country)	Design & Sample	Maternal Exposures	Offspring Outcomes	Findings	Covariates
Virk et al. 2018 (Denmark) [65]	Prospective cohort; 35,059 children in the DNBC	Folic acid and multivitamin supplementations from GW −4 to 8 assessed by questionnaire at GW 12	Hyperkinetic disorder and treatment for ADHD were identified from National Patient Register; children were 7 years of age. Hyperactivity-inattention symptoms assessed by SDQ at age 7 years based on parent reports, and a score ≥7 was defined as abnormal	Folic acid supplement was not associated with risk of hyperkinetic disorder diagnosis (HR = 0.87, 95% CI: 0.54, 1.41) or ADHD medication (HR = 0.96, 95% CI: 0.68, 1.37). Maternal multivitamin use was associated with lower risk of hyperkinetic disorder diagnosis (HR = 0.70, 95% CI: 0.52, 0.96) *, ADHD medication (HR = 0.78, 95% CI: 0.62, 0.98) *	Maternal age, household socio-economic status, maternal smoking and alcohol consumption during pregnancy, maternal prepregnancy body mass index, birth year, and offspring sex
Julvez et al. 2009 (Spain) [66]	Prospective cohort; 420 children in the Menorca cohort	Current folic acid and vitamin supplementations assessed by interviews at GW 12	ADHD assessed by ADHD Rating Scale-IV based on teacher report at 4 years of age; scores >80th percentile was defined abnormal	Folic acid with or without other vitamins compared to no folic acid or vitamins was not associated with ADHD risk (OR = 0.74, 95% CI: 0.38, 1.47). Vitamins without folic acid compared to no folic acid or vitamins was not associated with ADHD risk (OR = 0.26, 95% CI: 0.05, 1.31)	Parental social class and level of education, mother's parity at child's age four, mother's marital status, maternal tobacco smoking during pregnancy, maternal intake of supplementary calcium and iron at the same time as study determinants, gestational age at interview, child's gender, child's duration of breast feeding, child's age and school season during test assessment, evaluator and child's home location at age four
Folate and multivitamin-ADHD symptoms					
Schlotz et al. 2010 (UK) [67]	Prospective cohort; 139 children	Total folate intake from foods and supplements during early pregnancy assessed by FFQ at GW 14, and during late pregnancy assessed at GW 28	Hyperactivity-inattention symptoms assessed by SDQ based on mothers' report at 8 years	Maternal red cell folate concentration (beta per SD = −1.23, 95% CI: −2.20, −0.26) * and total folate intake from food and supplements (beta per SD = −0.75, 95% CI: −1.39, −0.11) * in early pregnancy were both associated with fewer hyperactivity-inattention symptoms. However, total folate intake from food and supplements in late pregnancy (beta per SD = 0.07, 95% CI: −0.80, 0.93) was not associated with hyperactivity-inattention symptoms	Analysis of red cell folate: child's sex, mother's smoking and drinking alcohol during pregnancy, and mother's educational attainment. Analysis of total folate intake: daily energy, child's sex

Table 2. *Cont.*

Source (Country)	Design & Sample	Maternal Exposures	Offspring Outcomes	Findings	Covariates
Iodine-ADHD diagnosis or cutoff and ADHD symptoms					
Abel et al. 2017 (Norway) [68]	Prospective cohort; 77,164 children in the MoBa	Iodine intake from foods and supplements assessed by FFQ at GW 22	ADHD identified from Norwegian Patient Registry; ADHD symptom assessed by the ADHD Rating Scale based on mother report at 8 years	Iodine from food was not associated with ADHD diagnosis (p-overall = 0.89). Iodine supplement was not associated with ADHD diagnosis, irrespective of food iodine intake. However, higher iodine from food was associated with fewer ADHD symptoms (beta [95% CI] for 25, 50, 75, 100, 125, 200, 225, 250, 300, 350, 400 vs. 160 mcg/day were 0.05 [−0.02, 0.12], 0.06 [0.01, 0.10], 0.06 [0.03, 0.09], 0.05 [0.02, 0.09], 0.03 [0.01, 0.05], −0.01 [-0.03, −0.00], -0.02 [-0.04, 0.01], −0.01 [-0.05, 0.02], −0.01 [-0.07, 0.05], −0.01 [−0.09, 0.08] and −0.00 [−0.12, 0.11], p-overall = 0.001) *. Higher iodine supplement was associated with higher ADHD score among women with less than 160 mcg/day of food iodine (beta [95% CI] for 1–200 and >200 mcg/day were 0.06 [0.03, 0.10] and 0.06 [−0.03, 0.16]) *, but not among women with more than 160 mcg/day of food iodine	Sibling clusters, total energy intake, maternal age, BMI, parity, education, smoking in pregnancy, and fiber intake

Table 2. *Cont.*

Source (Country)	Design & Sample	Maternal Exposures	Offspring Outcomes	Findings	Covariates
			PUFA and Seafood		
			PUFA-ADHD Diagnosis or Cutoff		
Miyake et al. 2018 (Japan) [69]	Prospective cohort; 1199 children in the KOMCHS	Fat intake from food in the past month assessed by FFQ at GW 5–39	Hyperactivity-inattention symptoms assessed by SDQ using mothers' report at 5 years of age; clinical cutoff was used to define abnormality	Total n-3 PUFA (ORs [95% CI] for quartile 2–4 were 0.82 [0.51, 1.31], 0.75 [0.46, 1.22], and 0.80 [0.49, 1.29], *p*-trend = 0.31), ALA (0.93 [0.59, 1.49], 0.73 [0.44, 1.20], and 0.72 [0.44, 1.18], *p*-trend = 0.13), EPA (0.90 [0.55, 1.46], 0.92 [0.56, 1.49], and 0.97 [0.59, 1.59], *p*-trend = 0.91), and DHA (0.85 [0.52, 1.39], 1.01 [0.62, 1.65], and 1.07 [0.66, 1.73], *p*-trend = 0.66) were not associated with hyperactivity-inattention problem. Total n-6 PUFA (1.05 [0.66, 1.68], 0.75 [0.45, 1.23], and 0.81 [0.49, 1.33], *p*-trend = 0.22), LA (1.03 [0.65, 1.64], 0.67 [0.40, 1.11], and 0.81 [0.49, 1.32], *p*-trend = 0.18), and AA (0.92 [0.56, 1.51], 1.10 [0.69, 1.77], and 0.91 [0.55, 1.50], *p*-trend = 0.92) were not associated with hyperactivity-inattention problem. Total n-3 to n-6 ratio (1.34 [0.83, 2.18], 1.24 [0.75, 2.04], and 0.97 [0.58, 1.63], p-trend = 0.84) was not associated with hyperactivity-inattention problem	Maternal age, gestation at baseline, region of residence at baseline, number of children at baseline, maternal and paternal education, household income, maternal depressive symptoms during pregnancy, maternal alcohol intake during pregnancy, maternal vitamin B complex supplement use during pregnancy, maternal smoking during pregnancy, child's birth weight, child's sex, breastfeeding duration, and smoking in the household during the first year of life
			PUFA-ADHD symptoms		
Ramakrishnan et al. 2016 (Mexico) [70]	Randomized controlled trial; 797 children in POSGRAD study	Interventions of 400 mg of DHA supplementation or placebo from GW 18–22 to delivery	Hyperactivity-inattention symptoms assessed by K-CPT at 5 years of age. >70th percentile was at clinical risk of suffering from a disorder such as ADHD	DHA supplement of 400 mg/day was not associated with overall K-CPT score >70 (7.2% and 8.1%, *p* = 0.62)	None

Table 2. *Cont.*

Source (Country)	Design & Sample	Maternal Exposures	Offspring Outcomes	Findings	Covariates
			Seafood-ADHD diagnosis or cutoff		
Gale et al. 2008 (UK) [71]	Prospective cohort; 219 children	Fish intake in the past 3 months assessed by FFQ at GW 15 and 32	Hyperactivity-inattention symptoms assessed by SDQ using mothers' report at 9 years of age; clinical cutoff was used to define abnormality	More frequent oily fish intake in early pregnancy (ORs [95% CI] for <1 and ≥1 time/week vs. no intake were 0.30 [0.12, 0.76] and 0.41 [0.15, 1.12]) * and late pregnancy (ORs [95% CI] for <1 and ≥1 time/week vs. no intake were 0.40 [0.16, 0.98] and 0.72 [0.26, 1.98]) * were both associated with lower risk of hyperactivity-inattention problem. Frequency of eating all types of fish was not associated with hyperactivity-inattention problem	Maternal social class, educational qualifications, age, IQ, smoking and drinking in pregnancy, duration of breastfeeding and birthweight
Hibbeln et al. 2007 (UK) [72]	Prospective cohort; 8946 children in ALSPAC	Seafood intake during pregnancy assessed by FFQ at GW 32	Hyperactivity-inattention symptoms assessed by SDQ using mothers' report at 7 years of age; highest quartile was defined as suboptimal outcome	Seafood intake was not associated with hyperactivity-inattention problem (ORs [95% CI] for none and 1–340 g/week vs. ≥340 g/week were 1.13 [0.84, 1.53] and 0.91 [0.73, 1.12], *p*-trend = 0.66)	Maternal education, housing, crowding at home, life events, partner, maternal age, maternal smoking in pregnancy, maternal alcohol use in pregnancy, parity, breastfeeding, gender, ethnic origin, birthweight, preterm delivery, 12 non-fish food groups
			Caffeine, coffee and tea		
			Caffeine-ADHD diagnosis or cutoff		
Miyake et al. 2018 (Japan) [73]	Prospective cohort; 1199 children in the KOMCHS	Caffeine intake from food in the past month assessed by FFQ at GW 5–39	Hyperactivity-inattention symptoms assessed by SDQ using mothers' report at 5 years of age; clinical cutoff was used to define abnormality	Caffeine was not associated with hyperactivity-inattention problem (ORs [95% CI] for quartile 2–4 were 1.04 [0.64, 1.68], 0.99 [0.61, 1.62], and 0.84 [0.51, 1.38], *p*-trend = 0.49)	Maternal age, gestation at baseline, region of residence at baseline, number of children at baseline, maternal and paternal education, household income, maternal depressive symptoms during pregnancy, maternal alcohol intake during pregnancy, maternal vitamin B complex supplement use during pregnancy, maternal smoking during pregnancy, child's birth weight, child's sex, breastfeeding duration, and smoking in the household during the first year of life

Table 2. *Cont.*

Source (Country)	Design & Sample	Maternal Exposures	Offspring Outcomes	Findings	Covariates
Del-Ponte et al. 2016 (Brazil) [74]	Prospective cohort; 3485 children	Caffeine intake during each trimester assessed in interviews after delivery	ADHD assessed by DAWBA based on mother's report at 11 years of age; clinical cutoff was used to define abnormality	Caffeine in the entire pregnancy was not associated with ADHD risk (ORs [95% CI] for 100–299 and ≥300 vs. <100 mg/day were 1.12 [0.68 to 1.84] and 0.90 [0.51 to 1.59]). Similar results were found in each of the three trimesters	Maternal mood symptoms during pregnancy, National Economic Index, paternal education level and maternal conjugal situation
Loomans et al. 2012 (The Netherlands) [75]	Prospective cohort; 3439 children in the ABCD study	Caffeine intake from coffee, tea and cola in the past week assessed by questionnaire at GW 16	Hyperactivity-inattention symptoms assessed by SDQ based on mothers' report at 5–6 years of age; clinical cutoff was used to define abnormality	Caffeine was not associated with hyperactivity-inattention problem (ORs [95% CI] for 86–255, 256–425, and >425 vs. 0–85 mg/day were 0.94 [0.68, 1.31], 0.87 [0.57, 1.33], and 1.08 [0.55, 2.12])	Maternal age, ethnicity, maternal education, maternal anxiety, cohabitant status, smoking, alcohol, child's gender, family size
Coffee and tea-ADHD diagnosis or cutoff					
Hvolgaard Mikkelsen et al. 2017 (Denmark) [76]	Prospective cohort; 47,491 children in the DNBC	Current coffee and tea intake assessed by interviews at GW 15 and 30	Hyperactivity-inattention symptoms assessed by SDQ based on children, parents and teachers' report at 11 years of age; computerized algorithms were used to identified ADHD	Higher coffee intake in the first trimester was associated with higher risk of hyperactivity-inattention problem (ORs [95% CI] for 1–3, 4–7 and ≥8 cups/day vs. no intake were 0.97 [0.88, 1.08], 1.09 [0.93, 1.27] and 1.47 [1.18, 1.83], *p*-trend = 0.03) *. In the third trimester, it was not associated (ORs [95% CI] for 1–3, 4–7 and ≥8 cups/day vs. no intake were 0.94 [0.85, 1.04], 0.96 [0.83, 1.13] and 1.21 [0.95, 1.55], *p*-trend = 0.88). Tea intake in the first trimester was not associated with hyperactivity-inattention problem (ORs [95% CI] for 1–3, 4–7 and ≥8 cups/day vs. no intake were 0.93 [0.85, 1.03], 0.97 [0.85, 1.12] and 1.21 [0.98, 1.49], *p*-trend = 0.57). In the third trimester, higher tea intake was associated with lower risk of hyperactivity-inattention problem (ORs [95% CI] for 1–3, 4–7 and ≥8 cups/day vs. no intake were 0.90 [0.81, 1.01], 0.79 [0.66, 0.94] and 0.84 [0.63, 1.11], *p*-trend = 0.01) *	Sex, birth year, smoking, socioeconomic status, maternal age, parity, maternal BMI, and mutually coffee or tea

Table 2. *Cont.*

Source (Country)	Design & Sample	Maternal Exposures	Offspring Outcomes	Findings	Covariates
Linnet et al. 2009 (Denmark) [77]	Prospective cohort; 24,068 children in the Aarhus Birth Cohort	Coffee intake during pregnancy assessed by a questionnaire prior to GW 16	Hyperkinetic disorder and ADHD recorded in Danish Psychiatric Central Register; children were 3–12 years of age	Coffee was not associated with ADHD risk (RRs [95% CI] for 1–3, 4–9 and ≥10 cups of coffee were 0.9 [0.5, 1.6], 1.3 [0.7, 2.3] and 2.3 [0.9, 5.9])	Smoking, alcohol, maternal age, gender of the child, parental years of schooling after basic school, employment status, cohabitant status and parental and sibling's psychiatric hospitalizations or contacts as outpatients
Dietary patterns					
Dietary patterns-ADHD diagnosis or cutoff					
Galera et al. 2018 (France) [78]	Prospective cohort; 1242 children in the EDEN mother-child cohort	Dietary patterns in the third trimester assessed by FFQ after delivery and derived using principle component analysis	Hyperactivity-inattention symptoms assessed by SDQ based on mother's report at 3, 5, and 8 years of age; clinical cutoff was used to define abnormality; longitudinal trajectories were derived based on mixture models	Lower scores of healthy dietary pattern (OR [95% CI] for quartile 1 vs. the rest was 1.61 [1.09, 2.37]) * and higher scores of Western dietary pattern (OR for quartile 4 vs. the rest was 1.67 [1.13, 2.47]) * were both associated with higher risk of high hyperactivity-inattention trajectory	Centre, child gender, maternal age, prepregnancy BMI, maternal smoking, maternal alcohol-drinking, gestational diabetes, multiparity, gestational length, birth weight, breastfeeding, prenatal maternal depressive symptoms, prenatal maternal anxiety, postnatal maternal depressive symptoms, parental separation, family income, maternal education, child dietary patterns at age 2, and mutual adjusted for healthy and Western dietary patterns
Dietary patterns-ADHD symptoms					
Rijlaarsdam et al. 2017 (UK) [56]	Prospective cohort; 83 youths with early-onset persistent conduct problems and 81 youths with low conduct problem in ALSPAC	Dietary patterns during pregnancy assessed by FFQ at GW 32 and derived using confirmatory factor analysis	ADHD symptoms assessed by DAWBA based on parent reports at 7 years of age	Unhealthy dietary pattern was indirectly associated with more ADHD symptoms through *IGF2* DNA methylation at birth among youths with early-onset persistent conduct problems (beta per SD = 0.069, 95% CI: 0.003, 0.206) *, but not among youths with low conduct problem (beta per SD = −0.015, 95% CI: −0.086, 0.019)	Cumulative risk index during pregnancy and in childhood, including life events, contextual risks, parental risks, interpersonal risks, direct victimization

* Statistically significant findings (p-value < 0.05). Abbreviates of research studies: ABCD—Amsterdam Born Children and their Development; ALSPAC—Avon Longitudinal Study of Parents and Children; DNBC—Danish National Birth Cohort; EDEN—Étude des Déterminants pré et postnatals du développement et de la santé de l'ENfant; KOMCHS—Kyushu Okinawa Maternal and Child Health Study; MoBa—Norwegian Mother and Child Cohort Study; POSGRAD—Prenatal Omega-3 Fatty Acid Supplementation and Child Growth and Development. Other abbreviations: ADHD—attention—deficit/hyperactivity disorder; BMI—body mass index; CI—confidence interval; DAWBA—Development and Well—Being Assessment; DHA—docosahexaenoic acid; FFQ—food frequency questionnaire; GW—gestational week; HR—hazard ratio; K-CPT—Conner's Kiddie Continuous Performance Test; OR—odds ratio; RR—relative risk; SD—standard deviation; SDQ—Strengths and Difficulties Questionnaire.

3.2.2. Maternal PUFA and Seafood Intake and Offspring ADHD Risk

Two studies examined maternal PUFA intake in relation to children's ADHD risk and findings did not support a significant association. More specifically, among the 1,199 children in the KOMCHS [69], neither maternal intake of total or specific n-3 and n-6 PUFA from food were associated with children's risk of the hyperactivity-inattention problems. In a randomized controlled trial among 797 children in Mexico [70], maternal DHA supplementation of 400 mg/day from mid-pregnancy to delivery was not associated with clinical risk of ADHD measured by the Conner's Kiddie Continuous Performance Test (K-CPT) core indicating (>70th percentile). Of note, the ability of the K-CPT to accurately identify children at risk for ADHD has been questioned [79].

Two studies examined maternal seafood intake in relation to children's risk of hyperactivity-inattention problems. Among 219 children in the UK [71], more frequent intake of oily fish during pregnancy was associated with lower risk of the hyperactivity-inattention problem, whereas intake of all types of fish was not. In contrast, among 8946 children in Avon Longitudinal Study of Parents and Children (ALSPAC) study in the UK [72], seafood intake was not associated with ADHD risk. However, results for oily fish intake were not reported. In summary, studies on the association between maternal PUFA or seafood intake and children's ADHD risk are inconsistent and provide little evidence for an association; differences in exposure assessments inhibits a clear interpretation of the findings. Future studies need to have a comprehensive assessment of maternal fish, seafood, and PUFA intake/status in relation to offspring ADHD risk.

3.2.3. Maternal Caffeine, Coffee, and Tea Intake and Offspring ADHD Risk

Three cohort studies, including 3485 children in Brazil [74], 3439 children in The Netherlands [75], and 1199 children in Japan [73], consistently found no association between maternal caffeine intake during pregnancy and hyperactivity-inattention problem in children. Across the three studies, the cutoff for the highest intake category was 300–384 mg/day, which is equivalent to three to four and a half cups of coffee/day (a cup coffee is defined as 8 oz). In the meta-analysis pooling all three studies, the overall effect estimate comparing the highest to the lowest category of caffeine intake was null (OR = 0.91, 95% CI: 0.66, 1.27; $I^2 = 0.0\%$, p for $I^2 = 0.84$).

On the other hand, two large prospective cohort studies [76,77] found suggestive evidence that extremely high levels of coffee intake in early pregnancy were associated with an increased risk of ADHD. Among 47,491 children in the DNBC [76], ≥8 cups/day of coffee in early pregnancy (OR = 1.47, 95% CI: 1.18, 1.83), but not late pregnancy (OR = 1.21, 95% CI: 0.95, 1.55), was associated with a significantly increased risk of hyperactivity inattention problems. Among 24,068 children in the Aarhus Birth Cohort in Denmark [77], ≥10 cups/day of coffee in early pregnancy was also associated with a substantial but non-significant increase in the risk for hyperkinetic disorders and ADHD diagnosis (OR = 2.3, 95% CI: 0.9, 5.9). Less coffee intake (<8 cups/day in the DNBC and <10 cups/day in the Aarhus Birth Cohort) was not associated with ADHD risk in either study. Of note, only about 3% of women had extremely high intake levels in both studies [76,77], and they appeared to be highly selective group, characterized by lower social class, much higher rate of cigarette smoking, and higher rate of hyperactivity themselves [76]. While the two studies adjusted for selected socioeconomic, lifestyle and psychological characteristic of the women [76,77], residual confounding from unmeasured variables cannot be ruled out. On the other hand, it is possible that only extreme levels of caffeine consumption affect fetal neurodevelopment [20]. The extreme levels of coffee intake were not captured in the studies examining caffeine intake. Taken together, these studies suggest a null association between moderate coffee intake and offspring ADHD risk. Further evaluation of extremely high levels of maternal coffee intake and ADHD risk is needed.

3.2.4. Maternal Dietary Patterns and Offspring ADHD Risk

Two cohort studies [56,78] suggested an association between poor dietary quality during pregnancy and increased risk of ADHD or ADHD symptoms in children. Among 1242 children in the EDEN mother-child cohort in France [56], the lowest quartile of "healthy dietary patterns" (i.e., high intake in fruit, vegetables, fish, and whole grain cereals) and the highest quartile of "western dietary pattern" (i.e., high intake in processed and snacking foods) were both associated with increased risk of hyperactivity-inattention trajectory between age three and eight years. In the ALSPAC [56], an "unhealthy dietary pattern" (i.e., high fat and sugar) score was positively associated with ADHD symptoms among 83 youths with early-onset persistent conduct problems, but not associated with ADHD symptoms among the 81 youths with low conduct problems; the association among youths with early-onset persistent conduct problems was mediated by higher levels of *IGF2* DNA methylation at birth. Of note, *IGF2* gene has important roles in regulating placental and fetal growth; genetic and epigenetic changes in the *IGF2* gene and changes in IGF2 hormonal levels has been linked to altered development in the cerebellum and hippocampus, both of which are relevant to ADHD [56]. The significant association between maternal dietary quality and children's ADHD risk should be further evaluated.

4. Methodological Issues and Future Directions

Two major methodological concerns among studies of maternal nutrition and offspring neurodevelopmental disorders merit further discussion. The first is potential measurement error in the exposure assessment. Studies that comprehensively characterized nutrients from both food and supplements are limited. This is relevant as the effect of the supplementation may depend on baseline nutrient sufficiency status before supplementation, as well as the supplementation dose. Similarly, the effects of a nutrient from food may be overwhelmed by supplementation. Moreover, most studies examined maternal nutritional exposures using questionnaires, including food frequency questionnaires, which are prone to recall bias. To address these concerns, future studies need to prospectively quantify nutrient intakes from both foods and dietary supplements, which may help to establish potential dose-response relations and sufficient dose to prevent offspring neurodevelopmental disorders. Future studies should also consider quantifying nutrient status using biomarkers, which complement dietary information from questionnaires and provide a source of validation.

A second methodological concern with regard to existing studies is potential bias due to residual confounding. Many maternal demographic, lifestyle, and psychosocial factors that contribute to poorer maternal nutritional status may also contribute to the risk of neurodevelopmental disorders in children [4,80]. Smaller studies frequently lack the power to adjust for a comprehensive list of potential confounders. Even in large studies where such adjustments were made, residual confounding from unknown risk factors are still possible, and a causal link cannot be established. Alternative study designs may help to ameliorate this concern and strengthen the evidence. For example, variants in *MTHFR* gene encoding methylenetetrahydrofolate reductase affect vulnerability to low folate intake [55]; variants in *FADS* gene encoding fatty acid desaturase are determinants of long change PUFA status [81]. These genetic variants have been found to modify the association between maternal intake of respective nutrients and offspring neurodevelopmental outcomes [15,44]. Futures studies may use these variants to implement Mendelian randomization in observational studies to further evaluate a potential causal effect of nutrients on offspring outcomes.

Besides these major methodological concerns, several others may merit consideration in designing future studies. First, the effect of a nutrient on neurodevelopmental disorders may vary by fetal developmental period, reflecting the underlying developmental processes affected. Many existing studies did not investigate the timing of the exposure explicitly. Future studies should have explicit hypotheses about the window of sensitivity, and use it inform study design and implementation and the interpretation of results. Longitudinal assessment of the exposures throughout relevant periods would be particularly suitable to identify the most relevant window of sensitivity to the nutrient. Knowledge of the sensitive window of exposure is essential for establishing evidence and designing interventions. Second, epigenetic modification is postulated to be major mechanism by which early life nutrition contributes to risk of health and disease later in life [82], and maternal intake of nutrients such as folate and DHA has been linked to differential DNA methylation patterns [8]. Two studies have reported promising findings where maternal diet has been simultaneously linked to altered methylation of specific genes and neurodevelopmental disorders [52,56]. More studies incorporating epigenetic data are needed to better understand the mechanism.

5. Conclusions

Maternal nutrition is a potentially modifiable factor important for fetal neurodevelopment. In the past decade, a body of research emerged examining the impact of maternal nutritional status and offspring developmental disorders. To our knowledge, this is the first comprehensive and systematic review of maternal nutrition during the preconception and perinatal period and offspring risk of neurodevelopmental disorders. This review included studies on maternal intake (or status) at multiple levels: nutrients (i.e., vitamins, minerals, PUFA, multivitamins), food (i.e., fish), and dietary patterns in relation to children's risk of ASD and ADHD. Findings from the review supported an inverse association between maternal folic acid or multivitamin intake and children's risk of ASD, although large heterogeneity existed across studies. Data on associations of other dietary factors and ASD, ADHD and related outcomes are inconclusive and warrant future investigation. Future studies that comprehensively quantify maternal nutrient intake from both food and supplements and integrate more objective measures of biomarkers reflecting intake and metabolism are warranted. In addition, incorporating genetic variants related to nutrient metabolism shall enable Mendelian randomization analyses to inform causal inferences and a better understanding of gene-diet interactions in relation to neurodevelopmental disorders. Understanding the sensitive window of exposure and gene-diet interactions may help inform precise intervention and prevention.

Author Contributions: C.Z., M.L. and S.N.H. conceptualized the study; M.L., S.N.H. and E.F. designed the study; M.L., E.F. and A.S.A. contributed to the acquisition, analysis, and interpretation of the data; M.L. wrote the first draft of the manuscript; all authors substantially revised the manuscript for important intellectual content and approved the submitted version of the manuscript.

References

1. King, J.C. A summary of pathways or mechanisms linking preconception maternal nutrition with birth outcomes. *J. Nutr.* **2016**, *146*, 1437s–1444s. [CrossRef] [PubMed]
2. Stephenson, J.; Heslehurst, N.; Hall, J.; Schoenaker, D.; Hutchinson, J.; Cade, J.E.; Poston, L.; Barrett, G.; Crozier, S.R.; Barker, M.; et al. Before the beginning: Nutrition and lifestyle in the preconception period and its importance for future health. *Lancet* **2018**, *391*, 1830–1841. [CrossRef]
3. Tau, G.Z.; Peterson, B.S. Normal development of brain circuits. *Neuropsychopharmacology* **2010**, *35*, 147–168. [CrossRef] [PubMed]
4. Lyall, K.; Schmidt, R.J.; Hertz-Picciotto, I. Maternal lifestyle and environmental risk factors for autism spectrum disorders. *Int. J. Epidemiol.* **2014**, *43*, 443–464. [CrossRef] [PubMed]
5. Linnet, K.M.; Dalsgaard, S.; Obel, C.; Wisborg, K.; Henriksen, T.B.; Rodriguez, A.; Kotimaa, A.; Moilanen, I.; Thomsen, P.H.; Olsen, J.; et al. Maternal lifestyle factors in pregnancy risk of attention deficit hyperactivity disorder and associated behaviors: review of the current evidence. *Am. J. Psychiatry* **2003**, *160*, 1028–1040. [CrossRef] [PubMed]
6. Prado, E.L.; Dewey, K.G. Nutrition and brain development in early life. *Nutr. Rev.* **2014**, *72*, 267–284. [CrossRef] [PubMed]

7. Bale, T.L.; Baram, T.Z.; Brown, A.S.; Goldstein, J.M.; Insel, T.R.; McCarthy, M.M.; Nemeroff, C.B.; Reyes, T.M.; Simerly, R.B.; Susser, E.S.; et al. Early life programming and neurodevelopmental disorders. *Biol. Psychiatry* **2010**, *68*, 314–319. [CrossRef] [PubMed]
8. Lee, H.S. Impact of maternal diet on the epigenome during in utero life and the developmental programming of diseases in childhood and adulthood. *Nutrients* **2015**, *7*, 9492–9507. [CrossRef] [PubMed]
9. Steegers-Theunissen, R.P.; Obermann-Borst, S.A.; Kremer, D.; Lindemans, J.; Siebel, C.; Steegers, E.A.; Slagboom, P.E.; Heijmans, B.T. Periconceptional maternal folic acid use of 400 microg per day is related to increased methylation of the *IGF2* gene in the very young child. *PLoS ONE* **2009**, *4*, e7845. [CrossRef]
10. Craciunescu, C.N.; Brown, E.C.; Mar, M.H.; Albright, C.D.; Nadeau, M.R.; Zeisel, S.H. Folic acid deficiency during late gestation decreases progenitor cell proliferation and increases apoptosis in fetal mouse brain. *J. Nutr.* **2004**, *134*, 162–166. [CrossRef]
11. Jadavji, N.M.; Deng, L.; Malysheva, O.; Caudill, M.A.; Rozen, R. MTHFR deficiency or reduced intake of folate or choline in pregnant mice results in impaired short-term memory and increased apoptosis in the hippocampus of wild-type offspring. *Neuroscience* **2015**, *300*, 1–9. [CrossRef] [PubMed]
12. Pitkin, R.M. Folate and neural tube defects. *Am. J. Clin. Nutr.* **2007**, *85*, 285s–288s. [CrossRef] [PubMed]
13. Yehuda, S.; Rabinovitz, S.; Mostofsky, D.I. Essential fatty acids are mediators of brain biochemistry and cognitive functions. *J. Neurosci. Res.* **1999**, *56*, 565–570. [CrossRef]
14. Martinez, M. Tissue levels of polyunsaturated fatty acids during early human development. *J. Pediatrics* **1992**, *120*, S129–S138. [CrossRef]
15. Lauritzen, L.; Brambilla, P.; Mazzocchi, A.; Harsløf, L.; Ciappolino, V.; Agostoni, C. DHA effects in brain development and function. *Nutrients* **2016**, *8*, 6. [CrossRef]
16. McCann, J.C.; Ames, B.N. Is docosahexaenoic acid, an n-3 long-chain polyunsaturated fatty acid, required for development of normal brain function? An overview of evidence from cognitive and behavioral tests in humans and animals. *Am. J. Clin. Nutr.* **2005**, *82*, 281–295. [CrossRef] [PubMed]
17. Carlson, S.E. Docosahexaenoic acid and arachidonic acid in infant development. *Semin. Neonatol.* **2001**, *6*, 437–449. [CrossRef]
18. Fretham, S.J.; Carlson, E.S.; Georgieff, M.K. The role of iron in learning and memory. *Adv. Nutr.* **2011**, *2*, 112–121. [CrossRef]
19. Skeaff, S.A. Iodine deficiency in pregnancy: The effect on neurodevelopment in the child. *Nutrients* **2011**, *3*, 265–273. [CrossRef]
20. Porciúncula, L.O.; Sallaberry, C.; Mioranzza, S.; Botton, P.H.S.; Rosemberg, D.B. The Janus face of caffeine. *Neurochem. Int.* **2013**, *63*, 594–609. [CrossRef]
21. Bougma, K.; Aboud, F.E.; Harding, K.B.; Marquis, G.S. Iodine and mental development of children 5 years old and under: A systematic review and meta-analysis. *Nutrients* **2013**, *5*, 1384–1416. [CrossRef] [PubMed]
22. Borge, T.C.; Aase, H.; Brantsaeter, A.L.; Biele, G. The importance of maternal diet quality during pregnancy on cognitive and behavioural outcomes in children: A systematic review and meta-analysis. *BMJ Open* **2017**, *7*, e016777. [CrossRef] [PubMed]
23. Freedman, R.; Hunter, S.K.; Hoffman, M.C. Prenatal primary prevention of mental illness by micronutrient supplements in pregnancy. *Am. J. Psychiatry* **2018**, *175*, 607–619. [CrossRef] [PubMed]
24. Starling, P.; Charlton, K.; McMahon, A.T.; Lucas, C. Fish intake during pregnancy and foetal neurodevelopment—A systematic review of the evidence. *Nutrients* **2015**, *7*, 2001–2014. [CrossRef] [PubMed]
25. Gould, J.F.; Smithers, L.G.; Makrides, M. The effect of maternal omega-3 (n-3) LCPUFA supplementation during pregnancy on early childhood cognitive and visual development: A systematic review and meta-analysis of randomized controlled trials. *Am. J. Clin. Nutr.* **2013**, *97*, 531–544. [CrossRef] [PubMed]
26. Wang, M.; Li, K.; Zhao, D.; Li, L. The association between maternal use of folic acid supplements during pregnancy and risk of autism spectrum disorders in children: A meta-analysis. *Mol. Autism* **2017**, *8*, 51. [CrossRef] [PubMed]
27. DeVilbiss, E.A.; Gardner, R.M.; Newschaffer, C.J.; Lee, B.K. Maternal folate status as a risk factor for autism spectrum disorders: A review of existing evidence. *Br. J. Nutr.* **2015**, *114*, 663–672. [CrossRef]
28. Bayer, S.A.; Altman, J.; Russo, R.J.; Zhang, X. Timetables of neurogenesis in the human brain based on experimentally determined patterns in the rat. *Neurotoxicology* **1993**, *14*, 83–144.

29. Centers for Disease Control and Prevention. Data & Statistics on Autism Spectrum Disorder. Available online: https://www.cdc.gov/ncbddd/autism/data.html (accessed on 5 June 2019).
30. Centers for Disease Control and Prevention. Data & Statistics about ADHD. Available online: https://www.cdc.gov/ncbddd/adhd/data.html (accessed on 5 June 2019).
31. Tierney, J.F.; Stewart, L.A.; Ghersi, D.; Burdett, S.; Sydes, M.R. Practical methods for incorporating summary time-to-event data into meta-analysis. *Trials* **2007**, *8*, 16. [CrossRef]
32. StataCorp LP. *Stata Statistical Software: Release 14. (computer program)*; StataCorp LP: College Station, TX, USA, 2015.
33. Schmidt, R.J.; Iosif, A.M.; Angel, E.G.; Ozonoff, S. Association of maternal prenatal vitamin use with risk for autism spectrum disorder recurrence in young siblings. *JAMA Psychiatry* **2019**, *76*, 391–398. [CrossRef]
34. Levine, S.Z.; Kodesh, A.; Viktorin, A.; Smith, L.; Uher, R.; Reichenberg, A.; Sandin, S. Association of maternal use of folic acid and multivitamin supplements in the periods before and during pregnancy with the risk of autism spectrum disorder in offspring. *JAMA Psychiatry* **2018**, *75*, 176–184. [CrossRef] [PubMed]
35. Li, Y.M.; Shen, Y.D.; Li, Y.J.; Xun, G.L.; Liu, H.; Wu, R.R.; Ou, J.J. Maternal dietary patterns, supplements intake and autism spectrum disorders: A preliminary case-control study. *Medicine* **2018**, *97*, e13902. [CrossRef] [PubMed]
36. Raghavan, R.; Riley, A.W.; Volk, H.; Caruso, D.; Hironaka, L.; Sices, L.; Hong, X.; Wang, G.; Ji, Y.; Brucato, M.; et al. Maternal multivitamin intake, plasma folate and vitamin B12 levels and autism spectrum disorder risk in offspring. *Paediatr. Perinat. Epidemiol.* **2018**, *32*, 100–111. [CrossRef]
37. Strom, M.G.C.; Lyall, K.; Ascherio, A.; Olsen, S.F. Research letter: Folic acid supplementation and intake of folate in pregnancy in relation to offspring risk of autism spectrum disorder. *Psychol. Med.* **2018**, *48*, 1048–1054. [CrossRef] [PubMed]
38. DeVilbiss, E.A.; Magnusson, C.; Gardner, R.M.; Rai, D.; Newschaffer, C.J.; Lyall, K.; Dalman, C.; Lee, B.K. Antenatal nutritional supplementation and autism spectrum disorders in the Stockholm youth cohort: Population based cohort study. *BMJ* **2017**, *359*, j4273. [CrossRef] [PubMed]
39. Virk, J.; Liew, Z.; Olsen, J.; Nohr, E.A.; Catov, J.M.; Ritz, B. Preconceptional and prenatal supplementary folic acid and multivitamin intake and autism spectrum disorders. *Autism* **2016**, *20*, 710–718. [CrossRef] [PubMed]
40. Braun, J.M.; Froehlich, T.; Kalkbrenner, A.; Pfeiffer, C.M.; Fazili, Z.; Yolton, K.; Lanphear, B.P. Brief report: Are autistic-behaviors in children related to prenatal vitamin use and maternal whole blood folate concentrations? *J. Autism Dev. Disord.* **2014**, *44*, 2602–2607. [CrossRef]
41. Nilsen, R.M.; Surén, P.; Gunnes, N.; Alsaker, E.R.; Bresnahan, M.; Hirtz, D.; Roth, C. Analysis of self-selection bias in a population-based cohort study of autism spectrum disorders. *Paediatr. Perinat. Epidemiol.* **2013**, *27*, 553–563. [CrossRef]
42. Suren, P.; Roth, C.; Bresnahan, M.; Haugen, M.; Hornig, M.; Hirtz, D.; Lie, K.K.; Lipkin, W.I.; Magnus, P.; Reichborn-Kjennerud, T.; et al. Association between maternal use of folic acid supplements and risk of autism spectrum disorders in children. *Jama* **2013**, *309*, 570–577. [CrossRef]
43. DeSoto, M.C.; Hitlan, R.T. Synthetic folic acid supplementation during pregnancy may increase the risk of developing autism. *J. Pediatric Biochem.* **2012**, *2*, 251–261.
44. Schmidt, R.J.; Tancredi, D.J.; Ozonoff, S.; Hansen, R.L.; Hartiala, J.; Allayee, H.; Schmidt, L.C.; Tassone, F.; Hertz-Picciotto, I. Maternal periconceptional folic acid intake and risk of autism spectrum disorders and developmental delay in the CHARGE (Childhood Autism Risks from Genetics and Environment) case-control study. *Am. J. Clin. Nutr.* **2012**, *96*, 80–89. [CrossRef] [PubMed]
45. Schmidt, R.J.; Hansen, R.L.; Hartiala, J.; Allayee, H.; Schmidt, L.C.; Tancredi, D.J.; Tassone, F.; Hertz-Picciotto, I. Prenatal vitamins, one-carbon metabolism gene variants, and risk for autism. *Epidemiology* **2011**, *22*, 476–485. [CrossRef] [PubMed]
46. Steenweg-de Graaff, J.; Ghassabian, A.; Jaddoe, V.W.; Tiemeier, H.; Roza, S.J. Folate concentrations during pregnancy and autistic traits in the offspring. The Generation R Study. *Eur. J. Public Health* **2015**, *25*, 431–433. [CrossRef] [PubMed]
47. Schmidt, R.J.; Tancredi, D.J.; Krakowiak, P.; Hansen, R.L.; Ozonoff, S. Maternal intake of supplemental iron and risk of autism spectrum disorder. *Am. J. Epidemiol.* **2014**, *180*, 890–900. [CrossRef] [PubMed]

48. Lyall, K.; Munger, K.L.; O'Reilly, E.J.; Santangelo, S.L.; Ascherio, A. Maternal dietary fat intake in association with autism spectrum disorders. *Am. J. Epidemiol.* **2013**, *178*, 209–220. [CrossRef]
49. Steenweg-De Graaff, J.; Tiemeier, H.; Ghassabian, A.; Rijlaarsdam, J.; Jaddoe, V.W.V.; Verhulst, F.C.; Roza, S.J. Maternal fatty acid status during pregnancy and child autistic traits: The Generation R Study. *Am. J. Epidemiol.* **2016**, *183*, 792–799. [CrossRef]
50. Gao, L.; Cui, S.S.; Han, Y.; Dai, W.; Su, Y.Y.; Zhang, X. Does periconceptional fish consumption by parents affect the incidence of autism spectrum disorder and intelligence deficiency? A Case-control study in Tianjin, China. *Biomed. Environ. Sci.* **2016**, *29*, 885–892. [CrossRef]
51. Julvez, J.; Mendez, M.; Fernandez-Barres, S.; Romaguera, D.; Vioque, J.; Llop, S.; Ibarluzea, J.; Guxens, M.; Avella-Garcia, C.; Tardon, A.; et al. Maternal consumption of seafood in pregnancy and child neuropsychological development: A longitudinal study based on a population with high consumption levels. *Am. J. Epidemiol.* **2016**, *183*, 169–182. [CrossRef]
52. House, J.S.; Mendez, M.; Maguire, R.L.; Gonzalez-Nahm, S.; Huang, Z.; Daniels, J.; Murphy, S.K.; Fuemmeler, B.F.; Wright, F.A.; Hoyo, C. Periconceptional maternal mediterranean diet is associated with favorable offspring behaviors and altered CpG methylation of imprinted genes. *Front. Cell Dev. Biol.* **2018**, *6*, 107. [CrossRef]
53. Schmidt, R.J.; Ozonoff, S.; Hansen, R.; Hartiala, J.; Allayee, H.; Schmidt, L.; Tassone, F.; Hertz-Picciotto, I. (old record 6424) Maternal periconceptional folic acid intake and risk for developmental delay and autism spectrum disorder: A case-control study. *Am. J. Epidemiol.* **2012**, *175*, S126. [CrossRef]
54. Li, Y.-M.; Ou, J.-J.; Liu, L.; Zhang, D.; Zhao, J.-P.; Tang, S.-Y. Association between maternal obesity and autism spectrum disorder in offspring: A meta-analysis. *J. Autism Dev. Disord.* **2016**, *46*, 95–102. [CrossRef] [PubMed]
55. Ueland, P.M.; Hustad, S.; Schneede, J.; Refsum, H.; Vollset, S.E. Biological and clinical implications of the *MTHFR* C677T polymorphism. *Trends Pharmacol. Sci.* **2001**, *22*, 195–201. [CrossRef]
56. Rijlaarsdam, J.; Cecil, C.A.; Walton, E.; Mesirow, M.S.; Relton, C.L.; Gaunt, T.R.; McArdle, W.; Barker, E.D. Prenatal unhealthy diet, *insulin-like growth factor* 2 gene (*IGF2*) methylation, and attention deficit hyperactivity disorder symptoms in youth with early-onset conduct problems. *J. Child Psychol. Psychiatry* **2017**, *58*, 19–27. [CrossRef] [PubMed]
57. Pidsley, R.; Dempster, E.; Troakes, C.; Al-Sarraj, S.; Mill, J. Epigenetic and genetic variation at the *IGF2/H19* imprinting control region on 11p15. 5 is associated with cerebellum weight. *Epigenetics* **2012**, *7*, 155–163. [CrossRef] [PubMed]
58. Office of Dietary Supplements; National Library of Medicine. Dietary Supplement Label Database. Available online: https://www.dsld.nlm.nih.gov/dsld/index.jsp (accessed on 7 February 2019).
59. Stamm, R.; Houghton, L. Nutrient intake values for folate during pregnancy and lactation vary widely around the world. *Nutrients* **2013**, *5*, 3920–3947. [CrossRef] [PubMed]
60. Wilcken, B.; Bamforth, F.; Li, Z.; Zhu, H.; Ritvanen, A.; Redlund, M.; Stoll, C.; Alembik, Y.; Dott, B.; Czeizel, A. Geographical and ethnic variation of the 677C> T allele of 5, 10 *methylenetetrahydrofolate reductase* (*MTHFR*): Findings from over 7000 newborns from 16 areas world wide. *J. Med Genet.* **2003**, *40*, 619–625. [CrossRef] [PubMed]
61. Schmitz, G.; Ecker, J. The opposing effects of n-3 and n-6 fatty acids. *Prog. Lipid Res.* **2008**, *47*, 147–155. [CrossRef]
62. Patterson, E.; Wall, R.; Fitzgerald, G.F.; Ross, R.P.; Stanton, C. Health implications of high dietary omega-6 polyunsaturated fatty acids. *J. Nutr. Metab.* **2012**, *2012*, 539426. [CrossRef]
63. D'Souza, S.W.; Waldie, K.E.; Peterson, E.R.; Underwood, L.; Morton, S.M.B. Antenatal and postnatal determinants of behavioural difficulties in early childhood: Evidence from growing up in New Zealand. *Child Psychiatry Hum. Dev.* **2019**, *50*, 45–60. [CrossRef]
64. Miyake, Y.T.K.; Okubo, H.; Sasaki, S.; Arakawa, M. Maternal B vitamin intake during pregnancy and childhood behavioral problems in Japan: The Kyushu Okinawa maternal and child health study. *Nutr. Neurosci.* **2018**, *19*, 1–8. [CrossRef]
65. Virk, J.; Liew, Z.; Olsen, J.; Nohr, E.A.; Catov, J.M.; Ritz, B. Pre-conceptual and prenatal supplementary folic acid and multivitamin intake, behavioral problems, and hyperkinetic disorders: A study based on the Danish National Birth Cohort (DNBC). *Nutr. Neurosci.* **2018**, *21*, 352–360. [CrossRef] [PubMed]

66. Julvez, J.; Fortuny, J.; Mendez, M.; Torrent, M.; Ribas-Fitó, N.; Sunyer, J. Maternal use of folic acid supplements during pregnancy and four-year-old neurodevelopment in a population-based birth cohort. *Paediatr. Perinat. Epidemiol.* **2009**, *23*, 199–206. [CrossRef] [PubMed]
67. Schlotz, W.; Jones, A.; Phillips, D.I.; Gale, C.R.; Robinson, S.M.; Godfrey, K.M. Lower maternal folate status in early pregnancy is associated with childhood hyperactivity and peer problems in offspring. *J. Child Psychol. Psychiatry* **2010**, *51*, 594–602. [CrossRef] [PubMed]
68. Abel, M.H.; Ystrom, E.; Caspersen, I.H.; Meltzer, H.M.; Aase, H.; Torheim, L.E.; Askeland, R.B.; Reichborn-Kjennerud, T.; Brantsaeter, A.L. Maternal iodine intake and offspring attention-deficit/hyperactivity disorder: Results from a large prospective cohort study. *Nutrients* **2017**, *9*, 1239. [CrossRef] [PubMed]
69. Miyake, Y.T.K.; Okubo, H.; Sasaki, S.; Arakawa, M. Maternal fat intake during pregnancy and behavioral problems in 5-y-old Japanese children. *Nutrition* **2018**, *50*, 91–96. [CrossRef]
70. Ramakrishnan, U.; Gonzalez-Casanova, I.; Schnaas, L.; DiGirolamo, A.; Quezada, A.D.; Pallo, B.C.; Hao, W.; Neufeld, L.M.; Rivera, J.A.; Stein, A.D.; et al. Prenatal supplementation with DHA improves attention at 5 years of age: A randomized controlled trial. *Am. J. Clin. Nutr.* **2016**, *104*, 1075–1082. [CrossRef] [PubMed]
71. Gale, C.R.; Robinson, S.M.; Godfrey, K.M.; Law, C.M.; Schlotz, W.; O'Callaghan, F.J. Oily fish intake during pregnancy—Association with lower hyperactivity but not with higher full-scale IQ in offspring. *J. Child Psychol. Psychiatry Allied Discip.* **2008**, *49*, 1061–1068. [CrossRef]
72. Hibbeln, J.R.; Davis, J.M.; Steer, C.; Emmett, P.; Rogers, I.; Williams, C.; Golding, J. Maternal seafood consumption in pregnancy and neurodevelopmental outcomes in childhood (ALSPAC study): An observational cohort study. *Lancet* **2007**, *369*, 578–585. [CrossRef]
73. Miyake, Y.T.K.; Okubo, H.; Sasaki, S.; Arakawa, M. Maternal caffeine intake in pregnancy is inversely related to childhood peer problems in Japan: The Kyushu Okinawa maternal and child health study. *Nutr. Neurosci.* **2018**, *13*, 1–8. [CrossRef]
74. Del-Ponte, B.; Santos, I.S.; Tovo-Rodrigues, L.; Anselmi, L.; Munhoz, T.N.; Matijasevich, A. Caffeine consumption during pregnancy and ADHD at the age of 11 years: A birth cohort study. *BMJ Open* **2016**, *6*, e012749. [CrossRef]
75. Loomans, E.M.; Hofland, L.; van der Stelt, O.; van der Wal, M.F.; Koot, H.M.; Van den Bergh, B.R.; Vrijkotte, T.G. Caffeine intake during pregnancy and risk of problem behavior in 5- to 6-year-old children. *Pediatrics* **2012**, *130*, e305–e313. [CrossRef] [PubMed]
76. Hvolgaard Mikkelsen, S.; Obel, C.; Olsen, J.; Niclasen, J.; Bech, B.H. Maternal caffeine consumption during pregnancy and behavioral disorders in 11-year-old offspring: A Danish National Birth Cohort study. *J. Pediatrics* **2017**, *189*, 120–127.e121. [CrossRef] [PubMed]
77. Linnet, K.M.; Wisborg, K.; Secher, N.J.; Thomsen, P.H.; Obel, C.; Dalsgaard, S.; Henriksen, T.B. Coffee consumption during pregnancy and the risk of hyperkinetic disorder and ADHD: A prospective cohort study. *Acta Paediatr.* **2009**, *98*, 173–179. [CrossRef] [PubMed]
78. Galera, C.; Heude, B.; Forhan, A.; Bernard, J.Y.; Peyre, H.; Van der Waerden, J.; Pryor, L.; Bouvard, M.P.; Melchior, M.; Lioret, S.; et al. Prenatal diet and children's trajectories of hyperactivity-inattention and conduct problems from 3 to 8 years: The EDEN mother-child cohort. *J. Child Psychol. Psychiatry* **2018**, *59*, 1003–1011. [CrossRef] [PubMed]
79. McGee, R.A.; Clark, S.E.; Symons, D.K. Does the conners' continuous performance test aid in ADHD diagnosis? *J. Abnorm. Child Psychol.* **2000**, *28*, 415–424. [CrossRef] [PubMed]
80. Thapar, A.; Cooper, M.; Jefferies, R.; Stergiakouli, E. What causes attention deficit hyperactivity disorder? *Arch. Dis. Child.* **2012**, *97*, 260–265. [CrossRef]
81. Mathias, R.A.; Pani, V.; Chilton, F.H. Genetic Variants in the FADS gene: Implications for dietary recommendations for fatty acid intake. *Curr. Nutr. Rep.* **2014**, *3*, 139–148. [CrossRef]
82. Symonds, M.E.; Sebert, S.P.; Hyatt, M.A.; Budge, H. Nutritional programming of the metabolic syndrome. *Nat. Rev. Endocrinol.* **2009**, *5*, 604–610. [CrossRef]

15

Effects of Vitamin D Supplementation During Pregnancy on Birth Size

Andrea Maugeri, Martina Barchitta, Isabella Blanco and Antonella Agodi *

Department of Medical and Surgical Sciences and Advanced Technologies "GF Ingrassia", University of Catania, Via S. Sofia 87, 95123 Catania, Italy; andreamaugeri88@gmail.com (A.M.); martina.barchitta@unict.it (M.B.); dott.ssa.blanco.isabella@gmail.com (I.B.)

* Correspondence: agodia@unict.it

Abstract: During pregnancy, vitamin D supplementation may be a feasible strategy to help prevent low birthweight (LBW) and small for gestational age (SGA) births. However, evidence from randomized controlled trials (RCTs) is inconclusive, probably due to heterogeneity in study design and type of intervention. A systematic literature search in the PubMed-Medline, EMBASE, and Cochrane Central Register of Controlled Trials databases was carried out to evaluate the effects of oral vitamin D supplementation during pregnancy on birthweight, birth length, head circumference, LBW, and SGA. The fixed-effects or random-effects models were used to calculate mean difference (MD), risk ratio (RR), and 95% Confidence Interval (CI). On a total of 13 RCTs, maternal vitamin D supplementation had a positive effect on birthweight (12 RCTs; MD = 103.17 g, 95% CI 62.29–144.04 g), length (6 RCTs; MD = 0.22 cm, 95% CI 0.11–0.33 cm), and head circumference (6 RCTs; MD:0.19 cm, 95% CI 0.13–0.24 cm). In line with these findings, we also demonstrated that maternal vitamin D supplementation reduced the risk of LBW (3 RCTs; RR = 0.40, 95% CI 0.22–0.74) and SGA (5 RCTS; RR = 0.69, 95% CI 0.51–0.92). The present systematic review and meta-analysis confirmed the well-established effect of maternal vitamin D supplementation on birth size. However, further research is required to better define risks and benefits associated with such interventions and the potential implications for public health.

Keywords: nutrition; diet; vitamin D; birthweight; birth length; head circumference; gestational age; pregnancy outcomes

---

1. Introduction

Nutrition in women of childbearing age has a critical role on their health as well as on infant outcomes. A balanced supply of maternal nutrients, before conception, during pregnancy, and during breastfeeding, promotes optimal growth and development both in fetus and offspring [1,2]. During pregnancy, the fetus is entirely dependent on maternal sources of vitamin D, which also regulates placental function [3]. Several observational studies have shown that pregnancy is a crucial period in which vitamin D deficiency may affect mother and neonatal outcomes, thereby influencing the risk of recurrent pregnancy losses, preeclampsia, gestational diabetes, maternal infections, preterm birth, low birthweight (LBW), small for gestational age (SGA), and poor offspring health [4]. Thus, hypovitaminosis D in pregnancy requires an adequate treatment, and vitamin D supplementation represents a valid strategy for preventing and controlling vitamin D deficiency [5]. The Food and Nutrition Board at the Institute of Medicine of the National Academies suggests that a proper integration of vitamin D in pregnancy and in lactation is 15 micrograms (600 IU) per day [6]. Recently, many randomized controlled trials (RCTs) have been conducted to evaluate the benefits of vitamin D supplementation in pregnancy. Although vitamin D supplementation may increase serum 25(OH)D levels in both mothers and infants [7], it remains unclear whether vitamin D supplementation is protective for LBW, SGA or intrauterine growth restriction, and generally for long-term offspring health. To our knowledge, the meta-analysis by Thorne-Lyman et al. was the first to summarize the effect of vitamin D on birthweight and LBW incidence [8]. Pooled estimates of observational studies showed a positive relationship between vitamin D status and birthweight [8]. However, pooled analysis of interventional studies suggested, on one hand, no significant effect on mean birthweight, but on the other hand a lower risk of LBW newborns in women supplemented with vitamin D [8]. A recent systematic review by Harvey et al. [4] partially confirmed these results: out of seven studies, three trials showed that maternal vitamin D supplementation significantly increased birthweight in infants [4]. Although this evidence was also corroborated by Perez-Lopez et al. in a meta-analysis of 8 RCTs, the authors did not demonstrate the influence on the risk of LBW and SGA (3 RCTs, respectively) [5]. In contrast, four trials included in the most recent systematic review by De-Regil et al. reported that maternal vitamin D supplementation significantly reduced the risk of LBW [7]. However, no difference was reported in the mean birthweight of infants [7]. Therefore, evidence is currently inconclusive to drawn convincing assumptions on the usefulness of maternal vitamin D supplementation against LBW and SGA births. Moreover, previous mentioned reviews [4,5,7,8] showed heterogeneity in dose, duration and timing of supplementation, and study design (i.e., observational studies, quasi-RCTs, and RCTs). Herein, we provide a systematic review and a meta-analysis of data from RCTs, to evaluate the effects of oral vitamin D supplementation during pregnancy on fetal growth as indicated by neonatal anthropometric measures and incidence of LBW and SGA births. Moreover, we also performed subgroup analyses to demonstrate whether alternative formulations and regimens had different effect on birth size.

2. Materials and Methods

2.1. Literature Search

A systematic literature search in the PubMed-Medline, EMBASE, and Cochrane Central Register of Controlled Trials databases was carried out for RCTs investigating the role of oral vitamin D supplementation during pregnancy on neonatal anthropometric measures and incidence of LBW and SGA. Literature search was conducted independently by two authors (A.M. and I.B.) using the following keywords: (vitamin d OR ergocalciferol OR cholecalciferol OR calcifediol OR vitamin d supplementation OR 25-hydroxyvitamin D) AND (birth size OR birth weight OR birth length OR head circumference OR low birth weight OR SGA OR neonatal anthropometric measures). Full details of literature search terms are included in Supplementary Materials. The databases were searched from inception to May 2017 without language restriction; abstracts and unpublished studies were not included. Moreover, the reference lists from selected articles, including relevant review papers, were searched to identify all relevant studies. The preferred reporting items for systematic reviews and meta-analysis (PRISMA) guidelines were followed [9].

2.2. Inclusion and Exclusion Criteria

Studies were selected only if they satisfied the following criteria: (1) RCTs, with randomization at either individual or cluster level, (2) of pregnant women of any gestational age (3) without pregnancy complications, (4) that assessed the effect of oral vitamin D supplementation, irrespective of dose, duration or time of commencement, on birthweight, birth length, head circumference, and incidence of LBW, and/or SGA. Eligible intervention groups included daily or single-intermitted vitamin D supplementation (vitamin D2 or D3), alone or in combination with calcium and/or other micronutrients. For studies with more than two intervention groups, we combined disaggregated data into subgroup category to create a single pair-wise group comparison [10]. Control groups included no treatment or placebo. Exclusion criteria were as follows: (1) systematic reviews or meta-analyses; (2) observational studies, cross-over trials, or quasi-RCTs; (3) no appropriate treatment group (pregnant women with pre-existing pregnancy complications); (4) no appropriate control group (i.e., vitamin D supplementation); (5) not available data on birth size and/or incidence of LBW and SGA.

2.3. *Study Selection and Data Extraction*

Two of the authors (A.M. and I.B.) independently assessed for inclusion all the references identified through the literature search. From all the eligible studies, two authors (A.M. and I.B.) independently extracted the following information in a standard format: first author's last name, year of publication, country, and latitude where the study was performed, season when the study was performed, number of participants, age and information about vitamin D intervention (i.e., Formulation, regimen, method of administration, and treatment duration). Primary outcomes were birthweight (g), birth length (cm), head circumference (cm), low birthweight (LBW; <2500 g) and SGA, defined as birthweight below the 10th percentile of a reference distribution of weights specific for sex and gestational age. Other outcomes were: maternal serum 25-OHD levels at baseline and at the end of the intervention, cord 25-OHD levels, gestational age, caesarean delivery, pregnancy complications (i.e., preterm birth, gestational diabetes, pre-eclampsia), and Apgar score. Cross-checked data were entered into Review Manager software (RevMan, version 5.3, Copenhagen, Denmark)) by A.M., and checked for accuracy by M.B. During study selection and data extraction, any disagreements between A.M. and M.B. were resolved by discussion and consensus with a third Author (A.A.).

2.4. *Risk-of-Bias and Quality Assessment*

The risk of bias from each eligible RCT was evaluated using the Cochrane's Collaboration tool for assessing risk of bias in randomized trials [10]. This tool includes the following items, which were assigned as either 'low risk of bias', 'unclear risk of bias' or 'high risk of bias': random sequence generation (selection bias); concealment of the allocation sequence (selection bias); blinding of participants and personnel (performance bias); blinding of outcome assessment (detection bias); incomplete outcome data (attrition bias); selective outcome reporting (reporting bias); and other biases [8]. Risk of bias was assessed by two of the authors (A.M. and M.B.) using the Review Manager software (RevMan, version 5.3), and presented as a risk-of-bias summary figure. Disagreements were resolved by consensus or discussion with a third Author (A.A.). For each outcome, two of the authors (A.M. and M.B.) independently assessed the quality of the evidence using the Grading of Recommendations Assessment, Development and Evaluation (GRADE) approach [11]. The GRADE system considers eight criteria for assessing the quality of evidence: risk of bias, inconsistency, indirectness, imprecision, publication bias, and other (large magnitude of effect, dose response, and no plausible confounding). Based on these criteria, the quality of evidence was classified as high, moderate, low, or very low. Disagreements were resolved by consensus or discussion with a third Author (A.A.).

2.5. *Statistical Analysis*

Data on dichotomous outcomes were combined and effect sizes were presented as RR with 95% confidence intervals (CIs). For continuous outcomes, we estimated mean differences (MDs) with 95% CI. Forest plots were generated to illustrate the study-specific effect sizes along with a 95% CI. The significance of pooled effect size was determined using the Z test, and $p < 0.05$ was considered significant. Heterogeneity across studies was assessed using the Q-test based on the $\chi 2$ statistic

($p < 0.1$ was considered statistically significant). To quantify heterogeneity, the I2 value was calculated and interpreted as follows: an I2 value of 0% indicates "no heterogeneity," whereas 25% is "low," 50% is "moderate," and 75% is "high" heterogeneity. We considered heterogeneity as significant if $p < 0.1$ for Q-test based on the $\chi 2$ statistic and I^2 was greater than 30% [12]. To calculate pooled effect estimates, the fixed-effects model (Mantel-Haenszel method) was used in absence of significant heterogeneity, otherwise the random-effects model (Der Simonian-Laird method). In the random effect model, the between-study variance was estimated using the tau-squared ($\tau 2$) statistic [10]. The leave-one-out sensitivity analysis was performed by the omission of a single study at a time, to assess whether a particular omission could affect effect sizes and heterogeneity across studies. Sensitivity analysis by the omission of studies with daily vitamin D dose of 200 IU [13,14] was also performed to assess whether they affected the pooled effect sizes. We also performed subgroup analyses by formulation (vitamin D alone vs. vitamin D in combination with calcium and/or other micronutrients) and supplementation regimen (daily vs. single/intermitted high dose). Since vitamin D might have a dose-dependent effect on birth sizes, we performed a meta-regression using the Comprehensive Meta-analysis software (Version 2.0; Biostat Inc., Englewood, NJ, USA). Particularly, meta-regression analyses were performed on those outcomes with at least three studies evaluating daily vitamin D supplementation alone [15]. Heterogeneity in formulation, dose, duration, and timing of supplementation, did not allow us to perform meta-regression of studies with single supplementation and/or combination of supplements. In those outcomes with at least two group comparisons for subgroup, we assessed subgroup differences by the $\chi 2$ statistic, and the interaction test I^2 value. In those outcomes with 10 or more group comparisons, the presence of publication bias was investigated by visually assessment of funnel plot asymmetry, followed by Begg's test and Egger's regression asymmetry test [16,17]. Except for the Q-test, $p < 0.05$ was considered statistically significant, and all tests were 2-sided. All statistical analyses were performed using the Review Manager software (RevMan, version 5.3).

3. Results

3.1. Study Selection

The detailed steps of the study selection are given as a PRISMA flow diagram in Figure 1. A total of 669 abstracts were retrieved from the databases; 542 were excluded after reading titles and/or abstracts, and 127 articles were subjected to a full-text review. From these, 114 studies were excluded according to selection criteria, whereas 13 RCTs, published between 1980 and 2016, were included in the meta-analysis [13,14,18–28]. However, since four articles showed more eligible intervention groups [19–21,28], the meta-analysis reported data on 17 group comparisons between eligible intervention ($n = 17$) and control groups ($n = 13$) (Table 1).

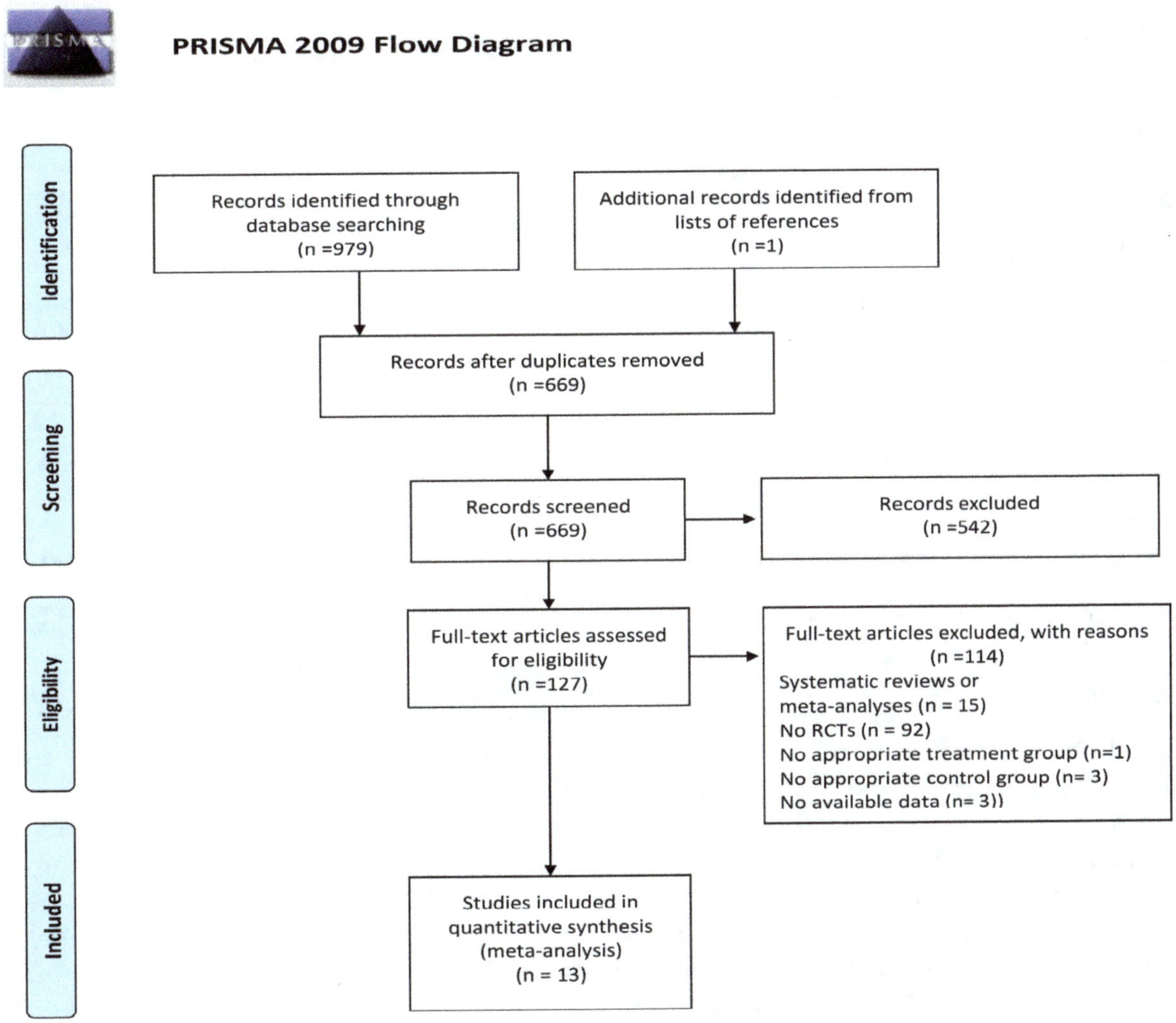

Figure 1. PRISMA flow diagram of study selection.

Table 1. Characteristics of randomized controlled trials included in the meta-analysis.

First Author, Year	Country	Treatment (Vitamin D Dosage)	CONTROL GROUP	Size of Intervention/ Control Groups	Treatment Duration (Week)	Outcomes
Asemi, 2016 [13]	Iran	Vit D3 + Ca (200 IU/day)	Placebo	21/21	9	Birthweight, birth length, head circumference
Brooke, 1980 [18]	UK	Vit D2 (1000 IU/day)	Placebo	59/67	8–12	Birthweight, birth length, head circumference, LBW, SGA
Brough, 2010 [14]	UK	Vit D3 + micronutrients (200 IU/day)	Placebo	88/61	NA	Birthweight, head circumference, LBW, SGA
Charandabi, 2015 [19]	Iran	Vit D + Ca (1000 IU/day) Vit D (1000 IU/day)	Placebo	40/42 42/42	9	Birthweight, birth length, head circumference
Goldring, 2013 [20]	UK	Vit D2 (800 IU/day) Vit D3 (single dose of 200000 IU)	No intervention	56/50	12	Birthweight
Hollis, 2011 [21]	USA	Vit D3 + micronutrients (1600 IU/day) Vit D3 + micronutrients (3600 IU/day)	Placebo	122/111 117/111	24–28	Birthweight

Table 1. *Cont.*

First Author, Year	Country	Treatment (Vitamin D Dosage)	CONTROL GROUP	Size of Intervention/ Control Groups	Treatment Duration (Week)	Outcomes
Hossain, 2014 [22]	Pakistan	Vit D3 (4000 IU/day)	No intervention	86/89	16	Birthweight, birth length, head circumference, SGA
Marya, 1988 [23]	India	Vit D3 (two doses of 600000 IU)	No intervention	100/100	12	Birthweight, birth length
Naghshineh, 2016 [24]	Iran	Vit D (600 IU/day)	No intervention	68/70	20	Birthweight
Roth, 2013 [25]	Bangladesh	Vit D3 (35,000 IU/week)	Placebo	80/80	12	Birthweight, birth length, head circumference
Sabet, 2012 [26]	Iran	Vit D3 (100000 IU/mol)	Placebo	25/25	12	Birthweight, birth length
Sablok, 2015 [27]	India	Vit D3 (single-intermitted dose depending upon the serum 25OHD levels)	No intervention	108/57	16	Birthweight, SGA
Yu, 2009 [28]	UK	Vit D2 (800 IU/d) Vit D2 (single dose of 200000 IU)	No intervention	60/59 60/59	13	LBW, SGA

Abbreviations: Ca, Calcium; IU, International Unit; 25-OHD, 25-hydroxyvitamin D; LBW, low birth weight; SGA, small for gestational age; NA, not available.

3.2. Systematic Review

A total of 8 studies were from Asian countries, 4 from European countries, and 1 from USA. Accordingly, the latitude of the setting was the Northern tropic in all the included studies. To avoid confounding due to seasonal variation in sunlight exposure, 6 RCTs were carried out in different seasons [14,18,22,24,26,27]. Otherwise, the seasons varied from winter [19] to spring-summer period [13,20,25,28]; this information was not available for 2 RCTs [21,23]. Overall, sample sizes ranged between 40 and 400 pregnant women, and neonatal outcomes of 2016 newborns were reported: 1184 from mothers in the intervention groups and 832 from controls. All the eligible studies were carried out using an individual randomization. Intervention groups were characterized by vitamin D2 (n = 4) or D3 (n = 10) supplementation alone (n = 12) or in combination with calcium (n = 2) or other micronutrients (n = 3). Two trials did not report the vitamin D form used in 3 intervention groups [19,24]. The duration of vitamin D intervention was 6–28 weeks of gestation. Women in 11 intervention groups were supplemented with daily dose of vitamin D, whereas subjects in the remaining 6 intervention groups were supplemented with single-intermitted high dose. The daily dose ranged from 200 IU to 4000 IU; among single-intermitted interventions, the high dose varied from 35000 IU to 600000 IU. Control groups included patients who received placebo (n = 8) or no treatment (n = 5). In those studies evaluating the effect of vitamin D supplementation on 25-hydroxyvitamin D levels, the intervention significantly increased 25-OHD concentration in both mothers [13,14,18,21–23,25–28] and infants [21,22,25–28]. Although 3 RCTs suggested that women who received vitamin D supplementation during pregnancy had a lower risk of preterm birth than controls [13,24,27], in other trials the intervention did not affect gestational age [13,14,20–22,24] and preterm birth risk [14,19,22].

3.3. Meta-Analysis

3.3.1. Birthweight

The effect of vitamin D supplementation on birthweight was assessed by 12 RCTs [13,14,18–27] and 15 group comparisons. Compared to controls, birthweight was significantly higher in the intervention groups (MD: 103.17 g, 95% CI 62.29–144.04 g; $p < 0.001$). *Q*-test and I2 statistics showed no significant heterogeneity across studies ($p > 0.1$; I2 = 7.0%). Particularly, vitamin D supplementation alone, but not in combination with other micronutrients, significantly increased birthweight (MD: 118.46 g,

95% CI 70.47–166.45 g, $p < 0.001$; MD: 62.76 g, 95% CI −15.24–140.77 g, $p = 0.520$, respectively) (Figure 2). The effect of vitamin D in combination with other micronutrients remained no significant also after the omission of studies with daily vitamin D dose of 200 IU [13,14] (MD: 49.30 g, 95% CI −43.52–142.11 g, $p = 0.300$). Particularly, meta-regression did not reveal a dose-dependent effect of vitamin D supplementation alone on birthweight ($p = 0.773$). Subgroup analysis by regimen showed that both daily and single-intermitted high dose supplementation significantly increased birthweight (MD: 74.66 g, 95% CI 18.80–130.52 g, $p < 0.001$; MD: 136.02 g, 95% CI 76.05–195.98 g, $p < 0.001$, respectively).

Study or Subgroup	Vitamin D supplementation Mean	SD	Total	Control Mean	SD	Total	Weight	Mean Difference IV, Fixed, 95% CI
1.1.1 Vitamin D								
Brooke 1980	3,157	469	59	3,034	524	67	5.6%	123.00 [-50.39, 296.39]
Charandabi 2015 (b)	3,225.6	473.3	40	3,192.1	392.4	42	4.7%	33.50 [-155.17, 222.17]
Goldring 2013 (a)	3,290	467	52	3,268	585	50	3.9%	22.00 [-183.92, 227.92]
Goldring 2013 (b)	3,321	525	56	3,268	585	50	3.7%	53.00 [-159.60, 265.60]
Hossain 2014	2,810	520	86	2,750	440	89	8.2%	60.00 [-82.95, 202.95]
Marya 1988	2,990	360	100	2,800	370	100	16.3%	190.00 [88.82, 291.18]
Naghshineh 2016	3,027.4	645.7	68	2,796.9	625.2	70	3.7%	230.50 [18.36, 442.64]
Roth 2013	2,802	543	80	2,788	378	80	7.9%	14.00 [-130.98, 158.98]
Sabet 2012	3,293	334	25	3,248	320	25	5.1%	45.00 [-136.32, 226.32]
Sablok 2015	2,600	410	108	2,400	310	57	13.4%	200.00 [88.39, 311.61]
Subtotal (95% CI)			**674**			**630**	**72.5%**	**118.46 [70.47, 166.45]**
Heterogeneity: Chi² = 10.30, df = 9 (P = 0.33); I² = 13%								
Test for overall effect: Z = 4.84 (P < 0.00001)								
1.1.2 Vitamin D + micronutrients								
Asemi 2016	3,322.1	414.2	21	3,302.4	438.3	21	2.5%	19.70 [-238.22, 277.62]
Brough 2010	3,270	591	88	3,141	485	61	5.6%	129.00 [-44.38, 302.38]
Charandabi 2015 (a)	3,150.2	325.8	42	3,192.1	392.4	42	7.0%	-41.90 [-196.15, 112.35]
Hollis 2011 (a)	3,360	585	122	3,222	675	111	6.3%	138.00 [-24.92, 300.92]
Hollis 2011 (b)	3,285	598	117	3,222	675	111	6.1%	63.00 [-102.86, 228.86]
Subtotal (95% CI)			**390**			**346**	**27.5%**	**62.76 [-15.24, 140.77]**
Heterogeneity: Chi² = 3.26, df = 4 (P = 0.52); I² = 0%								
Test for overall effect: Z = 1.58 (P = 0.11)								
Total (95% CI)			**1064**			**976**	**100.0%**	**103.17 [62.29, 144.04]**
Heterogeneity: Chi² = 14.97, df = 14 (P = 0.38); I² = 7%								
Test for overall effect: Z = 4.95 (P < 0.00001)								
Test for subgroup differences: Chi² = 1.42, df = 1 (P = 0.23), I² = 29.6%								

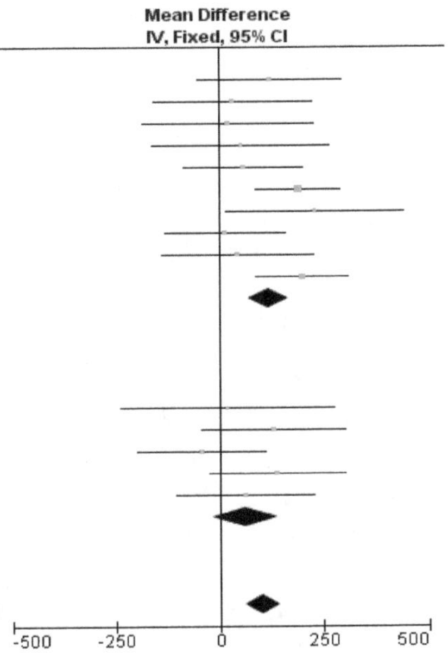

Figure 2. Forest plot of the effect of vitamin D intervention alone or in combination with micronutrients on birthweight (g), based on the fixed-effects model. Charandabi 2015 (**a**): Vit D + Ca (1000 IU/day); Charandabi 2015 (**b**): Vit D (1000 IU/day); Goldring 2013 (**a**): Vit D2 (800 IU/day); Goldring 2013 (**b**): Vit D3 (single dose of 200000 IU); Hollis 2011 (**a**): Vit D3 + micronutrients (1600 IU/day); Hollis 2011 (**b**): Vit D3 + micronutrients (3600 IU/day).

3.3.2. Birth Length

The effect of vitamin D supplementation on birth length was assessed by 7 RCTs [13,18,19,22,23,25,26] and 8 group comparisons. The Q-test and I2 statistics showed significant heterogeneity across studies ($p < 0.001$; I2 = 75.2%). Based on the random effect model, birth length was significantly higher in the intervention groups than in controls (MD: 0.50 cm, 95% CI 0.08–0.92 cm; $p = 0.020$). Moreover, we performed a leave-one-out sensitivity analysis to investigate the sources of heterogeneity across studies. The sensitivity analysis found that the study by Marya et al. [23] affected the heterogeneity across studies. When this study was omitted, the between-studies heterogeneity decreased ($p > 0.1$; I2 = 0.0%) and birth length remained significantly higher in the intervention groups than in controls (MD: 0.22 cm, 95% CI 0.10–0.34 cm; $p < 0.001$). Meta-regression did not reveal a dose-dependent effect of vitamin D supplementation alone on birth length ($p = 0.895$). Subgroup analysis by formulation showed that vitamin D supplementation alone, but not in combination with other micronutrients, significantly increased birth length (MD: 0.22 cm, 95% CI 0.10–0.34 cm, $p < 0.001$; MD: 0.21 cm, 95% CI −0.49–0.92 cm, $p = 0.700$, respectively) (Figure 3). Subgroup analysis by regimen showed that both daily and single-intermitted high dose supplementation significantly increased birth length (MD: 0.20 cm, 95% CI 0.08–0.32 cm; $p = 0.001$; MD: 0.50 cm, 95% CI 0.02–0.97 cm; $p = 0.041$, respectively).

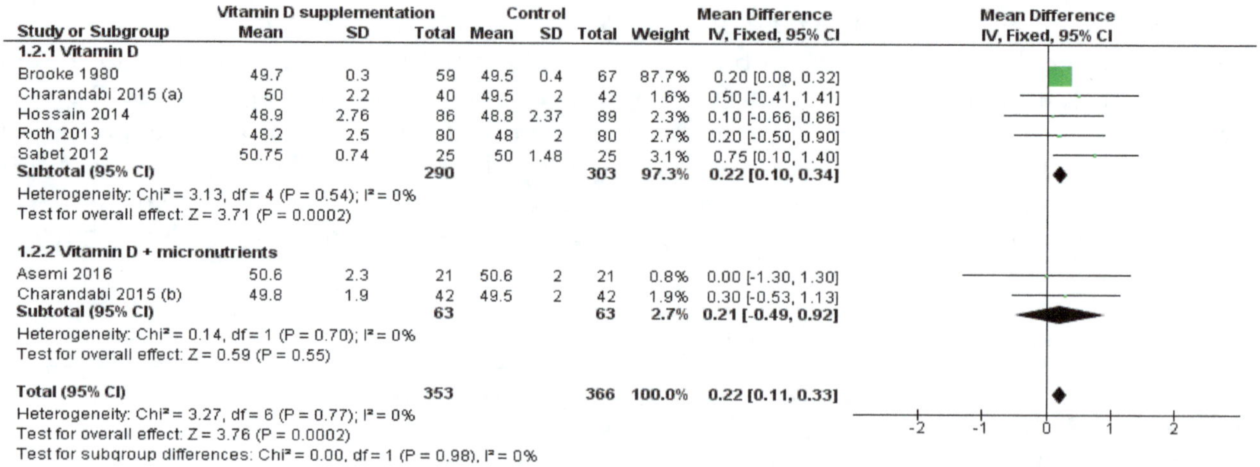

Figure 3. Forest plot of the effect of vitamin D intervention alone or in combination with micronutrients on birth length (cm), based on the fixed-effects model. Charandabi 2015 (**a**): Vit D + Ca (1000 IU/day); Charandabi 2015 (**b**): Vit D (1000 IU/day).

3.3.3. Head Circumference

The effect of vitamin D supplementation on head circumference was assessed by 6 RCTs [13,14,18,19,22,25] and 7 group comparisons. Compared to controls, head circumference was significantly greater in the intervention groups (MD: 0.19 cm, 95% CI 0.13–0.24 cm; $p < 0.001$). Q-test and I2 statistics showed no significant heterogeneity across studies ($p > 0.1$; I2 = 2.0%). Particularly, vitamin D supplementation alone, but not in combination with other micronutrients, significantly increased head circumference (MD: 0.19 cm, 95% CI 0.14–0.25 cm, $p < 0.001$; MD: −0.06 cm, 95% CI −0.41–0.28 cm, $p = 0.720$, respectively; Figure 4). Meta-regression did not reveal a dose-dependent effect of vitamin D supplementation alone on head circumference ($p = 0.746$). Subgroup analysis by regimen showed that daily maternal vitamin D supplementation significantly increased head circumference (MD: 0.19 cm, 95% CI 0.14–0.24 cm; $p < 0.001$). Regarding single-intermitted intervention, Roth et al. reported no significant effect [25].

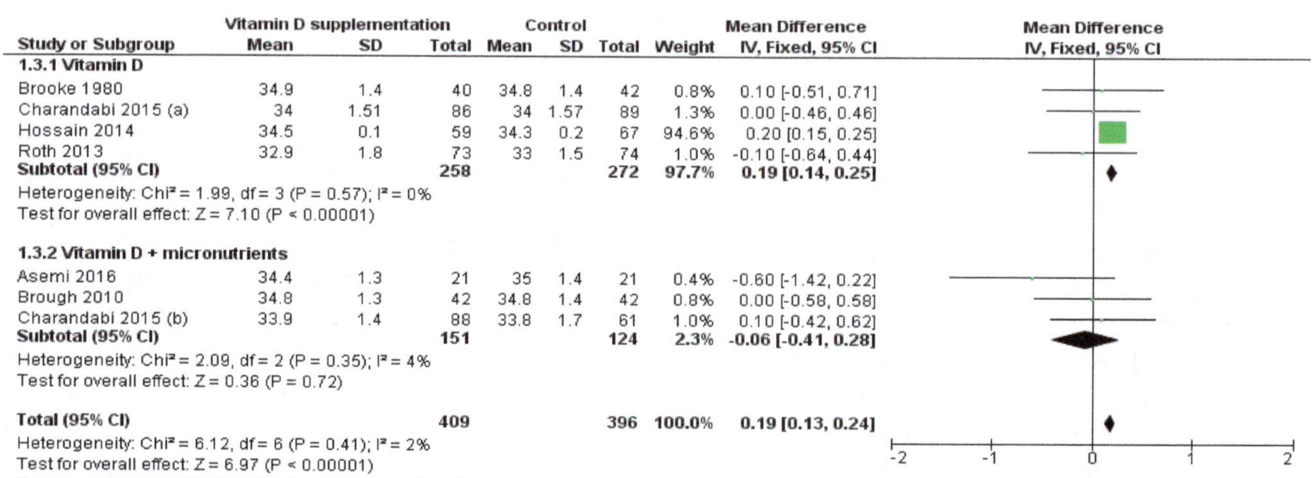

Figure 4. Forest plot of the effect of vitamin D intervention alone or in combination with micronutrients on head circumference (cm), based on the fixed-effects model. Charandabi 2015 (**a**): Vit D + Ca (1000 IU/day); Charandabi 2015 (**b**): Vit D (1000 IU/day).

3.3.4. Low Birthweight

The effect of vitamin D supplementation on incidence of LBW was assessed by 3 RCTs [14,18,28] and 4 group comparisons. Compared to control groups, the risk of LBW newborns was lower in the intervention groups (RR = 0.40, 95% CI 0.22–0.74; $p = 0.003$) (Figure 5). Interestingly, the omission of the study by Brough [14], showed that women supplemented with vitamin D alone had a lower risk of LBW than controls (RR = 0.47, 95% CI 0.23–0.97; $p = 0.040$). In contrast, Brough et al. reported no significant effect of vitamin D supplementation with micronutrients [14]. *Q*-test and I2 statistics showed no significant heterogeneity across studies ($p > 0.1$; I2 = 0%). Subgroup analysis by regimen showed that daily maternal vitamin D supplementation significantly reduced the risk of LBW (RR = 0.40, 95% CI 0.21–0.78; $p = 0.007$). Regarding single-intermitted intervention, Yu et al. reported no significant effect [28].

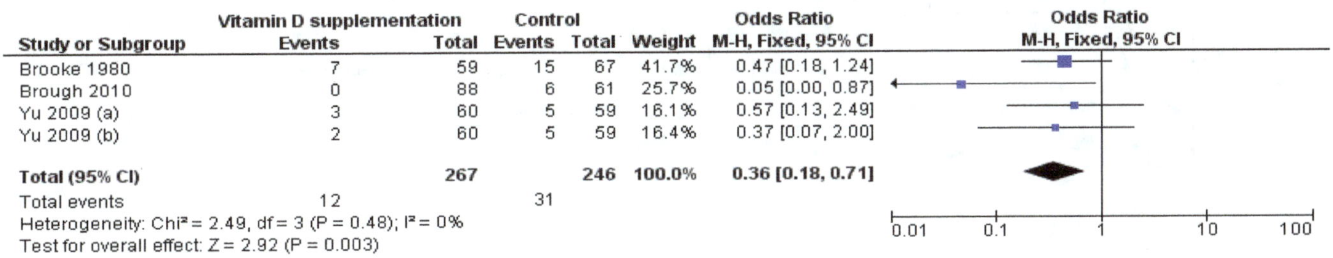

Figure 5. Forest plot of the effect of vitamin D intervention on the risk of low birthweight, based on the fixed-effects model. Yu 2009 (**a**): Vit D2 (800 IU/day); Yu 2009 (**b**): Vit D2 (single dose of 200000 IU).

3.3.5. Small for Gestational Age

The effect of vitamin D supplementation on incidence of SGA was assessed by 5 RCTs [14,18,22,27,28] and 6 group comparisons. Compared to control groups, the risk of SGA was lower in the intervention groups (RR = 0.69, 95% CI 0.51–0.92; $p = 0.018$) (Figure 6). Interestingly, the omission of the study by Brough [14], showed that women supplemented with vitamin D alone had a lower risk of SGA than controls (RR = 0.70, 95% CI 0.47–0.97; $p = 0.047$). In contrast, Brough et al. reported no significant effect of vitamin D supplementation with micronutrients [14]. *Q*-test and I2 statistics showed no significant heterogeneity across studies ($p > 0.1$; I2 = 16.2%). Meta-regression did not reveal a dose-dependent effect of vitamin D supplementation alone on SGA ($p = 0.903$). Subgroup analysis by regimen demonstrated that both daily and single-intermitted dose significantly reduced the risk of SGA (RR = 0.73, 95% CI 0.51–0.98; $p = 0.042$; RR = 0.58, 95% CI 0.32–0.99; $p = 0.048$).

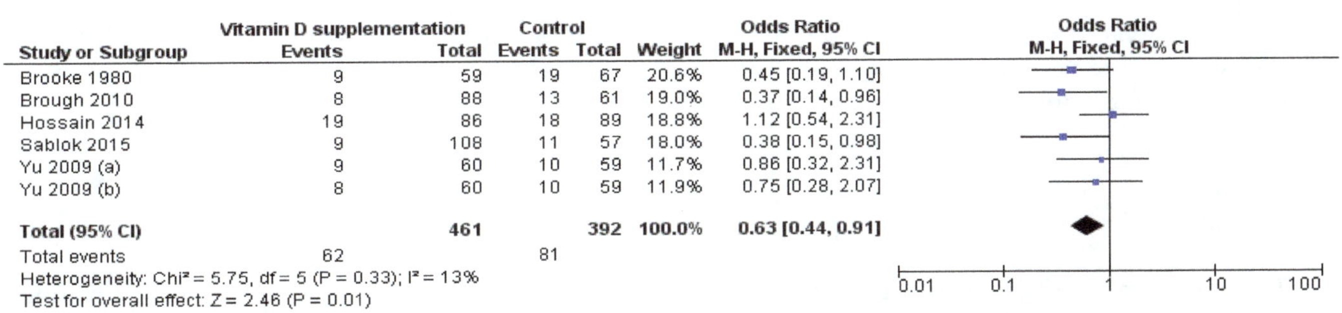

Figure 6. Forest plot of the effect of vitamin D intervention on the risk of small for gestational age, based on the fixed-effects model. Yu 2009 (**a**): Vit D2 (800 IU/day); Yu 2009 (**b**): Vit D2 (single dose of 200000 IU).

3.4. Risk-of-Bias and Quality Assessment

Risk-of-bias assessment was shown in Figure 7. Overall, we identified low risk of attrition and other biases; however, unclear and/or high risk of selection, performance, detection, and reporting biases cannot be excluded. Overall, the quality of evidence varied from very low (head circumference) to moderate (birthweight, birth length, LBW, and SGA). The main reasons for downgrading the quality of evidence were the risk of bias of RCTs (i.e., high risk of bias for blinding) and the imprecision (i.e., low sample size and/or number of events which resulted in wide 95% CI). Full details of risk-of-bias and quality assessment are included in Supplementary Materials.

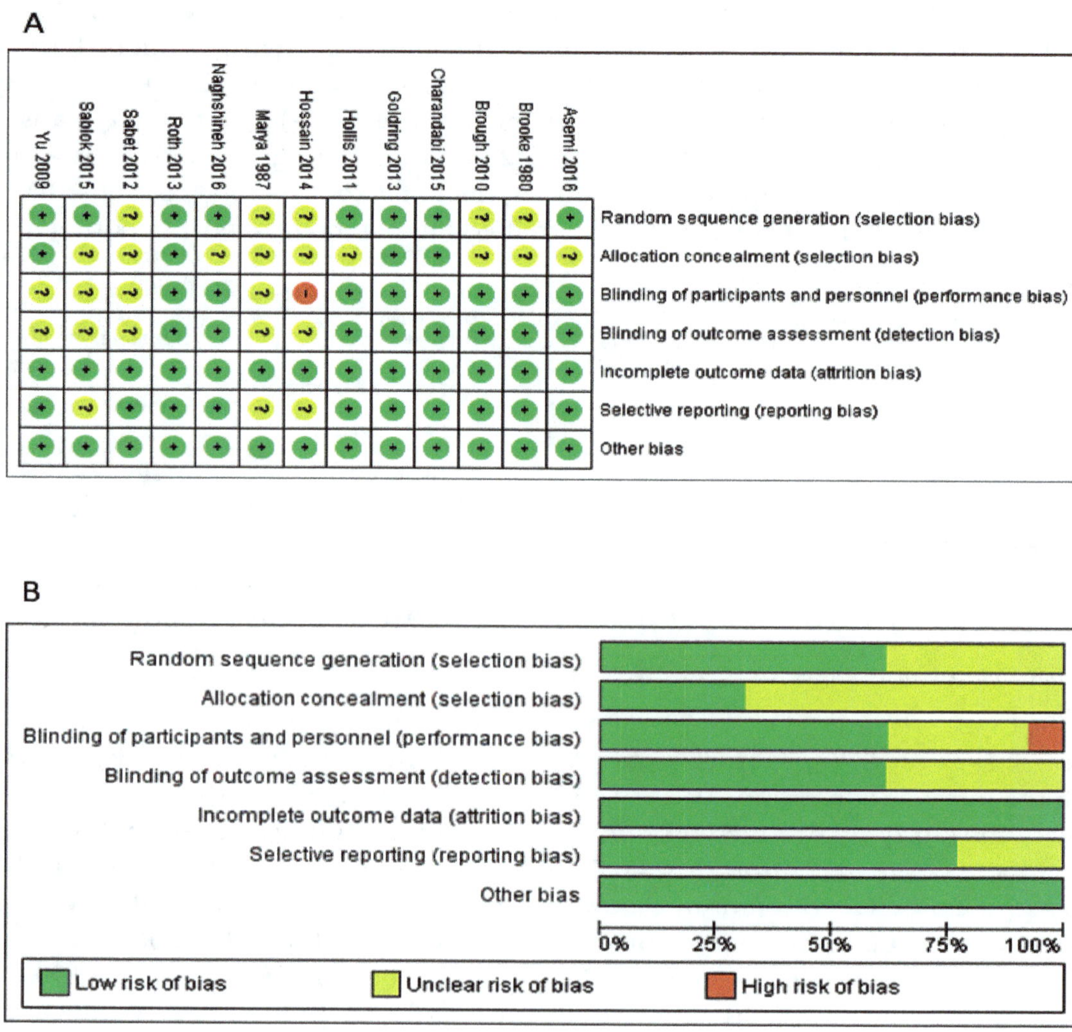

Figure 7. Risk-of-bias assessment of randomized controlled trials included in the meta-analysis. Risk-of-bias summary (**A**) and graph (**B**), according to the Cochrane's Collaboration tool for assessing risk of bias in randomized trials.

3.5. Publication Bias

The funnel plot of the effect of vitamin D supplementation on birthweight appeared symmetric (Figure 8). Accordingly, Begg's rank correlation method and Egger's weighted regression method showed no sources of publication bias (p-values > 0.05). Regarding other outcomes, due to the limited number of studies, the extent of publication biases cannot be excluded because the power of the tests for funnel plot asymmetry was too low to identify a real asymmetry [10].

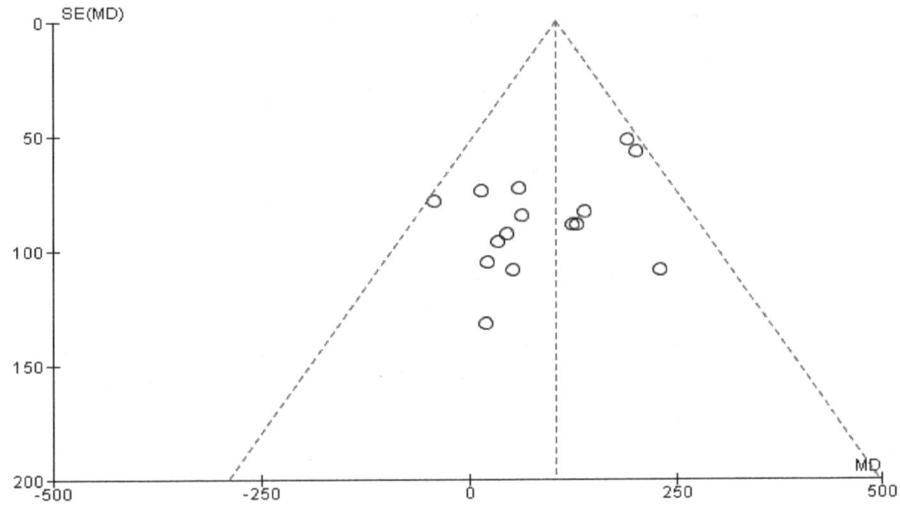

Figure 8. Funnel plot with estimated 95% confidence intervals for meta-analysis of the effect of vitamin D intervention on birthweight.

4. Discussion

When interpreting findings about the effect of maternal vitamin D supplementation on birth size, differences in study design and type of intervention should be considered. To reduce heterogeneity, we limited our analysis to RCTs of pregnant women without pregnancy complications, with randomization at either individual or cluster level. We excluded observational studies, cross-over trials, or quasi-RCTs. Moreover, to demonstrate whether alternative formulations and/or regimens had different effect on birth size, we performed subgroup analyses. Overall, we compared the effect of oral vitamin D (D2 or D3 form) supplementation, alone or in combination with other micronutrients, with placebo or no treatment. Most of the interventions provided daily vitamin supplementation, and to a lesser extent intermitted or single high doses. To date, the recommended dose of vitamin D supplementation, during pregnancy and lactation, is 600 IU per day [6]. This recommendation, based on outcomes related to skeletal health, was proposed as the amount of vitamin D to maintain blood levels of 25(OH)D above 50 nmol/L [29]. However, several lines of evidence argued that deficiency should be defined at thresholds of 75 nmol/L or higher [30–34]. The majority of RCTs included in our work evaluated the benefits of a supplementation greater than 600 IU per day. The daily doses ranged from 200 IU to 4000 IU while, among high single-intermitted interventions, the doses varied from 35000 IU to 600000 IU. During pregnancy, the tolerable upper intake level of vitamin D is now set at 4000 IU/day, although the adverse effects of higher levels are uncertain [30]. As suggested by several RCTs included in the present systematic review, interventions which reached or exceed the tolerable upper intake level did not manifest adverse effects [20,22,23,25,26,28]. However, due to inconclusive evidence, monitoring of toxicity and potential adverse effects of high intermittent dosages should be an important consideration in RCTs design [30].

Our findings add to the growing body of evidence about the effect of vitamin D supplementation on neonatal anthropometric measures and incidence of LBW and SGA births. Compared to previous meta-analyses [5,8], our work summarized data from 13 RCTs, published until May 2017, providing a larger number of group comparisons for each outcome of interest. We confirmed that vitamin D supplementation alone, but not in combination with other micronutrients, significantly increased birthweight, birth length, and head circumference. Compared to the most recent meta-analysis of RCTs by Perez-Lopez et al. [5], we also showed that newborns from women supplemented with vitamin D alone had a lower risk of LBW. This evidence was consistent with four trials included in the recent systematic review by De-Regil et al. [7] and pooled results by Thorne-Lyman et al. [8]. Although birthweight and length are the most used indicators for the assessment of intrauterine growth, the evaluation of weight distribution at birth is more adequate when it is adjusted for gestational age. Accordingly, the reduction of LBW is not the best goal of intervention of RCTs, because it does not distinguish between suboptimal fetal growth and shortened gestation [35]. Evidence about the effect of vitamin D supplementation on gestational age and preterm birth is controversial; De-Regil et al. reported that vitamin D supplementation alone may reduce the risk of preterm birth, while the combined supplementation with calcium increased the risk [7]. Findings from RCTs included in the present study suggested that women who received vitamin D supplementation alone [24,27] or in combination with calcium [13] had a lower risk of preterm birth. However, in other RCTs the intervention did not affect gestational age [13,14,20–22,24] and preterm birth incidence [14,19,22]. To our knowledge, the present study is the first demonstrating that maternal vitamin D supplementation alone significantly reduced the risk of SGA births, defined as birthweight below the 10th percentile for sex and gestational age. SGA newborns show a higher risk of neonatal and infant mortality, childhood malnutrition, neurocognitive disorders, and adulthood metabolic diseases [36]. Subgroup analysis by regimen showed that both daily and high single-intermitted dose significantly increased birthweight and length, reducing the risk of SGA births. In fact, the fat-soluble properties of vitamin D allow the single-intermitted dosage during pregnancy, which may be a feasible strategy against adverse neonatal outcomes in low income countries with poor health infrastructures [8].

Since we included studies with different interventions, we assessed the dose-dependent effect of vitamin D supplementation on birth size. For this purpose, we performed meta-regression analyses of those outcomes with at least three studies evaluating daily vitamin D supplementation alone. By contrast, heterogeneity in formulation, dose, duration, and timing of supplementation, did not allow us to perform meta-regression of studies with single supplementation and/or combination of supplements. However, our analysis did not reveal a dose-dependent effect of vitamin D on birth sizes, probably due to the limited number of studies. Moreover, very few studies investigated the effect of vitamin D supplementation with other micronutrients, and hence we were not able to understand whether the combination with other supplements might affect the efficacy of intervention. Although single and combination interventions were based on similar vitamin D doses, we cannot exclude an antagonistic effect of other micronutrients. Given these limitations, further research is needed to assess the dose-dependent effect of vitamin D alone or in combination with other micronutrients.

The positive effect of maternal vitamin D supplementation on birth size and risk of LBW and SGA might be mediated by changes in fetal cell mass and function, skeletal mineralization, and metabolism [37]. Moreover, maternal serum vitamin D insufficiency is associated with an increased risk of preterm birth [38–40]. The main role of vitamin D in the human body is to maintain adequate levels of calcium and phosphate, enabling the critical processes of bone mineralization and development during fetal life [37]. In many fetal tissues, the active form of vitamin D binds to the vitamin D receptors, regulating genes responsible for the proper implantation of the placenta [41], which is important for fetal growth. Moreover, vitamin D could influence the maternal immune response to the placenta [42] and the expression of human chorionic gonadotropin and sex steroids [43]. Some experimental studies have also proposed the role of vitamin D in glucose and insulin metabolism, affecting availability of energy to the fetus [44], as well as its influence on musculoskeletal growth [45].

Potential weaknesses of our work include the limited number of databases searched. According to selection criteria, some data, such as conference abstracts and/or unpublished reports, were excluded. Our reluctance to include unpublished results is based on: (i) the absence of peer-review of unpublished literature; (ii) the studies that can be located may be an unrepresentative sample of all unpublished studies; (iii) unpublished studies may be of lower methodological quality than published studies [10]. To address publication biases, we visually assessed funnel plot asymmetry followed by Begg's test and Egger's regression asymmetry test. However, in those outcomes with less than 10 intervention groups, the extent of publication bias cannot be completely excluded. Beyond potential reporting and publication biases, we assessed an unclear risk of bias for random sequence generation, allocation concealment, selective reporting and blinding (i.e., absence of blinding should be considered when interpreting results by Hossain et al. [22]). Accordingly, the quality of evidence varied from very low to moderate. The main reasons for downgrading the quality of evidence were the high risk of bias for blinding and the low sample size, which resulted in wide 95% CI. We also recognize that including more group comparisons could have the potential of overestimating or underestimating the effect of vitamin D supplementation. To solve this issue, where possible, we performed subgroup analyses that classified group comparison into different subgroups, whenever possible. Another weakness is the potential effect of confounders. To control for factors that could contribute to the effect of vitamin D supplementation on birth size, RCTs should be based on more standardized protocols [46]: dosage for vitamin D supplementation should be chosen upon the maternal serum 25OHD levels at baseline [8], as performed by Sablok et al. [27], and such trials should take into account risk factors for vitamin D deficiency (i.e., genetic factors, latitude, lifestyles, dietary intake and seasonality) [47–49]. To avoid confounding due to seasonal variation in sunlight exposure, several RCTs were carried out in different seasons [14,18,22,24,26,27]. Taking into account the abovementioned limitations, further research and large multicenter RCTs, evaluating the effect of genetic, environmental, sociodemographic, and life-style factors, is needed.

5. Conclusions

Despite growing interest in the relationship between vitamin D supplementation and pregnancy outcomes, previous evidence about the effect on birth size remained weak. Findings from these systematic review and meta-analysis confirm vitamin D as an essential nutrient for fetal growth and development, with well-established effects on birth size. Moreover, to our knowledge, this work represents the first meta-analysis of RCTs which demonstrates a significant positive effect of maternal vitamin D supplementation on the risk of SGA births. However, further RCTs of vitamin D supplementation during pregnancy are required to better define risks and benefits associated with such interventions and the potential implication as a feasible strategy to prevent adverse pregnancy outcomes.

Author Contributions: Conceptualization, A.A.; methodology, A.M., M.B., and I.B.; formal analysis, A.M., M.B., and I.B.; data curation, A.M., M.B., and I.B.; writing—original draft preparation, A.M., M.B., I.B., and A.A.; writing—review and editing, A.M., M.B., I.B., and A.A.; supervision, A.A.

References

1. Ramakrishnan, U.; Grant, F.; Goldenberg, T.; Zongrone, A.; Martorell, R. Effect of women's nutrition before and during early pregnancy on maternal and infant outcomes: A systematic review. *Paediatr. Perinat. Epidemiol.* **2012**, *26* (Suppl. 1), 285–301. [CrossRef] [PubMed]
2. Agodi, A.; Barchitta, M.; Valenti, G.; Marzagalli, R.; Frontini, V.; Marchese, A.E. Increase in the prevalence of the MTHFR 677 TT polymorphism in women born since 1959: Potential implications for folate requirements. *Eur. J. Clin. Nutr.* **2011**, *65*, 1302–1308. [CrossRef] [PubMed]
3. Holick, M.F. Vitamin D: A d-lightful solution for health. *J. Investig. Med.* **2011**, *59*, 872–880. [CrossRef] [PubMed]
4. Harvey, N.C.; Holroyd, C.; Ntani, G.; Javaid, K.; Cooper, P.; Moon, R.; Cole, Z.; Tinati, T.; Godfrey, K.; Dennison, E.; et al. Vitamin D supplementation in pregnancy: A systematic review. *Health Technol. Assess.* **2014**, *18*, 1–190. [CrossRef] [PubMed]
5. Pérez-López, F.R.; Pasupuleti, V.; Mezones-Holguin, E.; Benites-Zapata, V.A.; Thota, P.; Deshpande, A.; Hernandez, A.V. Effect of vitamin D supplementation during pregnancy on maternal and neonatal outcomes: A systematic review and meta-analysis of randomized controlled trials. *Fertil. Steril.* **2015**, *103*, 1278–1288. [CrossRef] [PubMed]

6. Ross, A.C. The 2011 report on dietary reference intakes for calcium and vitamin D. *Public Health Nutr.* **2011**, *14*, 938–939. [CrossRef] [PubMed]
7. De-Regil, L.M.; Palacios, C.; Lombardo, L.K.; Peña-Rosas, J.P. Vitamin D supplementation for women during pregnancy. *Sao Paulo Med. J.* **2016**, *134*, 274–275. [CrossRef] [PubMed]
8. Thorne-Lyman, A.; Fawzi, W.W. Vitamin D during pregnancy and maternal, neonatal and infant health outcomes: A systematic review and meta-analysis. *Paediatr. Perinat. Epidemiol.* **2012**, *26* (Suppl. 1), 75–90. [CrossRef] [PubMed]
9. Moher, D.; Shamseer, L.; Clarke, M.; Ghersi, D.; Liberati, A.; Petticrew, M.; Shekelle, P.; Stewart, L.A.; Group, P.-P. Preferred reporting items for systematic review and meta-analysis protocols (PRISMA-P) 2015 statement. *Syst. Rev.* **2015**, *4*, 1. [CrossRef] [PubMed]
10. Higgins, J.; Green, S. *Cochrane Handbook for Systematic Reviews of Interventions*, Version 5.1.0 ed.; The Cochrane Collaboration: London, UK, 2008.
11. Guyatt, G.; Oxman, A.D.; Akl, E.A.; Kunz, R.; Vist, G.; Brozek, J.; Norris, S.; Falck-Ytter, Y.; Glasziou, P.; DeBeer, H.; et al. GRADE guidelines: 1. Introduction-GRADE evidence profiles and summary of findings tables. *J. Clin. Epidemiol.* **2011**, *64*, 383–394. [CrossRef] [PubMed]
12. Higgins, J.P.; Thompson, S.G. Quantifying heterogeneity in a meta-analysis. *Stat. Med.* **2002**, *21*, 1539–1558. [CrossRef] [PubMed]
13. Asemi, Z.; Samimi, M.; Siavashani, M.A.; Mazloomi, M.; Tabassi, Z.; Karamali, M.; Jamilian, M.; Esmaillzadeh, A. Calcium-Vitamin D Co-supplementation Affects Metabolic Profiles, but not Pregnancy Outcomes, in Healthy Pregnant Women. *Int. J. Prev. Med.* **2016**, *7*, 49. [CrossRef] [PubMed]
14. Brough, L.; Rees, G.A.; Crawford, M.A.; Morton, R.H.; Dorman, E.K. Effect of multiple-micronutrient supplementation on maternal nutrient status, infant birth weight and gestational age at birth in a low-income, multi-ethnic population. *Br. J. Nutr.* **2010**, *104*, 437–445. [CrossRef] [PubMed]
15. Thompson, S.G.; Sharp, S.J. Explaining heterogeneity in meta-analysis: A comparison of methods. *Stat. Med.* **1999**, *18*, 2693–2708. [CrossRef]
16. Begg, C.B.; Mazumdar, M. Operating characteristics of a rank correlation test for publication bias. *Biometrics* **1994**, *50*, 1088–1101. [CrossRef] [PubMed]
17. Egger, M.; Davey Smith, G.; Schneider, M.; Minder, C. Bias in meta-analysis detected by a simple, graphical test. *BMJ* **1997**, *315*, 629–634. [CrossRef]
18. Brooke, O.G.; Brown, I.R.; Bone, C.D.; Carter, N.D.; Cleeve, H.J.; Maxwell, J.D.; Robinson, V.P.; Winder, S.M. Vitamin D supplements in pregnant Asian women: Effects on calcium status and fetal growth. *Br. Med. J.* **1980**, *280*, 751–754. [CrossRef]
19. Mohammad-Alizadeh-Charandabi, S.; Mirghafourvand, M.; Mansouri, A.; Najafi, M.; Khodabande, F. The Effect of Vitamin D and Calcium plus Vitamin D during Pregnancy on Pregnancy and Birth Outcomes: A Randomized Controlled Trial. *J. Caring Sci.* **2015**, *4*, 35–44. [CrossRef]
20. Goldring, S.T.; Griffiths, C.J.; Martineau, A.R.; Robinson, S.; Yu, C.; Poulton, S.; Kirkby, J.C.; Stocks, J.; Hooper, R.; Shaheen, S.O.; et al. Prenatal vitamin d supplementation and child respiratory health: A randomised controlled trial. *PLoS ONE* **2013**, *8*, e66627. [CrossRef]
21. Hollis, B.W.; Johnson, D.; Hulsey, T.C.; Ebeling, M.; Wagner, C.L. Vitamin D supplementation during pregnancy: Double-blind, randomized clinical trial of safety and effectiveness. *J. Bone Miner. Res.* **2011**, *26*, 2341–2357. [CrossRef]
22. Hossain, N.; Kanani, F.H.; Ramzan, S.; Kausar, R.; Ayaz, S.; Khanani, R.; Pal, L. Obstetric and neonatal outcomes of maternal vitamin D supplementation: Results of an open-label, randomized controlled trial of antenatal vitamin D supplementation in Pakistani women. *J. Clin. Endocrinol. Metab.* **2014**, *99*, 2448–2455. [CrossRef] [PubMed]
23. Marya, R.K.; Rathee, S.; Dua, V.; Sangwan, K. Effect of vitamin D supplementation during pregnancy on foetal growth. *Indian J. Med. Res.* **1988**, *88*, 488–492. [PubMed]
24. Naghshineh, E.; Sheikhaliyan, S. Effect of vitamin D supplementation in the reduce risk of preeclampsia in nulliparous women. *Adv. Biomed. Res.* **2016**, *5*, 7. [CrossRef] [PubMed]
25. Roth, D.E.; Al Mahmud, A.; Raqib, R.; Akhtar, E.; Perumal, N.; Pezzack, B.; Baqui, A.H. Randomized placebo-controlled trial of high-dose prenatal third-trimester vitamin D3 supplementation in Bangladesh: The AViDD trial. *Nutr. J.* **2013**, *12*, 47. [CrossRef]

26. Sabet, Z.; Ghazi, A.; Tohidi, M.; Oladi, B. Vitamin D supplementation in pregnant Iranian women: Effects on maternal and neonatal vitamin D and parathyroid hormone status. *Acta Endo* **2012**, *8*, 59–66. [CrossRef]
27. Sablok, A.; Batra, A.; Thariani, K.; Bharti, R.; Aggarwal, A.R.; Kabi, B.C.; Chellani, H. Supplementation of vitamin D in pregnancy and its correlation with feto-maternal outcome. *Clin. Endocrinol.* **2015**, *83*, 536–541. [CrossRef] [PubMed]
28. Yu, C.K.; Sykes, L.; Sethi, M.; Teoh, T.G.; Robinson, S. Vitamin D deficiency and supplementation during pregnancy. *Clin. Endocrinol.* **2009**, *70*, 685–690. [CrossRef] [PubMed]
29. Institute of Medicine. *Dietary Reference Intakes for Calcium and Vitamin D*; National Academies Press: Washington, DC, USA, 2011.
30. Heaney, R.P.; Davies, K.M.; Chen, T.C.; Holick, M.F.; Barger-Lux, M.J. Human serum 25-hydroxycholecalciferol response to extended oral dosing with cholecalciferol. *Am. J. Clin. Nutr.* **2003**, *77*, 204–210. [CrossRef] [PubMed]
31. Bischoff-Ferrari, H.A.; Giovannucci, E.; Willett, W.C.; Dietrich, T.; Dawson-Hughes, B. Estimation of optimal serum concentrations of 25-hydroxyvitamin D for multiple health outcomes. *Am. J. Clin. Nutr.* **2006**, *84*, 18–28. [CrossRef] [PubMed]
32. Visser, M.; Deeg, D.J.; Puts, M.T.; Seidell, J.C.; Lips, P. Low serum concentrations of 25-hydroxyvitamin D in older persons and the risk of nursing home admission. *Am. J. Clin. Nutr.* **2006**, *84*, 616–622. [CrossRef]
33. Norman, A.W.; Bouillon, R.; Whiting, S.J.; Vieth, R.; Lips, P. 13th Workshop consensus for vitamin D nutritional guidelines. *J. Steroid Biochem. Mol. Biol.* **2007**, *103*, 204–205. [CrossRef] [PubMed]
34. Henry, H.L.; Bouillon, R.; Norman, A.W.; Gallagher, J.C.; Lips, P.; Heaney, R.P.; Vieth, R.; Pettifor, J.M.; Dawson-Hughes, B.; Lamberg-Allardt, C.J.; et al. 14th Vitamin D Workshop consensus on vitamin D nutritional guidelines. *J. Steroid Biochem. Mol. Biol.* **2010**, *121*, 4–6. [CrossRef] [PubMed]
35. Steer, P. Small for Gestational Age: Causes and Consequences. *J. Anat.* **2009**, *215*, 224. [CrossRef]
36. Institute of Medicine (US) Committee on Improving Birth Outcomes. *Improving Birth Outcomes: Meeting the Challenge in the Developing World*; Bale, J.R., Stoll, B.J., Lucas, A.O., Eds.; National Academies Press: Washington, DC, USA, 2003.
37. Kovacs, C.S. Bone metabolism in the fetus and neonate. *Pediatr. Nephrol.* **2014**, *29*, 793–803. [CrossRef] [PubMed]
38. Qin, L.L.; Lu, F.G.; Yang, S.H.; Xu, H.L.; Luo, B.A. Does Maternal Vitamin D Deficiency Increase the Risk of Preterm Birth: A Meta-Analysis of Observational Studies. *Nutrients* **2016**, *8*, 301. [CrossRef]
39. McDonnell, S.L.; Baggerly, K.A.; Baggerly, C.A.; Aliano, J.L.; French, C.B.; Baggerly, L.L.; Ebeling, M.D.; Rittenberg, C.S.; Goodier, C.G.; Mateus Niño, J.F.; et al. Maternal 25(OH)D concentrations ≥40 ng/mL associated with 60% lower preterm birth risk among general obstetrical patients at an urban medical center. *PLoS ONE* **2017**, *12*, e0180483. [CrossRef]
40. Zhou, S.S.; Tao, Y.H.; Huang, K.; Zhu, B.B.; Tao, F.B. Vitamin D and risk of preterm birth: Up-to-date meta-analysis of randomized controlled trials and observational studies. *J. Obstet. Gynaecol. Res.* **2017**, *43*, 247–256. [CrossRef]
41. Evans, K.N.; Bulmer, J.N.; Kilby, M.D.; Hewison, M. Vitamin D and placental-decidual function. *J. Soc. Gynecol. Investig.* **2004**, *11*, 263–271. [CrossRef]
42. Bodnar, L.M.; Krohn, M.A.; Simhan, H.N. Maternal vitamin D deficiency is associated with bacterial vaginosis in the first trimester of pregnancy. *J. Nutr.* **2009**, *139*, 1157–1161. [CrossRef]
43. Barrera, D.; Avila, E.; Hernández, G.; Méndez, I.; González, L.; Halhali, A.; Larrea, F.; Morales, A.; Díaz, L. Calcitriol affects hCG gene transcription in cultured human syncytiotrophoblasts. *Reprod. Biol. Endocrinol.* **2008**, *6*, 3. [CrossRef]
44. Pittas, A.G.; Lau, J.; Hu, F.B.; Dawson-Hughes, B. The role of vitamin D and calcium in type 2 diabetes. A systematic review and meta-analysis. *J. Clin. Endocrinol. Metab.* **2007**, *92*, 2017–2029. [CrossRef] [PubMed]
45. Giuliani, D.L.; Boland, R.L. Effects of vitamin D3 metabolites on calcium fluxes in intact chicken skeletal muscle and myoblasts cultured in vitro. *Calcif. Tissue Int.* **1984**, *36*, 200–205. [CrossRef] [PubMed]
46. Papageorghiou, A.T.; Ohuma, E.O.; Altman, D.G.; Todros, T.; Cheikh Ismail, L.; Lambert, A.; Jaffer, Y.A.; Bertino, E.; Gravett, M.G.; Purwar, M.; et al. International standards for fetal growth based on serial ultrasound measurements: The Fetal Growth Longitudinal Study of the INTERGROWTH-21st Project. *Lancet* **2014**, *384*, 869–879. [CrossRef]

47. Karras, S.; Paschou, S.A.; Kandaraki, E.; Anagnostis, P.; Annweiler, C.; Tarlatzis, B.C.; Hollis, B.W.; Grant, W.B.; Goulis, D.G. Hypovitaminosis D in pregnancy in the Mediterranean region: A systematic review. *Eur. J. Clin. Nutr.* **2016**, *70*, 979–986. [CrossRef] [PubMed]
48. Wang, T.J.; Zhang, F.; Richards, J.B.; Kestenbaum, B.; van Meurs, J.B.; Berry, D.; Kiel, D.P.; Streeten, E.A.; Ohlsson, C.; Koller, D.L.; et al. Common genetic determinants of vitamin D insufficiency: A genome-wide association study. *Lancet* **2010**, *376*, 180–188. [CrossRef]
49. Barchitta, M.; Maugeri, A.; La Rosa, M.C.; Magnano San Lio, R.; Favara, G.; Panella, M.; Cianci, A.; Agodi, A. Single Nucleotide Polymorphisms in Vitamin D Receptor Gene Affect Birth Weight and the Risk of Preterm Birth: Results From the "Mamma & Bambino" Cohort and A Meta-Analysis. *Nutrients* **2018**, *10*, 1172. [CrossRef]

16

Maternal Choline Supplementation Modulates Placental Markers of Inflammation, Angiogenesis and Apoptosis in a Mouse Model of Placental Insufficiency

Julia H. King [1], Sze Ting (Cecilia) Kwan [1], Jian Yan [1], Xinyin Jiang [1,2], Vladislav G. Fomin [1], Samantha P. Levine [1], Emily Wei [1], Mark S. Roberson [3,*] and Marie A. Caudill [1,*]

1 Division of Nutritional Sciences, Cornell University, Ithaca, NY 14850, USA; jhk288@cornell.edu (J.H.K.); sk2563@cornell.edu (S.T.K.); jy435@cornell.edu (J.Y.); XinyinJiang@brooklyn.cuny.edu (X.J.); vgf6@cornell.edu (V.G.F.); spl63@cornell.edu (S.P.L.); ew376@cornell.edu (E.W.)
2 Department of Health and Nutrition Sciences, Brooklyn College, Brooklyn, NY 11210, USA
3 Department of Biomedical Sciences, Cornell University, Ithaca, NY 14850, USA
* Correspondence: msr14@cornell.edu (M.S.R.); mac379@cornell.edu (M.A.C.)

Abstract: *Dlx3* (distal-less homeobox 3) haploinsufficiency in mice has been shown to result in restricted fetal growth and placental defects. We previously showed that maternal choline supplementation (4X versus 1X choline) in the *Dlx3+/−* mouse increased fetal and placental growth in mid-gestation. The current study sought to test the hypothesis that prenatal choline would modulate indicators of placenta function and development. Pregnant *Dlx3+/−* mice consuming 1X (control), 2X, or 4X choline from conception were sacrificed at embryonic (E) days E10.5, E12.5, E15.5, and E18.5, and placentas and embryos were harvested. Data were analyzed separately for each gestational day controlling for litter size, fetal genotype (except for models including only +/− pups), and fetal sex (except when data were stratified by this variable). 4X choline tended to increase ($p < 0.1$) placental labyrinth size at E10.5 and decrease ($p < 0.05$) placental apoptosis at E12.5. Choline supplementation decreased ($p < 0.05$) expression of pro-angiogenic genes *Eng* (E10.5, E12.5, and E15.5), and *Vegf* (E12.5, E15.5); and pro-inflammatory genes *Il1b* (at E15.5 and 18.5), *Tnfα* (at E12.5) and *Nfκb* (at E15.5) in a fetal sex-dependent manner. These findings provide support for a modulatory effect of maternal choline supplementation on biomarkers of placental function and development in a mouse model of placental insufficiency.

Keywords: choline; Dlx3; placenta; placental insufficiency; inflammation; angiogenesis; apoptosis

1. Introduction

Abnormal placental development underlies many pathologies of pregnancy including preeclampsia, intrauterine growth restriction (IUGR), and spontaneous abortion [1]. These conditions have serious consequences for the mother and fetus, and few treatments are currently available for their prevention or treatment.

Although the etiology of placental insufficiency is not fully understood, an imbalance of pro- and anti-angiogenic and inflammatory factors may contribute to it [1,2]. The development of the placenta requires extensive angiogenesis and vasculogenesis, and the maternal uterine spiral arteries must be invaded and remodeled by extravillous trophoblasts to allow for increased blood flow to the fetus [3]. This process requires adequate expression of angiogenic and remodeling genes including the vascular endothelial growth factor (VEGF) family. Inadequate trophoblast invasion is a characteristic of many placental pathologies. When this process is incomplete, blood flow to the placenta is compromised, and oxygen supply may be sporadic, leading to placental injury from hypoxia/reoxygenation. Oxidative stress, excessive apoptosis, and inflammation result, compromising trophoblast function and preventing efficient transfer of nutrients [4]. Anti-angiogenic factors in the maternal circulation, including soluble fms-like tyrosine kinase-1 (sFlt-1) and soluble endoglin (sEng), may contribute to the pathogenesis of preeclampsia symptoms including hypertension and proteinuria, and can be used as biomarkers or predictors of risk when measured in early gestation [5,6]. Together, these dysregulated processes interact to contribute to the pathogenesis of placental disorders such as preeclampsia and IUGR.

The essential nutrient choline is required for the synthesis of the neurotransmitter acetylcholine, the membrane phospholipid phosphatidylcholine, and the methyl donor and osmolyte betaine [7]. These biomolecules have crucial roles in supporting pregnancy via their effects on cell growth, DNA methylation, and signaling processes [8]. Choline has previously been shown to reduce levels of sFlt-1 in a randomized dietary intervention trial of maternal choline supplementation during the third trimester of pregnancy in healthy women [9]. Further, choline deficiency has been shown to increase inflammation and apoptotic processes in a cell culture model of human placental trophoblasts [10]; meanwhile, supplementing the maternal diet with additional choline decreases biomarkers of both processes in wildtype mouse placenta [11]. We, thus, hypothesized that choline supplementation would be beneficial for pregnancies complicated by placental insufficiency.

Dlx3 (distal-less homeobox 3) haploinsufficiency in mice has been shown to result in restricted fetal growth and placental defects [12]. This homeodomain-containing transcription factor is required for the development of the maternal–fetal interface [13]. Placentas lacking one copy of this gene display inadequate vascularization and abnormal development of the placental labyrinth [12], which is the area of nutrient exchange between the mother and fetus. Heterozygous embryos are viable but their placentas display abnormalities including impaired remodeling of maternal spiral arteries as well as increased placental oxidative stress and apoptosis [12]. In mice that are homozygous null for *Dlx3*, placental failure occurs between embryonic days 9.5–12.5 resulting in extremely restricted fetal growth and subsequently death [13]. Notably, we have previously shown that maternal choline supplementation (4X versus 1X choline) in *Dlx3+/−* dams increases fetal weights during mid-gestation in wildtype, heterozygous, and null embryos [14]. Most important to this body of work is the evidence supporting a role of DLX3 in human placental insufficiency (reviewed in Reference [15]).

In the present study, we sought to use the *Dlx3+/−* mouse model of placental insufficiency to investigate the effects of maternal choline supplementation on biomarkers of placental function and development across gestation. To accomplish these aims, we used tissue samples that were previously collected from *Dlx3+/−* pregnant dams randomized to consume one of three levels of choline intake [14].

2. Materials and Methods

2.1. Mice and Diets

All animal protocols and procedures used in this study were approved by the Institutional Animal Care and Use Committees at Cornell University, and were conducted in accordance with the Guide for the Care and Use of Laboratory Animals. *Dlx3+/−* mice were genotyped using tail DNA with three-primer duplex PCR (Table S1). Primers were designed to amplify a wildtype band, a knockout band, or both (indicating a heterozygote). Mice were housed in microisolator cages (Ancare, Bellmore, NY, USA) in an environmentally-controlled room (22–25 °C and 70% humidity) with a 12-hour light–dark cycle. During breeding, mice were given ad libitum access to commercial rodent chow (Teklad, Madison, WI, USA) and water. *Dlx3+/−* females were mated with *Dlx3+/−* males in a pair-wise manner, and their offspring were genotyped at time of weaning (3 weeks of age). Heterozygous pups were given ad libitum access to the 1X choline control diet containing 1.4 g choline chloride/kg (Dyets #103345). *Dlx3*+/− female mice were then randomized five days before mating with *Dlx3*+/− male mice and received either the 1X choline control diet, the 2X choline diet containing 2.8 g choline chloride/kg (Dyets #103346), or the 4X choline diet containing 5.6 g choline chloride/kg (Dyets #103347); all provided ad libitum. Embryonic (E) day 0.5 was designated via the presence of a vaginal plug. Pregnant mice were euthanized via carbon dioxide asphyxiation at four different gestational time points: E10.5, E12.5, E15.5, and E18.5.

2.2. Tissue Collection and Processing

After pregnant dams were sacrificed, embryos and placentas were carefully dissected with minimal decidual contamination and weighed. For approximately 1/3 of the litter, the implantation site was fixed in 10% formalin for histological analyses after removal of the embryo for genotyping. For the remaining placentas, at gestational time points E12.5, E15.5, and E18.5, placentas were bisected across the chorionic plate; one half was stabilized in RNAlater for mRNA analysis, while the remaining half was immediately frozen in liquid nitrogen and stored at −80 °C for metabolite analysis. Due to the smaller tissue size, E10.5 placentas were designated for mRNA analysis or metabolite analysis, alternately. Fetal DNA was extracted for *Dlx3* genotyping and sex determination using a commercial kit (Qiagen Inc., Germantown, MD, USA). Sex genotyping was performed using PCR for the *Sry* gene with a commercial kit (Qiagen Inc., Germantown, MD, USA). Primers are listed in Table S1.

2.3. Quantitative Real-Time RT-PCR

RNA was extracted from placentas maintained in RNAlater using TRIzol reagent (Invitrogen, Waltham, MA, USA). Two to three *Dlx3* heterozygous placentas per dam were randomly selected for extraction. RNA concentration and quality were assessed with a NanoDrop ND-1000 instrument (Thermo Fisher Scientific, Waltham, MA, USA), and samples with an A260/A280 ratio above 1.8 were used for quantification. Reverse transcription was performed using the ImProm-II Reverse Transcription System (Promega, Madison, WI, USA). Quantitative PCR was performed using SYBR® Green in a Roche LightCycler480 (Roche, IN, USA). All primers for the targeted genes (*Vegfa, Pgf, Eng, Mmp14, Tnfα, NfκB, Il1b*) were designed using NCBI Primer-BLAST (Table S1). Reaction conditions were as follows: 95 °C for 5 min, followed by 40 cycles for 15 s at 95 °C, 30 s annealing (see Table S1 for annealing temperatures), and 30 s at 72 °C. PCR product specificity was monitored using melting curve analysis at the end of the amplification cycles. Fold changes were calculated using the ΔCt method [16] normalized to the expression level of the housekeeping gene *Tbp* (TATA box binding protein), which has previously been shown to be stable in placental tissue [17], and in response to varying choline supply [18]. At E10.5, both wildtype and heterozygous placentas were used due to limited tissue availability, and *Dlx3* genotype was included in the statistical model. All qPCR analyses were performed in triplicate.

2.4. LC-MS/MS

Concentrations of acetylcholine were measured in the placenta using LC-MS/MS according to the method of Holm et al. [19] with modifications based on our equipment [20].

2.5. Placental Morphometry

Placental tissues fixed in 10% formalin were paraffin embedded and sectioned at 10 μm. Immunohistochemistry was performed on formalin-fixed sections as described previously [21]. For the analysis of maternal spiral artery areas, placental sections were incubated with smooth muscle actin (SMA) antibody (1:50, DakoCytomatin, Glostrup, Denmark), followed by a secondary antibody. Slides were imaged using an Aperio Scanscope (Vista, CA, USA). Maternal spiral arteries were manually defined based on the staining location and the presence of non-nucleated red blood cells. Aperio ImageScope software, version 102.0.7.5, was used to quantify the area. Data are presented as the ratio of artery luminal area to total arterial area. For the analysis of the placental labyrinth area, placental sections were incubated with biotinylated GSL 1-isolectin B4 (1:100, Vector Laboratories, Burlingame, CA, USA) and 3-amino-9-ethylcarbazole (AEC; Invitrogen, Carlsbad, CA, USA), and counterstained with hematoxylin. Isolectin is a marker of endothelial cells and has been used previously to stain vasculature in other mouse tissues. The placental labyrinth compartment was defined manually based on staining location, and area was calculated using Aperio ImageScope software (Vista, CA, USA). Data are expressed as mm^2 of cross-sectional labyrinth area.

2.6. *Placental Apoptosis*

Placental apoptosis was assessed using the terminal deoxynucleotidyl transferase dUTP nick end labeling (TUNEL) assay. A commercial kit (Millipore, Billerica, MA, USA) was used according to the manufacturer's instructions. Sections were imaged using an Aperio ScanScope and the number of TUNEL-positive cells was determined in the decidua and labyrinth by the average number of TUNEL-positive cells in several randomly selected fields. Field sizes were as follows: for E10.5, five fields of $250 \times 250\ \mu m^2$; for E12.5, five fields of $350 \times 350\ \mu m^2$; and for E15.5 and E18.5, ten fields of $500 \times 500\ \mu m^2$.

2.7. *Statistical Analysis*

For all outcome variables, data were analyzed separately for each gestational day using a linear mixed model. All statistical models included choline treatment as a fixed effect, and a maternal identifier (ID) as a random effect. Litter size, fetal genotype (except for the gene expression outcomes at E12.5, E15.5, and E18.5, which only included heterozygous pups), and fetal sex (except when the data were stratified by fetal sex) were controlled for in the models as fixed effects. Normality of the data was assessed by evaluating the distribution of residuals. Due to the hypothesis-driven nature of the study and the relatively small sample sizes, corrections for multiple analyses were not performed and statistical interactions were not assessed. Data are presented as means ± SEM. $p \leq 0.05$ was considered statistically significant and $0.05 < p < 0.10$ was considered to indicate trends. All analyses were performed using SPSS software, Version 23 (IBM, Chicago, IL, USA).

3. Results

We previously reported that maternal choline supplementation increased placental and fetal weights at E10.5 in offspring of *Dlx3*+/− dams regardless of fetal genotype [14]. These data can also be found in Table S2 which depicts embryo weight, placental weight, crown rump length, placental efficiency, and litter size in *Dlx3*+/− dams in response to maternal choline intakes (1X control, 2X, and 4X) at E10.5, E12.5, E15.5, and E18.5.

3.1. *Placental Morphometry*

Because the *Dlx3* model is associated with labyrinth abnormalities, we sought to determine whether choline treatment increased placental weight by increasing the size of the labyrinth. At E10.5, 4X choline placentas had 73% larger labyrinth area versus 2X choline ($p = 0.014$), and tended to be ~46% larger than 1X control placentas ($p = 0.092$, Figure 1A and 1B). At E12.5 and E15.5, there were no significant differences in labyrinth size by choline treatment. At E18.5, 2X placental labyrinths were ~25% smaller compared to 1X controls ($p = 0.037$) and tended to be ~20% smaller than 4X choline placentas ($p = 0.081$, Figure 1A).

3.2. *Placental Apoptosis*

We performed the terminal deoxynucleotidyl transferase dUTP nick end labeling assay (TUNEL) to assess placental levels of apoptosis at all four gestational time points. At E10.5, choline treatment tended to result in ~49% lower TUNEL scores (average # TUNEL-positive cells per field) in the 4X choline placentas ($p = 0.053$ versus 1X controls) (Figure 2A). At E12.5, 4X choline placentas had ~58%

lower TUNEL scores ($p = 0.048$ versus 1X controls) (Figure 2A,B). No differences in TUNEL score were detected between choline treatment groups at E15.5 and E18.5 (Figure 2A).

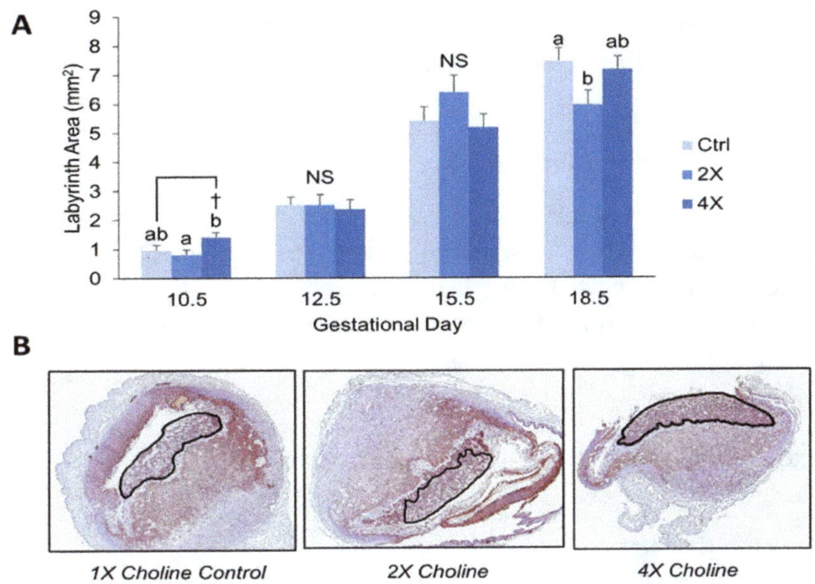

Figure 1. Placental labyrinth area at E10.5, E12.5, E15.5, and E18.5 by choline treatment (**A**). Representative images of placental labyrinths at E10.5 are shown in (**B**). Data were analyzed using mixed linear models with choline treatment as a fixed effect and maternal ID as a random effect. Litter size, fetal genotype, and fetal sex were controlled for in the models as fixed effects. Values are presented as mean ± SEM. Different letters denote significant differences between means of the treatments at $p \leq 0.05$. † denotes $p < 0.1$. $n = 7–12$ placentas per treatment per time point. NS, nonsignificant.

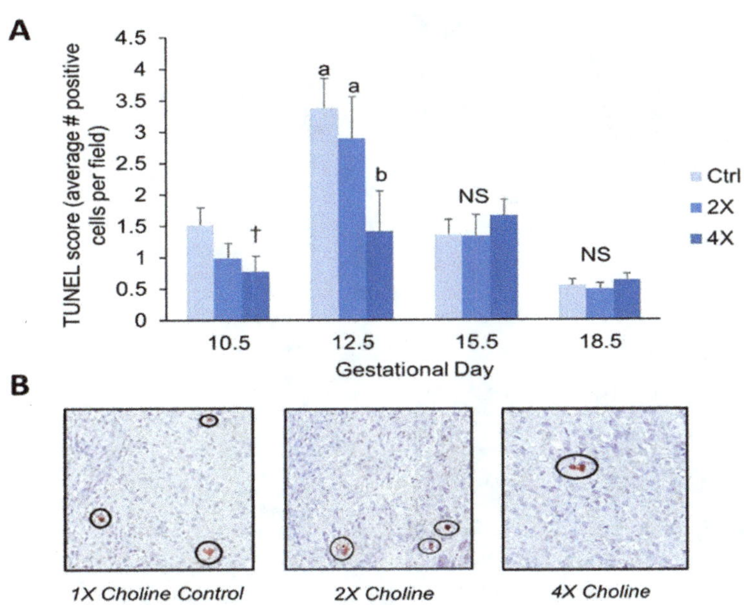

Figure 2. TUNEL score (calculated as the average number of TUNEL-positive cells per field) at E10.5, E12.5, E15.5, and E18.5 by maternal choline treatment (**A**). Representative images of TUNEL staining at E12.5 are shown in (**B**). Data were analyzed using mixed linear models with choline treatment as a fixed effect and maternal ID as a random effect. Litter size, fetal genotype, and fetal sex were controlled for in the models as fixed effects. Values are presented as mean ± SEM. Different letters denote significant differences between means of the treatments at $p \leq 0.05$. † denotes $p < 0.1$ versus 1X choline controls. $n = 7–15$ placentas per treatment per time point. NS, nonsignificant.

3.3. Placental Artery Remodeling

Because we had previously found an effect of maternal choline supplementation on spiral artery remodeling in wildtype mice [11], we investigated whether it would have a similar function in a model of placental insufficiency. We assessed the luminal ratio of maternal spiral arteries, defined as (luminal area)/total arterial area. Luminal ratio did not differ by choline treatment or *Dlx3* genotype at any gestational time point.

3.4. Placental Expression of Angiogenic Genes

Because altered levels of pro-angiogenic factors have been implicated in the development of preeclampsia and other pregnancy disorders, we measured mRNA expression of several key modulators of placental angiogenesis throughout pregnancy in *Dlx3*+/− placentas (Figure 3A–D). For this outcome, we stratified by fetal sex due to our previous findings showing effects of fetal sex on angiogenic gene expression [11].

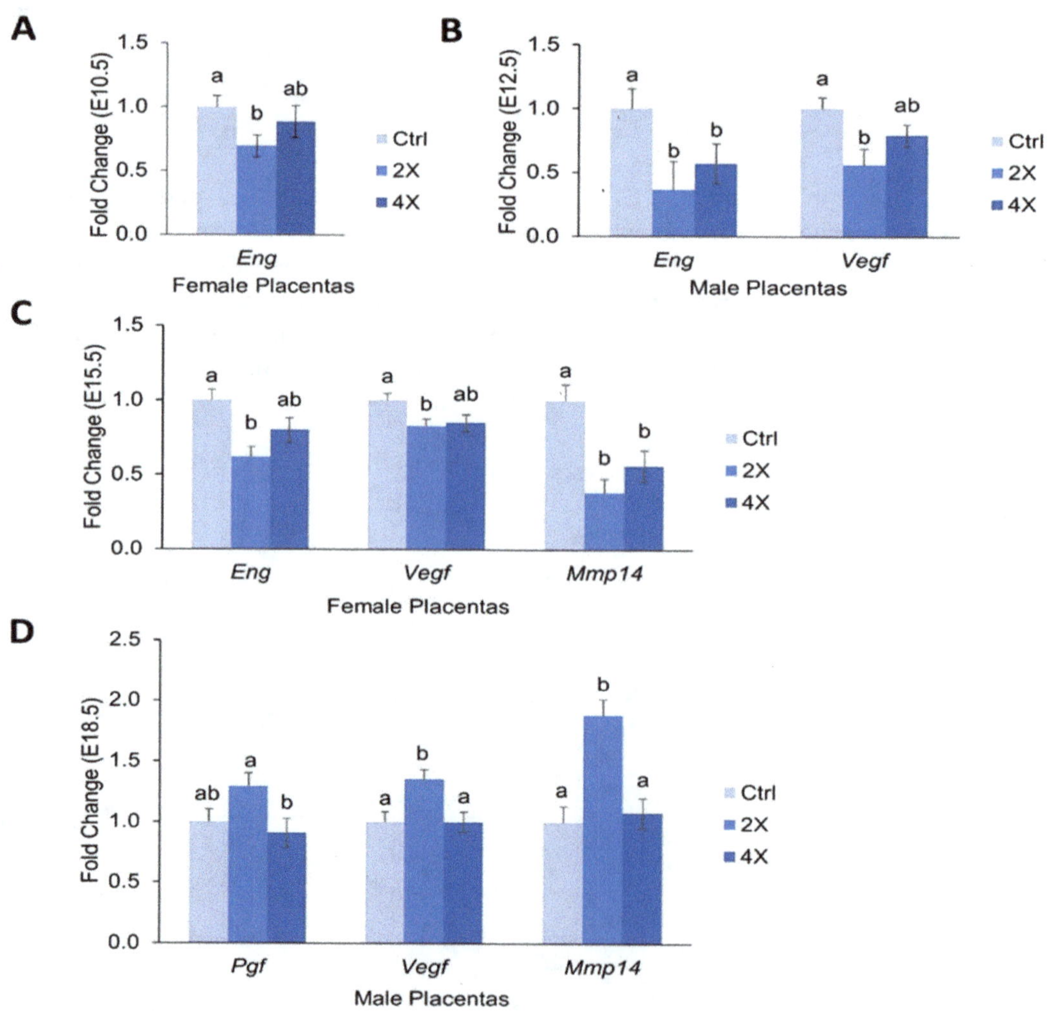

Figure 3. Placental mRNA abundance of angiogenic genes at (**A**) E10.5, (**B**) E12.5, (**C**) E15.5, and (**D**) E18.5 by maternal choline treatment. Data are expressed as the fold-change relative to the housekeeping gene *Tbp*. Data were analyzed using mixed linear models with choline treatment as a fixed effect and maternal ID as a random effect. Litter size and fetal genotype (for E10.5; heterozygous pups were used for E12.5, E15.5, and E18.5) were controlled for in the models as fixed effects. Values are presented as mean ± SEM. Different letters denote significant differences between means of the treatments at $p \leq 0.05$. $n = 20$ placentas per treatment per time point.

At E10.5, expression of *Eng* was ~31% lower in the female 2X choline placentas versus 1X controls ($p = 0.029$) (Figure 3A). No effects of choline treatment on *Eng* expression were detected for the male placentas, nor did choline treatment alter *Vegfa*, *Pgf*, or *Mmp14* expression at E10.5 in either sex.

At E12.5, 2X and 4X choline males had lower expression of *Eng* vs. 1X controls (~64% and ~43%, respectively, $p = 0.005, 0.013$) (Figure 3B). Similarly, male 2X choline placentas had ~44% lower expression of *Vegfa* ($p = 0.026$ versus 1X) (Figure 3B). No significant effects of choline treatment on these angiogenic factors were detected in females; nor did choline treatment influence *Pgf* or *Mmp14* expression at E12.5.

At E15.5, expression of *Eng* in female placentas was ~38% lower in the 2X choline group ($p = 0.002$ vs. 1X). Similarly, 2X choline female placentas had ~17% lower expression of *Vegfa* vs. 1X controls ($p = 0.031$) (Figure 3C). Expression of *Mmp14* was ~42% lower in female 2X choline placentas ($p = 0.019$, vs. 1X) and ~41% lower in 4X choline placentas ($p = 0.015$, vs. 1X) (Figure 3C). No effects of choline treatment on these angiogenic factors were detected in males; nor did choline treatment influence *Pgf* expression in either fetal sex at E15.5.

At E18.5, male placentas in the 2X choline group had ~35% higher expression of *Vegfa* versus 1X controls and 4X choline groups ($p = 0.011$ and 0.01, respectively). Similarly, expression of *Pgf* tended to be ~29% higher in 2X choline males versus 1X control males ($p = 0.091$) and was ~42% higher versus 4X choline ($p = 0.091$). Male 2X choline placentas also had ~62% higher expression of *Mmp14* versus 1X placentas ($p = 0.006$) (Figure 3D). No effects of choline treatment on these angiogenic factors were detected in females; nor did *Eng* expression differ by choline treatment at E18.5 in either fetal sex.

3.5. Placental Expression of Inflammatory Genes

Abnormal regulation of inflammation has been shown in various placental pathologies; therefore, we also measured mRNA expression of several major inflammatory regulators in the *Dlx3+/−* placentas (Figure 4A–C). Again, data were stratified by fetal sex due to our previous work showing the strong effects of fetal sex on inflammatory processes [11].

At E10.5, there were no significant differences in *Tnfα*, *Nfκb*, or *Il1b* expression among choline treatment groups. At E12.5, 2X choline male placentas had a lower expression of Tnfα (~57% versus 1X) and tended to have lower expression of *Nfκb* (~50%, $p = 0.096$ versus 1X) (Figure 4A). No effects of choline treatment on these inflammatory genes were detected in females; nor did expression of *Il1b* differ by treatment.

At E15.5, female 2X choline placentas had ~33% lower expression of *Nfκb* versus 1X controls ($p = 0.020$). Expression of *Il1b* was ~36% lower in 2X choline placentas of both sexes versus 1X controls ($p = 0.034$, Figure 4B), and also in males alone ($p = 0.031$).

At E18.5, expression of *Il1b* was ~32% lower in 4X choline pups of male and female placentas combined ($p = 0.02$) (Figure 4C), a finding that did not reach statistically significant levels in either sex alone. Female 4X choline placentas tended to have ~39% lower expression of *Nfκb* versus 1X control females ($p = 0.058$) (Figure 4C). No differences in Tnfα expression were seen among choline groups at E15.5 or E18.5.

3.6. Placental Acetylcholine

Because acetylcholine has been linked to angiogenic and inflammatory signaling in the placenta [22,23], we measured concentrations of placental acetylcholine throughout gestation. At E12.5, 2X choline placentas had ~136% higher concentrations of acetylcholine versus 1X controls ($p = 0.011$), and ~107% higher concentrations versus 4X choline placentas ($p = 0.020$). At E10.5, E15.5, and E18.5, acetylcholine concentrations did not differ by choline treatment (Figure 5).

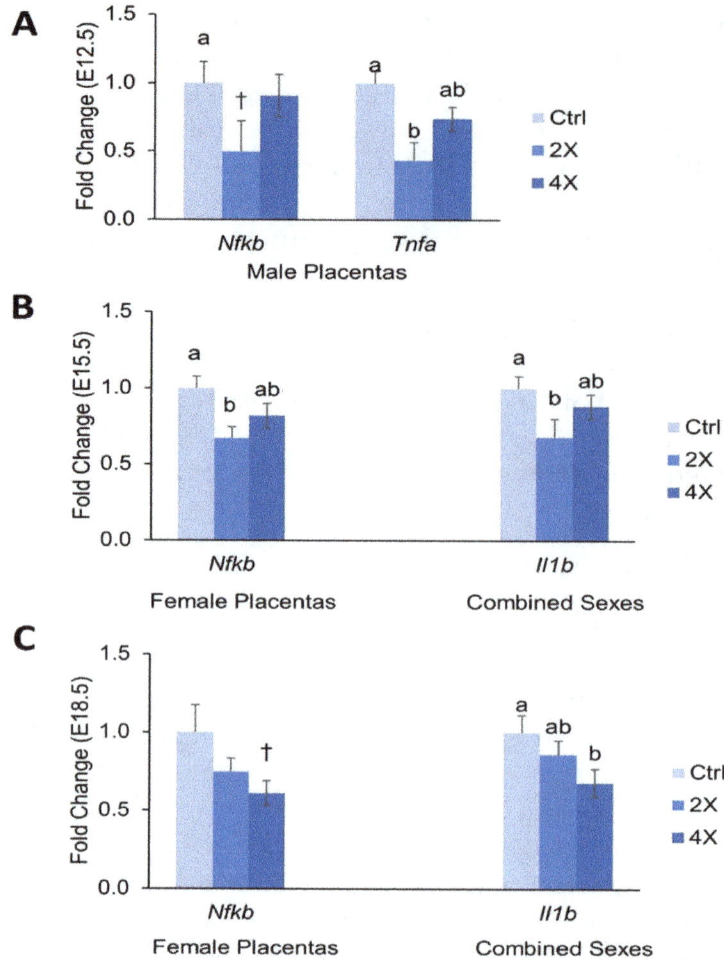

Figure 4. Placental mRNA abundance of inflammatory genes at (**A**) E12.5, (**B**) E15.5, and (**C**) E18.5 by maternal choline treatment. Data are expressed as the fold-change relative to the housekeeping gene *Tbp*. Data were analyzed using mixed linear models with choline treatment as a fixed effect and maternal ID as a random effect. Litter size and fetal genotype (for E10.5; heterozygous pups were used for E12.5, E15.5, and E18.5) were controlled for in the models as fixed effects. Values are presented as mean ± SEM. Different letters denote significant differences between means of the treatments at $p \leq 0.05$. † denotes $p < 0.1$ versus 1X choline controls. $n = 20$ placentas per treatment per time point.

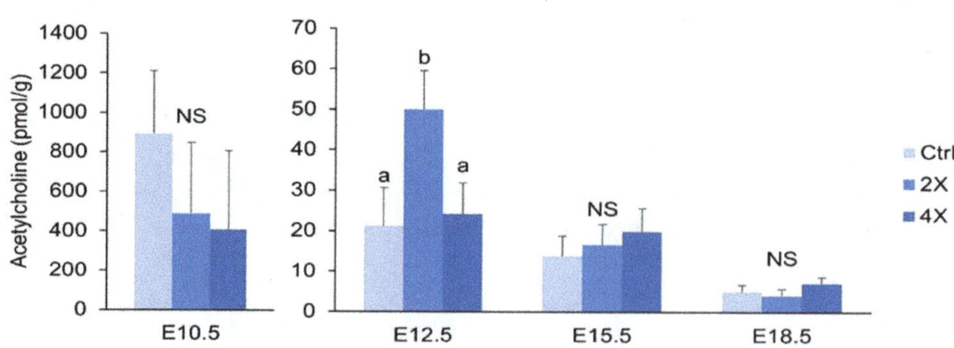

Figure 5. Placental acetylcholine concentrations (pmol/gram tissue) at E10.5, E12.5, 15.5, and 18.5 by maternal choline treatment (1X, 2X, and 4X choline). Data were analyzed using mixed linear models with choline treatment as a fixed effect and maternal ID as a random effect. Litter size, fetal genotype, and fetal sex were controlled for in the models as fixed effects. Values are presented as mean ± SEM. Different letters denote significant differences between means of the treatments at $p \leq 0.05$. $n = 20$ placentas per treatment per time point. NS, nonsignificant.

4. Discussion

4.1. Maternal Choline Supplementation in the Dlx3+/− Pregnant Dam Increases Placental Labyrinth Size and Decreases Placental Apoptosis in Mid-Gestation

Because we had previously reported a higher placental weight at E10.5 with maternal choline supplementation in *Dlx3+/−* dams [14], we sought to determine whether this effect could be explained by alterations in the size of the placental labyrinth or apoptosis levels. Development of the labyrinth region, which facilitates nutrient transfer between mother and fetus, is defective in *Dlx3−/−* animals [13]. At E10.5, a high dose of choline (4X the recommended intake) yielded a larger labyrinth size compared to the 2X choline dose, and tended to yield a larger labyrinth size compared to the 1X choline dose. Thus, an increase in surface area for nutrient transfer may have contributed to the larger embryo weights we previously reported in offspring (both +/− and +/+) of *Dlx3+/−* mothers whom received 4X choline supplementation [14].

An additional explanation for the larger placental weights could be through reductions in apoptosis. For example, 4X (versus 1X) choline placentas had ~58% lower TUNEL scores at E12.5, and a tendency for lower scores (49% lower) at E10.5. These findings concur with previous results showing reductions in apoptosis with choline supplementation in human trophoblast cells [10] and in placentas of wildtype mice [11]. Although apoptosis is required for normal placental development, elevated levels of apoptosis have been reported in preeclamptic and IUGR placentas [24–26]. Notably, the elevated levels of apoptosis in *Dlx3+/−* placentas had previously been rescued using a strong antioxidant, TEMPOL [12]. Therefore, a reduction in placental apoptosis in mid-gestation via maternal choline supplementation may have beneficial effects in reducing the risk of developing placental complications later in gestation.

In a preliminary histological examination of spiral artery remodeling, we did not find evidence that maternal choline supplementation altered arterial luminal area percentage in the *Dlx3+/−* mouse. This is in contrast to our previous findings in wildtype dams, where 4X choline significantly increased luminal area percentage at E10.5, E12.5, E15.5, and E18.5 [11]. It is possible that the pathological phenotype of spiral artery remodeling in the *Dlx3+/−* dam was too severe to be ameliorated by choline supplementation. However, due to the small size of our histology cohort, this finding should be confirmed in a larger study.

Although prior work has shown that *Dlx3* is required for normal placental morphogenesis (13) and reduced *Dlx3* gene dose results in elevated placental cell oxidative stress and apoptosis coincident with altered vascular remodeling (12), we did not detect any differences in labyrinth size, apoptosis levels, or spiral artery remodeling between *Dlx3+/+* and *Dlx3+/−* placentas. We previously found that *Dlx3+/−* fetuses had comparable weights, but a higher expression of growth factor genes versus their *Dlx3+/+* littermates when their mothers consumed a high-quality pregnancy diet [14], suggesting that the *Dlx3+/−* placenta may activate compensatory mechanisms that lead to results similar to wildtype placentas for certain outcomes.

4.2. Effects of Maternal Choline Supplementation on Placental Inflammatory and Angiogenic Gene Expression Vary by Gestational Time Point and Fetal Sex

Inflammation and angiogenesis have been shown to be dysregulated in pregnancy complications including preeclampsia, IUGR, and spontaneous abortion [1,27,28]. Because of this, we measured placental mRNA expression of major modulators of these processes to determine whether choline can influence their placental expression in the *Dlx3+/−* mouse.

Overall patterns seen included the tendency for pro-inflammatory and pro-angiogenic markers to be downregulated in response to choline supplementation, with the 2X dose frequently having a larger effect than that of 4X. For example, compared to 1X choline, 2X choline significantly reduced the expression of the proinflammatory factors *Tnfα*, *Nfκb*, and *Il1b* at various gestational time points of pregnancy; a finding that was not consistently observed with 4X choline. Previous studies have shown that choline deficiency increases the expression of pro-inflammatory cytokines in a human placental trophoblast cell culture model [10], and that maternal choline supplementation reduces inflammatory response in pregnant rats challenged with lipopolysaccharide [29]. The results seen in the current study with a 2X choline dose provide additional support for a role of choline in mitigating inflammation, and suggest that efforts to increase maternal choline intake may be a nutritional strategy to reduce placental inflammation and improve pregnancy outcomes especially since less than ten percent of U.S. pregnant women meet choline intake recommendations [30].

The weakening of the choline-induced anti-inflammatory effects with the 4X treatment may suggest variability whereby maternal choline supplementation has an anti-inflammatory effect up to a certain concentration, beyond which its effects are attenuated. Alternatively, a strong growth-promoting effect of 4X maternal choline supplementation was detected in these mice at E10.5 [14], which was followed by a gradual slowing of growth such that only minor differences were detected in fetal weights in late gestation (E18.5). Thus, the effects of 4X choline on inflammatory (and angiogenic) processes in the placenta may have been weakened by compensatory mechanisms engaged to prevent exaggerated fetal growth.

We also observed downregulation of placental expression of the proangiogenic factor endoglin with maternal choline supplementation at E10.5 and E15.5 in female placentas and at E12.5 in males. These effects were mirrored by similar downregulation of proangiogenic *Vegfa*, which has been shown to be elevated or decreased in preeclamptic patients depending on the study [31–33]. It is possible that the larger labyrinth observed at E10.5 in the current study, combined with the superior placenta efficiency observed previously in these mice [14], resulted in a decreased need for placental angiogenesis, leading to a downregulation of pro-angiogenic factors.

Endoglin also serves as the precursor to soluble VEGF receptor endoglin (sEng), an anti-angiogenic factor that prevents VEGF from acting on target tissues [5], and contributes to the development of placental dysfunction. In the current study, expression of *Mmp14*, the matrix metalloproteinase that cleaves endoglin into its pathogenic soluble form [34], was significantly lower at E15.5 in females with choline supplementation, which is suggestive of decreased generation of sENG. In males, however, placental expression of *Mmp14* was higher at E18.5 with 2X choline supplementation, suggesting greater generation of sENG. This putative increase in sENG in late gestation could have a beneficial role in preventing preterm birth by blunting the parturition promoting effects of VEGF signaling through PGF and VEGF [31,32], both of which also were upregulated at this time point.

The effects of maternal choline supplementation on placental gene expression were sex specific, as previously reported in wildtype mouse pregnancy [11]. Differential expression of angiogenic factors according to fetal sex has been reported in both normal [33] and preeclamptic [35] human pregnancies. Although the mechanisms remain unclear, sex-specific differences in epigenetic regulation and hormonal environment have been suggested to be contributing factors [36,37]. Our findings add to the body of evidence demonstrating that fetal sex should be accounted for when examining placental and fetal outcomes during pregnancy.

4.3. Placental Concentrations of Acetylcholine are Minimally Affected by Maternal Choline Supplementation

Because acetylcholine has been reported to play a role in angiogenic [23] and inflammatory [22] signaling in the placenta, we hypothesized that choline may be modulating gene expression by altering acetylcholine levels. Surprisingly, we did not detect an increase in placental acetylcholine concentrations in response to maternal choline supplementation at E10.5, E15.5, or E18.5. At E12.5, acetylcholine levels were higher in the 2X, but not 4X, choline group. The overall lack of effect of maternal choline supplementation on placental acetylcholine concentrations could reflect rapid uptake of the acetylcholine molecule by the developing fetus as we previously reported that 4X choline increased acetylcholine concentrations in the fetal brain of wildtype mice [38].

4.4. Strengths and Limitations

The study strengths include: (i) the use of a standardized diet and three choline intake levels; (ii) the inclusion of four gestational time points, which allows for a dynamic view of the changes that occur in the placenta throughout gestation; and (iii) the use of an animal model with a hemochorial structure similar to the primate placenta. Nonetheless, several limitations should be noted. The small sample size combined with the relatively high degree of variability for most of the outcome data precluded our ability to assess the interactive effects of fetal genotype and fetal sex with choline treatment. An additional limitation of the current study was the analyses of mRNA abundance without concurrent analyses of proteins. Finally, our histological analyses were included as a hypothesis-generating examination of choline's effects in compromised pregnancies, and should be confirmed in larger cohorts.

5. Conclusions

In conclusion, maternal choline supplementation modulated placental development and function in a mouse model of placental insufficiency, providing some evidence that choline may be a useful therapy during pregnancy to prevent or overcome development of placental disorders that impact fetal and maternal health. Decreases in pro-inflammatory gene expression and placental apoptosis are especially encouraging and align with previous results showing similar effects of choline in different experimental models. Since many pregnant women do not currently meet the recommended intake levels of choline [30], further research is warranted to investigate the effects of increased maternal choline intake on human placental function.

Author Contributions: The author contributions were as follows: conceptualization, J.H.K., X.J., M.S.R. and M.A.C.; investigation, J.H.K, S.T.K. and J.Y.; data curation, J.H.K, V.G.F., S.P.L. and E.W.; formal analysis, J.H.K.; writing—original draft preparation, J.H.K.; writing—review and editing, M.S.R. and M.A.C.; supervision, M.S.R. and M.A.C.; funding acquisition, X.J., M.S.R. and M.A.C.

References

1. Chaddha, V.; Viero, S.; Huppertz, B.; Kingdom, J. Developmental biology of the placenta and the origins of placental insufficiency. *Semin. Fetal Neonatal Med.* **2004**, *9*, 357–369. [CrossRef] [PubMed]
2. Azizieh, F.; Raghupathy, R.; Makhseed, M. Maternal Cytokine Production Patterns in Women with Pre-eclampsia. *Am. J. Reprod. Immunol.* **2005**, *54*, 30–37. [CrossRef] [PubMed]
3. Cartwright, J.E.; Whitley, G.S.J. Trophoblast-mediated spiral artery remodelling: A role for apoptosis. *J. Anat.* **2009**, *215*, 21–26.
4. Cheng, M.-H.; Wang, P.-H. Placentation abnormalities in the pathophysiology of preeclampsia. *Expert Rev. Mol. Diagn.* **2009**, *9*, 37–49. [CrossRef] [PubMed]
5. Venkatesha, S.; Toporsian, M.; Lam, C.; Hanai, J.-I.; Mammoto, T.; Kim, Y.M.; Bdolah, Y.; Lim, K.-H.; Yuan, H.-T.; Libermann, T.A.; et al. Soluble endoglin contributes to the pathogenesis of preeclampsia. *Nat. Med.* **2006**, *12*, 642–649. [CrossRef] [PubMed]
6. Boij, R.; Svensson-Arvelund, J.; Nilsson-Ekdahl, K.; Sandholm, K.; Lindahl, T.L.; Pálonek, E.; Garle, M.; Berg, G.; Ernerudh, J.; Jenmalm, M.; et al. Biomarkers of Coagulation, Inflammation, and Angiogenesis are Independently Associated with Preeclampsia. *Am. J. Reprod. Immunol.* **2012**, *68*, 258–270. [CrossRef] [PubMed]
7. Jiang, X.; West, A.A.; Caudill, M.A. Maternal choline supplementation: A nutritional approach for improving offspring health? *Trends Endocrinol. Metab.* **2014**, *25*, 263–273. [CrossRef] [PubMed]
8. Caudill, M.A. Pre- and Postnatal Health: Evidence of Increased Choline Needs. *J. Am. Diet. Assoc.* **2010**, *110*, 1198–1206. [CrossRef]
9. Jiang, X.; Bar, H.Y.; Yan, J.; Jones, S.; Brannon, P.M.; West, A.A.; Perry, C.A.; Ganti, A.; Pressman, E.; Devapatla, S.; et al. A higher maternal choline intake among third-trimester pregnant women lowers

placental and circulating concentrations of the antiangiogenic factor fms-like tyrosine kinase-1 (sFLT1). *FASEB J.* **2013**, *27*, 1245–1253. [CrossRef]
10. Jiang, X.; Jones, S.; Andrew, B.Y.; Ganti, A.; Malysheva, O.V.; Giallourou, N.; Brannon, P.M.; Roberson, M.S.; Caudill, M.A. Choline Inadequacy Impairs Trophoblast Function and Vascularization in Cultured Human Placental Trophoblasts. *J. Cell. Physiol.* **2014**, *229*, 1016–1027. [CrossRef]
11. Kwan, S.T. (Cecilia); King, J.H.; Yan, J.; Jiang, X.; Wei, E.; Fomin, V.G.; Roberson, M.S.; Caudill, M.A. Maternal choline supplementation during murine pregnancy modulates placental markers of inflammation, apoptosis and vascularization in a fetal sex-dependent manner. *Placenta* **2017**, *53*, 57–65. [PubMed]
12. Clark, P.; Brown, J.; Li, S.; Woods, A.; Han, L.; Sones, J.; Preston, R.; Southard, T.; Davisson, R.; Roberson, M.; et al. Distal-less 3 haploinsufficiency results in elevated placental oxidative stress and altered fetal growth kinetics in the mouse. *Placenta* **2012**, *33*, 830–838. [CrossRef]
13. Morasso, M.I.; Grinberg, A.; Robinson, G.; Sargent, T.D.; Mahon, K.A. Placental failure in mice lacking the homeobox gene Dlx3. *Proc. Natl. Acad. Sci. USA* **1999**, *96*, 162–167. [CrossRef] [PubMed]
14. King, J.H.; Kwan, S.T.C.; Yan, J.; Klatt, K.C.; Roberson, M.S.; Caudill, M.A. Maternal Choline Supplementation Alters Fetal Growth Patterns in a Mouse Model of Placental Insufficiency. *Nutrients* **2017**, *9*, 765. [CrossRef] [PubMed]
15. Murthi, P.; Kalionis, B.; Rajaraman, G.; Keogh, R.J.; Costa, F.D.S. The Role of Homeobox Genes in the Development of Placental Insufficiency. *Fetal Diagn. Ther.* **2012**, *32*, 225–230. [CrossRef] [PubMed]
16. Schmittgen, T.D.; Livak, K.J. Analyzing real-time PCR data by the comparative CT method. *Nat. Protoc.* **2008**, *3*, 1101–1108. [CrossRef] [PubMed]
17. Meller, M.; Vadachkoria, S.; Luthy, D.; Williams, M. Evaluation of housekeeping genes in placental comparative expression studies. *Placenta* **2005**, *26*, 601–607. [CrossRef] [PubMed]
18. Mehedint, M.G.; Craciunescu, C.N.; Zeisel, S.H. Maternal dietary choline deficiency alters angiogenesis in fetal mouse hippocampus. *Proc. Natl. Acad. Sci. USA* **2010**, *107*, 12834–12839. [CrossRef]
19. Holm, P.I.; Ueland, P.M.; Kvalheim, G.; Lien, E.A. Determination of Choline, Betaine, and Dimethylglycine in Plasma by a High-Throughput Method Based on Normal-Phase Chromatography-Tandem Mass Spectrometry. *Clin. Chem.* **2003**, *49*, 286–294. [CrossRef]
20. Yan, J.; Wang, W.; Gregory, J.F., III; Malysheva, O.; Brenna, J.T.; Stabler, S.P.; Allen, R.H.; Caudill, M.A. MTHFR C677T genotype influences the isotopic enrichment of one-carbon metabolites in folate-compromised men consuming d9-choline. *Am. J. Clin. Nutr.* **2011**, *93*, 348–355. [CrossRef]
21. Berghorn, K.A.; Clark, P.A.; Encarnacion, B.; DeRegis, C.J.; Folger, J.K.; I Morasso, M.; Soares, M.J.; Wolfe, M.W.; Roberson, M.S. Developmental expression of the homeobox protein Distal-less 3 and its relationship to progesterone production in mouse placenta. *J. Endocrinol.* **2005**, *186*, 315–323. [CrossRef] [PubMed]
22. Jonge, W.J.; Ulloa, L. The alpha7 nicotinic acetylcholine receptor as a pharmacological target for inflammation. *Br. J. Pharmacol.* **2009**, *151*, 915–929. [CrossRef] [PubMed]
23. Arias, H.R.; Richards, V.E.; Ng, D.; Ghafoori, M.E.; Le, V.; Mousa, S.A. Role of non-neuronal nicotinic acetylcholine receptors in angiogenesis. *Int. J. Biochem. Cell Biol.* **2009**, *41*, 1441–1451. [CrossRef] [PubMed]
24. DiFederico, E.; Genbacev, O.; Fisher, S.J. Preeclampsia Is Associated with Widespread Apoptosis of Placental Cytotrophoblasts within the Uterine Wall. *Am. J. Pathol.* **1999**, *155*, 293–301. [CrossRef]
25. Allaire, A. Placental apoptosis in preeclampsia. *Obstet. Gynecol.* **2000**, *96*, 271–276. [PubMed]
26. Ishihara, N.; Matsuo, H.; Murakoshi, H.; Laoag-Fernandez, J.B.; Samoto, T.; Maruo, T. Increased apoptosis in the syncytiotrophoblast in human term placentas complicated by either preeclampsia or intrauterine growth retardation. *Am. J. Obstet. Gynecol.* **2002**, *186*, 158–166. [CrossRef] [PubMed]
27. Mestan, K.; Yu, Y.; Matoba, N.; Cerda, S.; Demmin, B.; Pearson, C.; Ortiz, K.; Wang, X. Placental Inflammatory Response Is Associated with Poor Neonatal Growth: Preterm Birth Cohort Study. *Pediatrics* **2010**, *125*, 891–898. [CrossRef] [PubMed]
28. Christiansen, O.B.; Nielsen, H.S.; Kolte, A.M. Inflammation and miscarriage. *Semin. Fetal Neonatal Med.* **2006**, *11*, 302–308. [CrossRef]
29. Zhang, M.; Han, X.; Bao, J.; Yang, J.; Shi, S.-Q.; Garfield, R.E.; Liu, H. Choline Supplementation During Pregnancy Protects Against Gestational Lipopolysaccharide-Induced Inflammatory Responses. *Reprod. Sci.* **2017**, *25*, 74–85. [CrossRef]

30. Wallace, T.C.; Fulgoni, V.L. Usual Choline Intakes Are Associated with Egg and Protein Food Consumption in the United States. *Nutrients* **2017**, *9*, 839. [CrossRef]
31. Wada, Y.; Ozaki, H.; Abe, N.; Mori, A.; Sakamoto, K.; Nagamitsu, T.; Nakahara, T.; Ishii, K. Role of Vascular Endothelial Growth Factor in Maintenance of Pregnancy in Mice. *Endocrinology* **2013**, *154*, 900–910. [CrossRef] [PubMed]
32. Lappas, M. Nuclear factor- B mediates placental growth factor induced pro-labour mediators in human placenta. *Mol. Hum. Reprod.* **2012**, *18*, 354–361. [CrossRef] [PubMed]
33. Scott, N.M.; Hodyl, N.A.; Murphy, V.E.; Osei-Kumah, A.; Wyper, H.; Hodgson, D.M.; Smith, R.; Clifton, V.L. Placental Cytokine Expression Covaries with Maternal Asthma Severity and Fetal Sex. *J. Immunol.* **2009**, *182*, 1411–1420. [CrossRef] [PubMed]
34. Kaitu'U-Lino, T.J.; Palmer, K.R.; Whitehead, C.L.; Williams, E.; Lappas, M.; Tong, S. MMP-14 Is Expressed in Preeclamptic Placentas and Mediates Release of Soluble Endoglin. *Am. J. Pathol.* **2012**, *180*, 888–894. [CrossRef] [PubMed]
35. Muralimanoharan, S.; Maloyan, A.; Myatt, L. Evidence of sexual dimorphism in the placental function with severe preeclampsia. *Placenta* **2013**, *34*, 1183–1189. [CrossRef] [PubMed]
36. Martin, E.; Smeester, L.; Bommarito, P.A.; Grace, M.R.; Boggess, K.; Kuban, K.; Karagas, M.R.; Marsit, C.J.; O'Shea, T.M.; Fry, R.C.; et al. Sexual epigenetic dimorphism in the human placenta: Implications for susceptibility during the prenatal period. *Epigenomics* **2017**, *9*, 267–278. [CrossRef] [PubMed]
37. Yang, X.; Schadt, E.E.; Wang, S.; Wang, H.; Arnold, A.P.; Ingram-Drake, L.; Drake, T.A.; Lusis, A.J. Tissue-specific expression and regulation of sexually dimorphic genes in mice. *Genome Res.* **2006**, *16*, 995–1004. [CrossRef]
38. Kwan, S.T. (Cecilia); King, J.H.; Yan, J.; Wang, Z.; Jiang, X.; Hutzler, J.S.; Klein, H.R.; Brenna, J.T.; Roberson, M.S.; Caudill, M.A.; et al. Maternal Choline Supplementation Modulates Placental Nutrient Transport and Metabolism in Late Gestation of Mouse Pregnancy. *J. Nutr.* **2017**, *147*, 2083–2092.

Permissions

All chapters in this book were first published by MDPI; hereby published with permission under the Creative Commons Attribution License or equivalent. Every chapter published in this book has been scrutinized by our experts. Their significance has been extensively debated. The topics covered herein carry significant findings which will fuel the growth of the discipline. They may even be implemented as practical applications or may be referred to as a beginning point for another development.

The contributors of this book come from diverse backgrounds, making this book a truly international effort. This book will bring forth new frontiers with its revolutionizing research information and detailed analysis of the nascent developments around the world.

We would like to thank all the contributing authors for lending their expertise to make the book truly unique. They have played a crucial role in the development of this book. Without their invaluable contributions this book wouldn't have been possible. They have made vital efforts to compile up to date information on the varied aspects of this subject to make this book a valuable addition to the collection of many professionals and students.

This book was conceptualized with the vision of imparting up-to-date information and advanced data in this field. To ensure the same, a matchless editorial board was set up. Every individual on the board went through rigorous rounds of assessment to prove their worth. After which they invested a large part of their time researching and compiling the most relevant data for our readers.

The editorial board has been involved in producing this book since its inception. They have spent rigorous hours researching and exploring the diverse topics which have resulted in the successful publishing of this book. They have passed on their knowledge of decades through this book. To expedite this challenging task, the publisher supported the team at every step. A small team of assistant editors was also appointed to further simplify the editing procedure and attain best results for the readers.

Apart from the editorial board, the designing team has also invested a significant amount of their time in understanding the subject and creating the most relevant covers. They scrutinized every image to scout for the most suitable representation of the subject and create an appropriate cover for the book.

The publishing team has been an ardent support to the editorial, designing and production team. Their endless efforts to recruit the best for this project, has resulted in the accomplishment of this book. They are a veteran in the field of academics and their pool of knowledge is as vast as their experience in printing. Their expertise and guidance has proved useful at every step. Their uncompromising quality standards have made this book an exceptional effort. Their encouragement from time to time has been an inspiration for everyone.

The publisher and the editorial board hope that this book will prove to be a valuable piece of knowledge for researchers, students, practitioners and scholars across the globe.

List of Contributors

Charles J. P. Snart, Elizabeth Taylor, Diane E. Threapleton and Laura J. Hardie
Department of Clinical and Population Science, Leeds Institute of Cardiovascular and Metabolic Medicine, School of Medicine, University of Leeds, Leeds LS2 9JT, UK

Darren C. Greenwood
Department of Clinical and Population Science, Leeds Institute of Cardiovascular and Metabolic Medicine, School of Medicine, University of Leeds, Leeds LS2 9JT, UK
Leeds Institute for Data Analytics, University of Leeds, Leeds LS2 9JT, UK
Division of Biostatistics, Centre for Epidemiology and Biostatistics, University of Leeds, Leeds LS2 9JT, UK

Claire Keeble
Leeds Institute for Data Analytics, University of Leeds, Leeds LS2 9JT, UK

Janet E. Cade
Nutritional Epidemiology Group, School of Food Science & Nutrition, University of Leeds, Leeds LS2 9JT, UK

Paul M. Stewart
Faculty of Medicine and Health, University of Leeds, Leeds LS2 9JT, UK

Michael Zimmermann
Laboratory for Human Nutrition, Institute of Food, Nutrition and Health, Swiss Federal Institute of Technology (ETH), 8092 Zürich, Switzerland

Stephen Reid
Earth Surface Science Institute, School of Earth and Environment, University of Leeds, Leeds LS2 9JT, UK

Lucilla Poston
Division of Women's Health, Women's Health Academic Centre, King's College London, London SE1 7EH, UK

Jenny E. Myers
Maternal and Fetal Health Research Centre, Institute of Human Development, University of Manchester, Manchester M13 0JH, UK

Nigel A. B. Simpson
Division of Women's and Children's Health, School of Medicine, University of Leeds, Leeds LS2 9JT, UK

Jonathan G. Mun, LeeCole L. Legette, Chioma J. Ikonte and Susan H. Mitmesser
Science & Technology, Pharmavite LLC, West Hills, CA 91304, USA

Camilla Nykjaer
Nutritional Epidemiology Group, School of Food Science and Nutrition, University of Leeds, Leeds LS2 9JT, UK
School of Biomedical Sciences, Faculty of Biological Sciences, University of Leeds, Leeds LS2 9JT, UK

Nigel A.B. Simpson and Charlotte Higgs
Department of Obstetrics and Gynaecology, University of Leeds, Leeds LS2 9JT, UK

Nisreen A. Alwan
School of Primary Care and Population Sciences, Faculty of Medicine, University of Southampton, Southampton General Hospital, Southampton SO16 6YD, UK
NIHR Southampton Biomedical Research Centre, University of Southampton and University Hospital Southampton NHS Foundation Trust, Southampton SO16 6YD, UK

Muna J. Tahir, Jacob L. Haapala, Laurie P. Foster, David R. Jacobs Jr., Lisa J. Harnack and Ellen W. Demerath
Division of Epidemiology and Community Health, University of Minnesota, Minneapolis, MN 55454, USA

Katy M. Duncan, April M. Teague and David A. Fields
Department of Pediatrics, University of Oklahoma Health Sciences Center, Oklahoma City, OK 73104, USA

Elyse O. Kharbanda
Health Partners Institute, Minneapolis, MN 55425, USA

Patricia M. McGovern
Division of Environmental Health Sciences, University of Minnesota, Minneapolis, MN 55455, USA

Kara M. Whitaker
Department of Health and Human Physiology, University of Iowa, Iowa City, IA 52242, USA
Department of Epidemiology, University of Iowa, Iowa City, IA 52246, USA

Carole Rougé
Bledina Limonest, 69410 Champagne-au-Mont-d'Or, France

Kathleen M. Rasmussen
Division of Nutritional Sciences, Cornell University, Ithaca, NY 14850, USA
Division of Nutritional Sciences, Cornell University, Ithaca, NY 14853, USA

Fanney Thorsteinsdottir, Peder Frederiksen and Amélie Keller
Fanney Thorsteinsdottir, Research Unit for Dietary Studies, The Parker Institute, Bisbebjerg og Frederiksberg Hospital, Nordre Fasanvej 57, 2000 Frederiksberg, Denmark

Ekaterina Maslova
Department of Primary Care and Public Health, Imperial College London, London W6 8RP, UK
Centre for Fetal Programming, Department of Epidemiology Research, Statens Serum Institut, 2300 Copenhagen, Denmark

Ramune Jacobsen
Fanney Thorsteinsdottir, Research Unit for Dietary Studies, The Parker Institute, Bisbebjerg og Frederiksberg Hospital, Nordre Fasanvej 57, 2000 Frederiksberg, Denmark
Department of Pharmacy, University of Copenhagen, 2100 Copenhagen, Denmark

Vibeke Backer
Department of Respiratory Medicine, Bispebjerg University Hospital, 2400 Copenhagen, Denmark

Berit Lilienthal Heitmann
Fanney Thorsteinsdottir, Research Unit for Dietary Studies, The Parker Institute, Bisbebjerg og Frederiksberg Hospital, Nordre Fasanvej 57, 2000 Frederiksberg, Denmark
The Boden Institute of Obesity, Nutrition, Exercise & Eating Disorders, University of Sydney, Sydney, NSW 2006, Australia
The Department of Public Health, Section for General Practice, University of Copenhagen, 2100 Copenhagen, Denmark

Elisa Anleu, Marcela Reyes and María Luisa Garmendia
Institute of Nutrition and Food Technology (INTA), University of Chile, 7830490 Santiago, Chile

Marcela Araya B
Department of Women and Newborn Health Promotion, Faculty of Medicine, University of Chile, 8380453 Santiago, Chile

Marcela Flores
Corporación de Salud Municipal de Puente Alto, 8210269 Santiago, Chile

Ricardo Uauy
Institute of Nutrition and Food Technology (INTA), University of Chile, 7830490 Santiago, Chile
Department of Pediatrics, School of Medicine, Pontificia Universidad Católica de Chile, 8330023 Santiago, Chile

Muna J. Tahir, Jacob L. Haapala, Laurie P. Foster, Lisa J. Harnack, David R. Jacobs Jr. and Ellen W. Demerath
Division of Epidemiology and Community Health, University of Minnesota, Minneapolis, MN 55454, USA

Patricia M. McGovern
Division of Environmental Health Sciences, University of Minnesota, Minneapolis, MN 55455, USA

Julia L. Finkelstein, Amy Fothergill, Heather M. Guetterman, Tera R. Kent and Kimberly O. O'Brien
Division of Nutritional Sciences, Cornell University, Ithaca, NY 14853, USA

Ronnie Guillet and Eva K. Pressman
University of Rochester Medical Center, Rochester, NY 14642, USA

Ummu D. Erliana and Alyce D. Fly
Indiana University Bloomington School of Public Health, Bloomington, IN 47405, USA

Julia Günther, Julia Hoffmann, Monika Spies, Dorothy Meyer, Julia Kunath, Lynne Stecher and Hans Hauner
Else Kröner-Fresenius-Centre for Nutritional Medicine, School of Medicine, Klinikum rechts der Isar, Technical University of Munich, Georg-Brauchle-Ring 62, 80992 Munich, Germany

Kathrin Rauh
Else Kröner-Fresenius-Centre for Nutritional Medicine, School of Medicine, Klinikum rechts der Isar, Technical University of Munich, Georg-Brauchle-Ring 62, 80992 Munich, Germany
Competence Centre for Nutrition (KErn), Am Gereuth 4, 85354 Freising, Germany

Eva Rosenfeld and Luzia Kick
Competence Centre for Nutrition (KErn), Am Gereuth 4, 85354 Freising, Germany

Shiro Kubota
Kubota Life Science Laboratory Co., Ltd., Saga 840-0535, Japan
Kubota Maternity Clinic, Fukuoka 810-0014, Japan

Tatsuya Yoshihara
Kubota Maternity Clinic, Fukuoka 810-0014, Japan
Clinical Research Center, Fukuoka Mirai Hospital, Fukuoka 813-0017, Japan

Masayoshi Zaitsu
Department of Social and Behavioral Sciences, Harvard T.H. Chan School of Public Health, Boston, MA 02115, USA
Department of Public Health, Graduate School of Medicine, The University of Tokyo, Tokyo 113-0033, Japan

Sébastien Skweres
Department of Neonatology, Maternite Regionale, CHRU Nancy, 54035 Nancy, France

Jean-Michel Hascoët
Department of Neonatology, Maternite Regionale, CHRU Nancy, 54035 Nancy, France
DevAH, Lorraine University, 54500 Vandoeuvre les Nancy, France

Martine Chauvin and Christine Pierret
Dietetic and Nutrition Unit, CHRU Nancy, 54035 Nancy, France

Mengying Li, Ellen Francis, Stefanie N. Hinkle, Aparna S. Ajjarapu and Cuilin Zhang
Division of Intramural Population Health Research, Eunice Kennedy Shriver National Institute of Child Health and Human Development, National Institutes of Health, Bethesda, MD 20817, USA

Gabriele Piuri and Attilio Francesco Speciani
Inflammation Society, 18 Woodlands Park, Bexley DA52EL, UK

Louis-Dominique Van Egroo
Saint Cloud Hospital, 92210 Paris, France

Enrico Ferrazzi
Inflammation Society, 18 Woodlands Park, Bexley DA52EL, UK
Fondazione IRCCS Cà Granda, Ospedale Maggiore Policlinico, Department of Clinical Sciences and Community Health, University of Milan, 20122 Milan, Italy

Patricia Franck
Biology Laboratory, CHRU Nancy, 54035 Nancy, France

Andrea Maugeri, Martina Barchitta, Isabella Blanco and Antonella Agodi
Department of Medical and Surgical Sciences and Advanced Technologies "GF Ingrassia", University of Catania, Via S. Sofia 87, 95123 Catania, Italy

Julia H. King, Sze Ting (Cecilia) Kwan, Jian Yan, Vladislav G. Fomin, Samantha P. Levine, Emily Wei and Marie A. Caudill
Division of Nutritional Sciences, Cornell University, Ithaca, NY 14850, USA

Xinyin Jiang
Division of Nutritional Sciences, Cornell University, Ithaca, NY 14850, USA
Department of Health and Nutrition Sciences, Brooklyn College, Brooklyn, NY 11210, USA

Mark S. Roberson
Department of Biomedical Sciences, Cornell University, Ithaca, NY 14850, USA

Index

www.ingramcontent.com/pod-product-compliance
Lightning Source LLC
LaVergne TN
LVHW081013210926
848485LV00004B/853